Updates in Hypertension and Cardiovascular Protection

Series Editors
Giuseppe Mancia, Milan, Italy
Enrico Agabiti-Rosei, Brescia, Brescia, Italy

The aim of this series is to provide informative updates on both the knowledge and the clinical management of a disease that, if uncontrolled, can very seriously damage the human body and is still among the leading causes of death worldwide. Although hypertension is associated mainly with cardiovascular, endocrine, and renal disorders, it is highly relevant to a wide range of medical specialties and fields – from family medicine to physiology, genetics, and pharmacology. The topics addressed by volumes in the series *Updates in Hypertension and Cardiovascular Protection* have been selected for their broad significance and will be of interest to all who are involved with this disease, whether residents, fellows, practitioners, or researchers.

Paolo Palatini
Enrico Agabiti-Rosei • Giuseppe Mancia
Editors

Exercise, Sports and Hypertension

Springer

Editors
Paolo Palatini
Studium Patavinum
University of Padova
Padova, Italy

Enrico Agabiti-Rosei
Dept of Clinical and Experimental Sci
University of Brescia
Brescia, Italy

Giuseppe Mancia
Emeritus Professor
University of Milano-Bicocca
Milano, Italy

ISSN 2366-4606 ISSN 2366-4614 (electronic)
Updates in Hypertension and Cardiovascular Protection
ISBN 978-3-031-07957-3 ISBN 978-3-031-07958-0 (eBook)
https://doi.org/10.1007/978-3-031-07958-0

This Springer imprint is published by the registered company Springer Nature Switzerland AG
The registered company address is: Gewerbestrasse 11, 6330 Cham, Switzerland

Contents

Haemodynamics of Exercise Testing and Sports Activities

1

Paolo Palatini

1.1 Introduction

The long-term efficacy of regular physical activity in decreasing blood pressure (BP) has been documented by a large number of studies [1–3]. This is why sports activities have gained a relevant place among other non-pharmacological measures for the prevention of hypertension and its complications. However, the use of exercise in the management of the hypertensive patient requires a deep knowledge of the BP changes which actually occur during dynamic and resistance sports activities.

For obvious methodological reasons, the BP and cardiac output changes caused by exercise in human beings have been studied almost exclusively during laboratory tests. However, the standard methodology does not appears suitable for studying exercise haemodynamics in the athletes, as the laboratory test should better simulate the type of physical activity one practises. Indeed, BP recordings performed "in the field" have shown that the BP behaviour during real sports activities can hardly be reproduced with the use of laboratory exercise testing [4, 5]. The aim of this chapter is to describe the left ventricular (LV) and BP changes that occur during laboratory ergometric tests and dynamic and heavy resistance sports, highlighting the haemodynamic differences between the two different settings.

1.2 Dynamic Exercise

During dynamic exercise local vasodilatation is the key mechanism that provides increased oxygen delivery to the working muscles [6–8]. This is accompanied by a simultaneous vasoconstriction in the non-working muscles and splanchnic bed. As

P. Palatini (✉)
Studium Patavinum, Department of Medicine, University of Padova, Padova, Italy
e-mail: palatini@unipd.it

P. Palatini et al. (eds.), *Exercise, Sports and Hypertension*, Updates in Hypertension and Cardiovascular Protection,
https://doi.org/10.1007/978-3-031-07958-0_1

a consequence, the venous return rapidly increases with a consequent rise in cardiac filling. Sympathetic activation causes a simultaneous increase in stroke volume (SV) and heart rate and a marked rise in cardiac output (CO). These haemodynamic changes together with the progressive decline in total peripheral resistance (TPR) produce changes in BP which differ according to the type and length of exercise.

1.2.1 BP Changes During Traditional Dynamic Ergometric Tests

When dynamic exercise is performed according to standard protocols with incremental workload a progressive rise in systolic BP and little changes in diastolic BP are recorded [7–9]. Bicycle ergometry is the most common form of stress test performed in European countries. Bicycling causes a progressive increase in systolic BP usually ranging from 50 to 70 mmHg and a slight increase in diastolic BP. Treadmill exercise, which is more popular in the USA, causes similar changes of systolic BP whereas diastolic BP remains substantially unchanged or even declines [8, 10]. However, a wide subject-to-subject variability has been reported.

In hypertensive subjects, during both types of testing systolic BP reaches higher levels than in normotensive subjects [7–10], but the absolute increase in BP is similar in the two groups.

It has to be pointed out that the level of systolic BP varies according to the site of measurement. As the BP measurement site moves distally, from the aorta to the radial artery, systolic BP increases due to wave reflection [11, 12]. The peripheral augmentation of systolic BP is further increased by exercise as shown by experimental studies performed with intra-arterial measurement [11–13]. In contrast, mean BP remains constant from central to peripheral sites.

1.2.2 BP Changes During Prolonged Steady-State Exercise

BP changes during prolonged exercise differ from those during exercise testing at incremental workload. BP during exercise is regulated by the action of receptors in the contracting muscles, which indicate whether the existing level of blood flow satisfies the metabolic demands of the muscles [14]. Homoeostatic reflexes originating from arterial and LV baroreceptors contribute to the regulation of the BP changes [15]. The regulation of BP during prolonged exercise is more complex and has not been fully investigated, due to the difficulty of reproducing in the laboratory the different types of dynamic physical activities. However, available evidence suggests that the rise in BP observed soon after the onset of exercise is caused by a "central command", originating in the cerebellum, basal ganglia, and spinal cord [16]. Initially, CO is raised by vagal withdrawal especially at low exercise intensities [6]. At higher levels of exercise, first-order heterostatic pressure-raising reflexes arise from nerve fibres within the skeletal muscles in response to ischaemia [17, 18]. The net effect of this mechanism is the restauration of an adequate muscle blood flow through an increase in heart rate, vasoconstrictor outflow and BP [6, 17, 18]. In the second phase of prolonged steady state exercise, second-order heterostatic reflexes, originating from receptors in the heart and the descending thoracic aorta, come into action [19, 20], thereby amplifying the circulatory effects of the exercise stimulus. The role of another heterostatic reflex, the Bainbridge reflex, in the initial phases of exercise, is more controversial [21–23]. During high-intensity prolonged exercise, BP is maintained constant by vasoconstriction in visceral organs, non-working muscles and other regions to prevent deleterious falls in BP. According to Rowell [6], muscle chemoreflexes are the most powerful controllers of BP levels during strenuous exercise especially in individuals with limited ability to raise CO during exercise [6]. Circulatory adjustments during exercise are regulated by the activity of the autonomic nervous system, which integrates thermal and the other afferent signals into a common neural outflow to the cardiovascular effectors [24, 25]. These mechanisms are of paramount importance in hypertensive individuals to prevent excessive BP increases as well as dangerous precipitous BP falls during the final phases of exercise and during the recovery.

Intra-arterial BP changes during prolonged exercise at the anaerobic threshold were recorded in our laboratory in two groups of normotensive (Fig. 1.1) and hypertensive (Fig. 1.2) athletes and were compared with those occurring during traditional bicycle ergometry [26, 27]. During the traditional ergometric test to exhaustion we observed parallel changes in systolic and diastolic BP in the two groups, characterized by a gradual BP increase up to peak exercise. During prolonged exercise, a parallel rise in systolic BP was observed only during the initial phase of exercise. BP reached maximum values during the first minutes of exercise. Thereafter, there was a progressive BP decline throughout the rest of the test with a larger drop among the hypertensive subjects. Soon after stopping exercise a sudden and large drop in

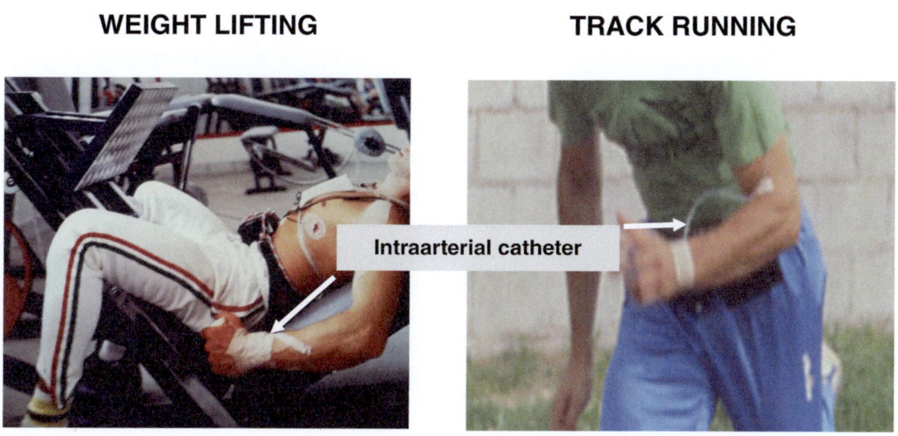

Fig. 1.1 Two athletes performing sports activities during intra-arterial blood pressure recording. An indwelling catheter was inserted into the radial artery and was connected to a pressure transducer through a cannula. The blood pressure signals were transmitted to a mini-recorder worn around the waist

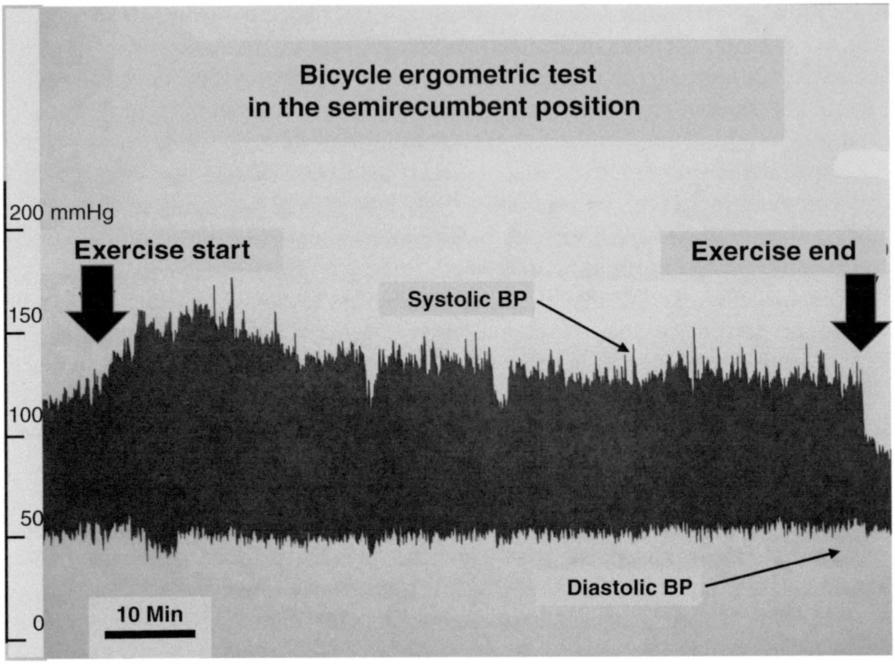

Fig. 1.2 Prolonged dynamic exercise performed in the laboratory in steady-state condition in a normotensive athlete. Blood pressure reached maximum values during the first minutes of exercise. Thereafter, there was a progressive decline of blood pressure and then blood pressure remained stable up to the end of exercise. A large blood pressure drop can be observed soon after the end of the effort

BP can be observed which is usually greater among the hypertensive subjects. In addition, a weak relationship was found between BP at baseline and BP at peak exercise. Thus, the main findings of this investigation were that (1) during a type of exercise simulating a true sport activity, a smaller BP increase occurs in hypertensive individuals than in normotensive subjects at peak exercise, (2) the BP level reached by a subject at peak exercise is not proportional to BP measured in resting conditions.

To clarify the reasons for the different BP behaviour in the normotensive and hypertensive subjects we investigated LV dimensions and performance during a session of prolonged strenuous exercise using the echocardiographic technique [27]. The main aim of this study was to assess whether there was a decline in LV systolic function in the hypertensive patients compared to a group of normotensive subjects of control. In resting conditions, a dysfunction of LV chamber may occur in hypertension but this is usually observed in an advanced stage of the disease after LV hypertrophy develops. Indeed, LV function has been found to be normal or even supernormal in the early stage of hypertension [28]. However, our hypothesis was that subtle abnormalities of LV performance may be detected during strenuous exercise which would account for the smaller BP increase observed during long-lasting strenuous effort in the hypertensive individuals. Our echocardiographic study showed that a greater LV ejection fraction ($P = 0.018$), systolic BP/end-systolic volume ($P < 0.0001$) and stress/end-systolic volume ($P = 0.027$) were present in young hypertensive individuals during strenuous exercise in a semi-recumbent position than in normotensive subjects of control, documenting the existence of an increased ejective performance in the former [27]. However, the above parameters were calculated from measurements performed at the endocardium which may overestimate actual LV contractility [29–31] as shown by previous studies at rest [32–34]. Indeed, we found that LV ejective performance was the key factor for preserving a high SV and CO during effort but LV contractility measured at midwall at peak exercise was actually depressed [35]. These findings indicate that increased LV ejective performance on a background of LV remodelling and depressed LV contractility can preserve an adequate flow to the exercising muscles. However, this unfavourable structural LV pattern may have deleterious consequences in the long run leading to overt LV dysfunction.

1.2.3 Factors Affecting LV Performance During Exercise

The exercise induced increase in LV ejection fraction is mainly determined by a decrease in end-systolic volume. Less is known about the role of the Frank–Starling mechanism during exercise which may be influenced by a series of several clinical variables that can affect LV dimensions.

Sex differences. Maximal exercise CO has been found to be greater in men than in women over a wide age range [36], due to a greater increase in LV ejection fraction from rest to peak exercise [37]. A lower decrease in end-systolic volume with exercise in female subjects seems to account for this difference. The behaviour of end-diastolic volume during exercise is more controversial. According to some authors, diastolic volume tends to decline in men and have constant dimensions in women [37].

Position of the body during exercise testing. When assuming the upright posture the end-diastolic volume and SV decline compared to the supine position, mainly due to peripheral pooling. However, during exercise both variables rapidly increase [38]. During supine exercise, the increase in CO is predominantly due to an increase in heart rate, with little change in SV and end-diastolic volume [38, 39], even though some authors observed a small increase also in end-diastolic volume [40].

Age. A large body of evidence has shown that ageing is associated with a progressive decline in CO during exercise [41, 42]. While in young subjects CO during exercise appears to be increased and then maintained elevated chiefly by the increase in heart rate, in older individuals also the Frank–Starling mechanism seems to contribute to the increase in CO [39, 40]. This mechanism seems to compensate for the well-known age-related decrease in LV compliance and LV filling in older individuals [43, 44].

Physical training. Controversy still exists as to whether LV end-diastolic diameter is subject to different changes in trained and untrained individuals [45].

According to some authors [40] the end-diastolic volume increases more in sedentary than in trained individuals, whereas according to others [46] only rises in the sedentary subject, and according to yet others [47] only increases in the athlete. There is general agreement that end-systolic LV diameter decreases to the same extent in trained and untrained individuals during exercise [45].

Hypertensive status. The results of our studies reported above suggest that in young subjects in the early phase of hypertension increased inotropic function is present during strenuous exercise as a consequence of enhanced sympathetic activity. However, in the long run this mechanism would lead to LV hypertrophy to reduce the LV wall stress. The following gradual deterioration of LV pump function may be the consequence of a series of adverse factors including inadequate LV filling, increased afterload, and impaired coronary reserve [29, 48].

Duration of exercise. There is general agreement that CO increases more during a short dynamic exercise than during prolonged steady-state exercise [30, 31]. According to some investigators [49], the lower CO at the end of prolonged exercise is due to a lower utilization of the Frank–Starling mechanism rather than to a lower LV systolic performance. However, according to other authors [30, 31] the decreased LV performance observed during the recovery from prolonged exercise suggests that prolonged strenuous exercise may cause an impairment of LV function. However, it should be pointed out that data obtained during the recovery can hardly be extrapolated to LV performance assessed during exercise. Studies assessing LV performance throughout 1 h-long vigorous exercise session [27] found that, after an initial increase, LV systolic function remained stable up to the end of exercise, without a tendency to decline and that a sharp fall in LV performance occurred soon after stopping exercise.

1.2.4 BP Changes During Endurance Sports

As mentioned above, the present knowledge on BP changes during sports activities is almost exclusively based on data obtained with laboratory stress testing which can only give a rough estimate of the actual BP changes that occur during physical activities performed in real life. However, measuring BP during physical activity in ambulatory subjects is not possible with current non-invasive techniques, because the cuffing method requires a stationary position of the subject during the measurement. Only a method using intra-arterial recording coupled to a Holter device or a telemetering system can acquire BP measurements in unrestricted subjects. The first invasive recordings during endurance sports were performed long ago by Bachmann et al. using a telemetering system [50]. However, a true systematic investigation on the BP behaviour during endurance sports was performed by means of a portable invasive technique, the Oxford system [4, 5]. This technique consisted of a miniaturized transducer-peristaltic-pump unit connected to the radial artery through an indwelling catheter (Fig. 1.3). The sphygmic waves were recorded on a Holter mini-recorder worn around the waist [51, 52].

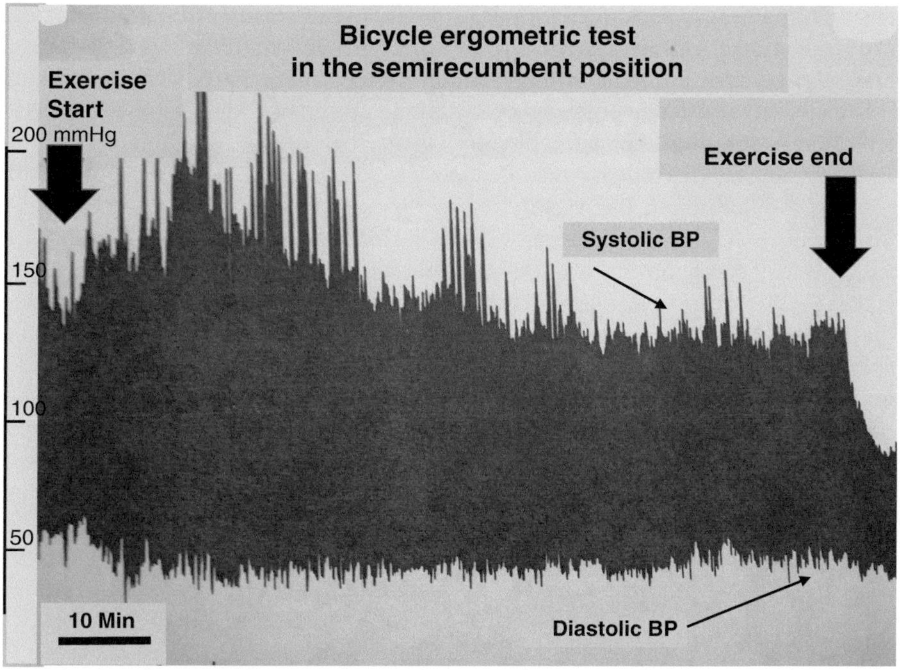

Fig. 1.3 Prolonged dynamic exercise performed in the laboratory in a hypertensive athlete. In this athlete, blood pressure reached a higher level than in the normotensive subject during the first phase of the test. However, a greater blood pressure decline was observed during the submaximal phases of the exercise. A larger blood pressure drop can be seen during the recovery compared to the normotensive subject of Fig. 1.1

Using the telemetering technique, Bachmann et al. measured BP levels of 262/100 mmHg [50] during running, 221/136 mmHg during swimming, and 158/80 mmHg during cross-country skiing. However, these data can only be considered anecdotal because the length and the intensity of the effort made by the subjects were not reported by the authors and were thus not comparable. Obviously, the pressor effect of different sports activities cannot be compared at different relative intensities, exercise duration, and heart rate levels. More comparable data were obtained by Rost and Kronig [53, 54], who measured BP during running and swimming at the same oxygen uptake and heart rate. According to these authors, BP is 20 mmHg greater in swimming than running whereas CO is similar during the two activities.

1.2.5 BP Changes During Running

Jogging and running are the most frequent physical activities performed by human beings since the dawn of time. Yet, the BP behaviour during running remained unknown till recently. A thorough investigation of beat-by-beat intra-arterial BP during running was performed by our group at the university of Padova using the above mentioned Oxford system [51, 52]. In 23 volunteer athletes we performed a bicycle ergometric test in the sitting position starting from a 50-W work load, which was increased by 20-W increments every 2 min until exhaustion. Systolic BP gradually increased during the test, whereas diastolic BP showed only minor changes. Both systolic and diastolic BP recorded at peak exercise were highly correlated with resting BP values (both $P < 0.001$).

On a different day, the same participants performed a run on a 400-m tartan track for an overall duration of 28 to over 60 min according to the individual capacity (Fig. 1.3). A warm-up was performed by running at a low speed (Fig. 1.4) and then the athletes gradually increased their running velocity until a steady submaximal speed was attained (Figs. 1.5 and 1.6). Before completing the run a brief final sprint was performed (Fig. 1.7). A peculiar behaviour of the pressure phasic waves was observed throughout the run (Figs. 1.4, 1.5, 1.6 and 1.7). Pulse pressure oscillations

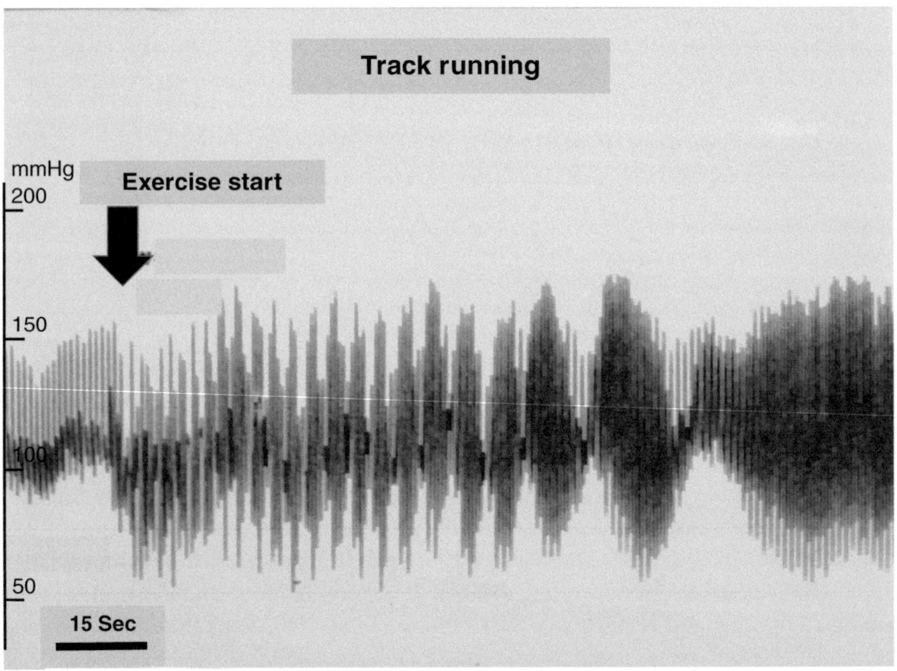

Fig. 1.4 Blood pressure changes during track running. Soon after the beginning of the exercise a peculiar behaviour of blood pressure can be observed characterized by marked oscillations reflecting a periodic widening and narrowing of pulse pressure. The shape of these cyclic pulse pressure changes led us to investigate whether they were "beats". Beats are generated when two waves of nearly equal frequency propagate through a fluid: b eat frequency is determined by the difference in frequency of the two component waves. During running besides the normal sphygmic wave a second wave is periodically generated in the arterial tree as a consequence of the impact of the runner's foot with the ground

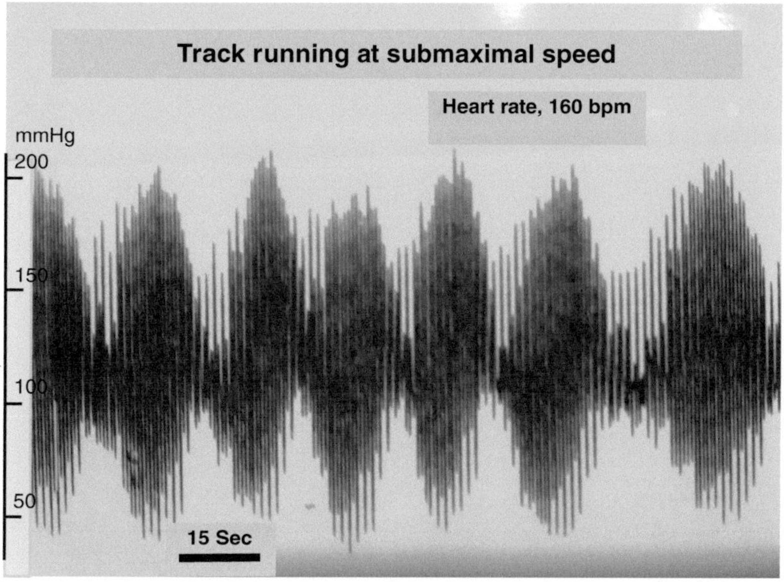

Fig. 1.5 Blood pressure changes during track running at submaximal speed. Here, the frequency of pulse pressure oscillations is 4/min and corresponds to the difference between heart rate (160 bpm) and stride frequency (164/min)

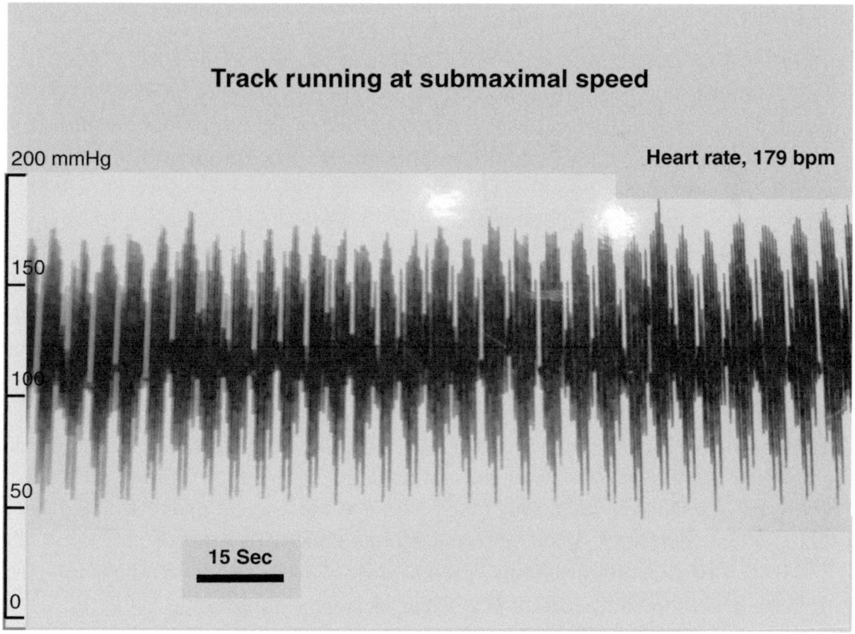

Fig. 1.6 Blood pressure changes during track running at submaximal speed. Compared to Fig. 1.5, here a higher heart rate was recorded (179 bpm) with a stride frequency of 165/min. The frequency of beats during this phase of the run was 14/min

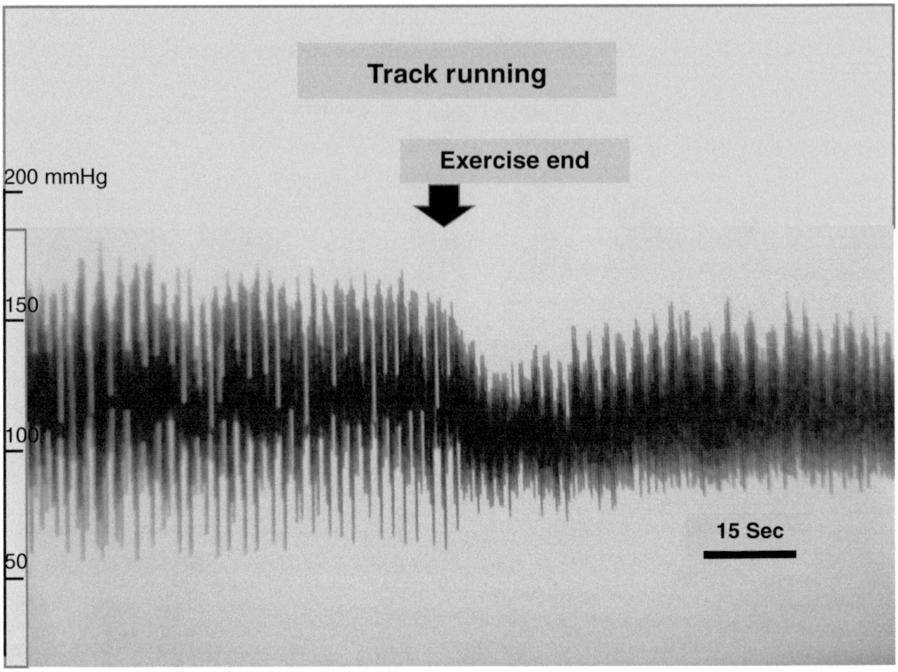

Fig. 1.7 Blood pressure changes at the end of track running. Soon after the end of the exercise a drop in blood pressure can be observed and the oscillatory pulse pressure pattern tends to disappear

varying from 4 to 28 cycles/min according to running velocity and heart rate were recorded. These changes were observed in all athletes although their amplitude varied from subject to subject. The main finding was that the frequency of the running-induced pulse pressure fluctuations almost always equalled the difference between heart rate and stepping frequency. Because of these wide oscillations, in some cases diastolic BP approached zero level. Despite the high variability of pulse pressure, mean BP remained rather stable throughout the bout of exercise. We could establish that the source of these pressure oscillations were the periodic shakes received by the heart and the great vessels during the run whose frequency was similar to that of heart rate, thereby generating a "beat phenomenon" [51, 52]. Maximum BP values during running were attained during the first minutes of warm-up, in spite of the lower running velocity. Subsequently, due to the vasodilatation a progressive decrease in BP could be observed, so that after 20–30 min of running, BP declined to below pre-exercise values. Our study showed for the first time that a periodic widening and narrowing of pulse pressure occurs during running and that these rhythmic oscillations are unrelated to respiration. Rhythmic aortic shakings during the run give source to an accessory wave, which summing up with the normal sphygmic wave generate "beats".

The BP level during track running varied according to hypertensive status. In agreement with previous results obtained in the laboratory during prolonged semi-supine bicycle ergometry [27, 28], the BP difference between the normotensive and the hypertensive group present at rest gradually flattened throughout the exercise period, so that at the end of the effort the two pressure curves were almost superimposed. This may be due to a depressed left ventricular diastolic filling in the hypertensive subjects during strenuous effort.

A totally different BP pattern was observed in sprinters in whom a sudden and short-lasting marked increase in systolic and diastolic BP was observed during the run, similar to that caused by heavy-resistance exercises (see below) [4, 5].

1.2.6 BP Changes During Cycling

Cycling implies a mix of dynamic and isometric exercise. The contribution of these two components to muscle contraction depends on the force applied to the pedals. The isometric component is more important when the subjects pedal uphill or at high speed on the flat. During competitive events a greater muscular force is developed during cycling than running and this accounts for the greater LV mass and the more concentric oriented remodelling of the left ventricle of cyclists compared to runners [55]. During cycling there is a larger compression of the vessels due to muscle contractions, and TPR cannot fall to the same extent as in running. This is attested to by the higher increase in diastolic BP that has been recorded with the intra-arterial method during road cycling than during track running [56]. As expected, the highest BP levels were recorded when the subjects exercised at high workloads. The BP levels achieved by cyclists exercising in outdoor conditions turned out to be much higher than those recorded during standard laboratory stress testing, confirming that the laboratory test is not a good predictor of the haemodynamic changes occurring during sports activities.

1.3 Isometric Exercise

Contrary to dynamic exercise, isometric exercise produces a rise in both systolic and diastolic BP [57–61] (Fig. 1.8). The main mechanisms responsible for this increase is the activation of the sympathetic nervous system triggered by earlier recruitment of type II fibres [12]. The main haemodynamic changes are a rise in cardiac output and heart rate [60] while stroke volume shows only a slight increase [62]. TPR is only marginally affected by isometric exercise [60, 62]. The level of work load is the main factor responsible for the BP elevation [63, 64]. Several clinical characteristics have been found to be important in predicting the BP response to isometric exercise including age, the level of resting BP, the duration of exercise, and strength [65, 66]. More controversial is the role of the size of the actively contracted muscle mass [67, 68].

1.3.1 Laboratory Testing

BP changes during isometric exercise have been studied mainly with the use of the hand grip test which is performed grasping a dynamometer using 30% to 50% of the maximal voluntary contraction [57, 58]. The average systolic BP increase ranges from 25 to 40 mmHg in normotensives and from 35 to 55 mmHg in hypertensives [62–65]. The increase in diastolic BP ranges from 28 to 39 mmHg in hypertensives and from 14 to 32 mmHg in normotensives. It should be pointed out that in real life situations most isometric activities are performed with concomitant isotonic activities such as walking while carrying heavy weights. In these activities the increase in diastolic BP is completely offset [69]. It should also be considered that during sports activities any predominantly isometric activity is preceded by an appropriate warm-up session, to allow an adequate vasodilatation of the exercising muscles. Vasodilatation has an important effect on the pressor response to isometric exercise as shown by Silke et al. [69]. When lifting and holding a weight was carried out while exercising on a treadmill, the increase in diastolic BP was progressively offset to fall to below pre-exercise values at the end of exercise. These results indicate that the typical isometric BP pattern changes when a concomitant isotonic activity is carried out.

1.3.2 Heavy-Resistance Sports

Heavy resistance exercises may cause marked increases in both systolic and diastolic BP whose magnitude depend on the workload and the modality of the effort. These short-lasting BP changes have been investigated with the use of intra-arterial recording mainly in athletes performing weight-lifting [70, 71]. In weight-lifters performing exercises involving the legs at the maximum workload, average values of 320/250 mmHg have been recorded by a Canadian group of investigators with peak values as high as 480/390 mmHg [70]. We performed intra-arterial recordings in 5 normotensive and 3 hypertensive weightlifters who exercised with the non-catheterized arm or with the legs (leg press and squatting) [71]. The load was progressively increased till the 100% maximum lift was reached. Marked BP increases were recorded which were proportional to the load, ranging from 197/156 mmHg to 345/245 mmHg [71]. The BP levels reached by the athletes were proportional to the muscle mass employed in the exercises and were higher when the effort was carried out in the upright position than in the supine. Before starting the exercises the participants also performed a maximal Valsalva manoeuvre in triplicate blowing into a tube against a mercury column. During the Valsalva, mouth pressures ranging from 40 to 155 mmHg were recorded. This was done because the potent Valsalva manoeuvre which accompanies heavy weight lifts is considered to be the main determinant for the remarkable BP rises during this type of sport (Fig. 1.8). The Valsalva manoeuvre is thought to cause sharp increases in intrathoracic and intraabdominal pressures [72]. To verify this hypothesis,

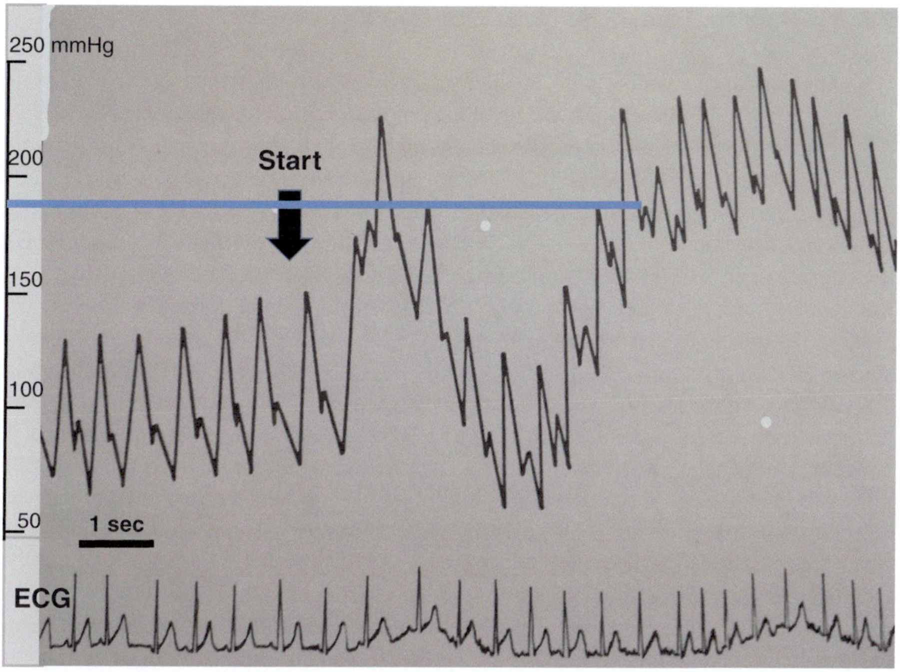

Fig. 1.8 Blood pressure changes in a weight lifter during a single leg-press exercise. Soon after the beginning of the exercise a sudden rise in blood pressure can be observed followed by a drop and by a subsequent more sustained blood pressure increase up to a maximum of 250/180 mmHg. These blood pressure fluctuations were due to the concomitant potent Valsalva manoeuvre performed by the subject while making the effort

intrathoracic and abdominal pressures were simultaneously measured by two balloon catheter systems (positioned one in the midoesophagus and one in the stomach) [71]. Remarkable intrathoracic and intraabdominal pressure elevations, proportional to the loads, were recorded. Intraabdominal pressure always reached higher values than intrathoracic pressure (maximum values of 170 and 75 mmHg, respectively). When the Valsalva manoeuvre was abolished, much lower BP levels and little or no increase in intracavitary pressures were recorded. These findings provided a direct evidence that the increase in intracavitary pressures is the main determinant of the BP elevations caused by weight-lifting. However, it should be borne in mind that intra-cavitary pressures are transmitted to the cerebrospinal fluid through the intervertebral foramina, a mechanism that reduces the actual transmural pressure across the cerebral vessels [72, 73]. Thus, the remarkable increases in abdominal pressure caused by heavy weight-lifting would exert a protective effect on the cerebral vessels. Other factors that contribute to elevating BP during heavy-resistance exercise are the potent pressor reflex originating from tendons stretching and the mechanical compression of the arteries by the contracting muscles [68, 69].

1.3.3 How to Assess the Hypertensive Athlete

When assessing the athlete with borderline or overt hypertension, the first problem remains to correctly assess the BP level at rest, which may be elevated because of a pronounced alerting reaction during the doctor's visit. To this purpose four different procedures are currently being used: (a) a long period of observation with repeated visits, (b) encouraging self BP measurement at home, (c) performing ambulatory BP monitoring, and (d) assessment of BP response to stress test. Ambulatory BP monitoring seems to be the best method to make an appropriate diagnosis in sports medicine where an objective evaluation performed in a short period of time is necessary. The purpose of exercise testing in the laboratory is to assess the subject's pressor response under conditions which are like those which occur during the sport activity performed by the subject under investigation. However, as earlier reported, an ergometric test does not elicit the same BP changes as do sports performed in outdoor conditions, but for obvious reasons a field test cannot be used for screening purposes. Therefore, in spite of its limitations the ergometric stress test either performed on a treadmill or a bicycle ergometer remains an essential evaluation to assess the athlete's BP response to exercise [74]. If possible, the subject should be evaluated on an ergometer where the athlete's specific physical activity can be reproduced. The procedure should differ from the protocols currently used in clinical practice for detecting coronary artery disease and should include an adequate warm-up period [4, 5]. The workload, steps, and duration of the exercise should be tailored according to the discipline and the athletic level of the subject. Overground testing requires a complex medical equipment and specific expertise and cannot be routinely performed. It should thus be performed only in controversial cases in which routine clinical assessment did not provide conclusive data. An important limitation of traditional stress testing is the BP level that should be considered abnormal [75]. Several different cut points have been proposed in the literature but none was based on objective criteria [74, 75]. When defining a BP cut point as abnormal we mean that this BP level is the top normal value detectable in normotensive healthy subjects. However, this does not necessarily imply that this BP level should be considered harmful especially in a young individual. Obviously, caution should be exerted when deciding whether an athlete with high BP should be considered fit for competition. If high BP is confirmed by out of office BP assessment, the first step should be the normalization of BP with antihypertensive therapy and the search for hypertension mediated organ damage. However, the presence of a mild LV hypertrophy is difficult to interpret because it may be the consequence of intense physical training. Physical training promotes an increase in LV mass and in this circumstance it is extremely difficult to discriminate between the physiological changes produced by athletic training and those produced by the chronic pressure overload in hypertension. Echocardiographic investigations of normotensive athletes have provided conflicting data on the chamber dimension and wall thickness changes, dependent on the type, intensity and duration of exercise training and on the presence of a hypertensive status [76]. Regular physical activity could facilitate the development of LV hypertrophy exposing the athlete to an increased risk of coronary artery disease and/or sudden death. However, in recent years several studies have shown a paradoxical effect of endurance training on the LV structure of hypertensive patients, with a reduction of LV mass after a period of aerobic training. One first study was performed by Baglivo et al., who observed a decrease of LV mass in middle-aged hypertensive subjects after 16 months of endurance exercise training [77]. A more structured study was performed by Kokkinos et al. in a group of African-American men with severe hypertension performing 16 weeks of aerobic training [78]. Also in this study a decrease in LV mass was observed after training. These findings were later confirmed by other authors who observed a reduction in both LV mass and wall thickness in patients with mild hypertension after training [79]. The results we obtained in young hypertensive individuals from the HARVEST study are in keeping with those previous findings [80]. We observed that the physically active subjects were less likely to develop LV hypertrophy than their sedentary counterparts during a median follow-up of 8.3 years, and that no athlete involved in competitions developed LV hypertrophy. Similar results were found in the LIFE study [81]. Although these results were not confirmed by some investigators [82] the majority of the published studies have shown a favourable effect of physical training on LV structure and mass in hypertension. This paradoxical effect may be due to the reduction in BP, heart rate, TPR, large artery stiffness, blood volume and CO [83, 84]. Also, the favourable effect of physical activity on several humoral factors including endothelial function, renin-angiotensin-aldosterone system, insulin and reduction of sympathetic nervous system activity may contribute to decreasing LV mass [83–86]. The reduction of the sympathetic tone probably is the main mechanism for the beneficial effect of exercise on the hypertensive heart because of the reduction of heart rate and BP and the improvement of the metabolic syndrome [85–88].

Because of the present lack of information about the risk of adverse events in the athlete with hypertension, a rather restrictive policy should be adopted especially in the presence of LV hypertrophy [74]. Studies of sports activities in the field would probably provide useful information on the actual BP changes occurring during different sports disciplines. Long lasting longitudinal observations will be very important to shed new light on this still controversial issue.

Acknowledgments None.

Funding None.

Author Contributions PP performed the design of the study, data collection and analysis, manuscript writing and revision.

Conflict of Interest None.

Statement All human studies whose data have been used for the present article have been reviewed by the appropriate ethics committees and have been performed in accordance with the ethical standards of the 1964 Declaration of Helsinki.

References

1. Fagard RH. Exercise therapy in hypertensive cardiovascular disease. Prog Cardiovasc Dis. 2011;53:404–11.
2. Palatini P, Graniero G, Mormino P, Nicolosi L, Mos L, Visentin P, et al. Relation between physical training and ambulatory blood pressure in stage I hypertensive subjects. Results of the HARVEST trial. Circulation. 1994;90:2870–6.
3. Williams B, Mancia G, Spiering W, Agabiti Rosei E, Azizi M, Burnier M, et al. ESC/ESH Guidelines for the management of arterial hypertension: The Task Force for the management of arterial hypertension of the European Society of Cardiology and the European Society of Hypertension. J Hypertens. 2018;36:1953–2041.
4. Palatini P. Blood pressure behaviour during physical activity. Sports Med. 1988;5:353–74.
5. Palatini P. Exercise haemodynamics in the normotensive and the hypertensive subject. Clin Sci (Lond). 1994;87:75–87.
6. Rowell LA. Blood pressure regulation during exercise. Ann Med. 1991;23:329–33.
7. Irving IB, Bruce TA, DeRouen TA. Variations in the significance of systolic pressure during maximal exercise (treadmill) testing. Am J Cardiol. 1977;33:841–8.
8. Levy AM, Tabakin BS, Hanson IS. Hemodynamic responses to graded treadmill exercise in young untreated labile hypertensive patients. Circulation. 1967;35:1063–72.
9. Radice M, Alli C, Avanzini F, Di Tullio M, Mariotti G, Taioli E, et al. Role of blood pressure response to provocative tests in the prediction of hypertension in adolescents. Eur Heart J. 1985;6:490–6.
10. Bruce RA, Gey GO Jr, Cooper MN, Fisher LD, Peterson DR. Seattle heart watch: initial clinical circulatory and electrocardiographic responses to maximal exercise. Am Heart J. 1974;33:459–69.
11. Rowell LB. Human cardiovascular adjustments to exercise and thermal stress. Physiol Rev. 1974;54:75–159.
12. Mitchell JH, Reardon WC, McLosky I. Reflex effects on circulation and respiration from contracting skeletal muscle. Am J Physiol. 1977;233:H374–8.
13. Rowell LB, Brengelmann GL, Blackmon JR, Bruce RA, Murray JA. Disparities between aortic and peripheral pulse pressures induced by upright exercise and vasomotor changes in man. Circulation. 1968;37:954–64.
14. Mitchell JH. The exercise pressor reflex: its cardiovascular effects. Afferent mechanisms, and central pathways. Annu Rev Physiol. 1983;45:229–42.
15. Melcher A, Donald DE. Maintained ability of carotid baroreflex to regulate arterial pressure during exercise. Am J Physiol. 1981;241:H838–49.
16. Hobbs SF. Central command during exercise: parallel activation of the cardiovascular and motor system by descending command signals. In: Smith OA, Galosy RA, Weirs SM, editors. Circulation, neurobiology and behavior. New York: Elsevier; 1982. p. 117–31.
17. Mitchell JH, Schmidt RF. Cardiovascular reflex control by afferent fibers from skeletal muscle receptors. In: Shepherd JT, Aboud FM, editors. Handbook of physiology. Section 1. The cardiovascular system. Peripheral circulation and organ blood flow, vol. 3. Bethesda: American Physiological Society; 1983. p. 623–58.
18. Sheriff DD, Wyss CR, La R, Scher AM. Does inadequate 0_2, delivery trigger the pressor response to muscle hypoperfusion during exercise? Am J Physiol. 1987;253:H1199–07.
19. Coleridge HM, Coleridge JCG. Cardiovascular afferents involved in regulation of peripheral vessels. Annu Rev Physiol. 1980;41:413–27.
20. Malliani A, Pagani M, Bergamaschi M. Positive feedback sympathetic reflexes and hypertension. Am J Cardiol. 1979;44:860–5.
21. Kappagoda CT, Linden RJ, Sivananthan N. The nature of the atrial receptors responsible for a reflex increase in heart rate in the dog. J Physiol (Lond). 1979;291:393–411.
22. Vatner SF, Boettcher DH, Heyndrickx GR, McRitchie RJ. Reduced baroreflex sensitivity with volume loading in conscious dogs at rest and during exercise. Circ Res. 1975;37:495–503.

23. Ludbrook J. Reflex control of blood pressure during exercise. Annu Rev Physiol. 1983;45:155–68.
24. Brengelman G. Circulatory adjustments to exercise and heat stress. Annu Rev Physiol. 1983;45:191–212.
25. Thauer R. Circulatory adjustments to climatic requirements. In: Hamilton WF, Dow P, editors. Handbook of physiology. Circulation, vol. 3. Washington, DC: American Society of Physiology; 1965. p. 1921–66.
26. Palatini P, Mos L, Mormino P, Munari L, Del Torre M, Valle F, et al. Intra-arterial blood pressure monitoring in the evaluation of the hypertensive athlete. Eur Heart J. 1990;11:348–54.
27. Palatini P, Bongiovì S, Mario L, Schiraldi C, Mos L, Pessina AC. Above normal left ventricular performance is present during exercise in young subjects with mild hypertension. Eur Heart J. 1995;16:232–42.
28. Palatini P, Visentin PA, Mormino P, Pietra M, Piccolo D, Cozzutti E, et al. Left ventricular performance in the early stages of systemic hypertension. Am J Cardiol. 1998;81:418–23.
29. Cuocolo A, Sax FL, Brush JE, Maron BJ, Bacharach SL, Eonow RO. Left ventricular hypertrophy and impaired diastolic filling in essential hypertension. Circulation. 1990;81:978–86.
30. Vanoverschelde JLJ, Younis LT, Melin JA, Vanbutsele R, Leclercq B, Robert AR, et al. Prolonged exercise inducesleft ventricular dysfunction in healthy subjects. J Appl Physiol. 1991;70:1356–63.
31. Seals DR, Rogers MA, Hagberg JM, Yamamoto C, Cryer P, Ehsani AA. Left ventricular dysfunction after prolonged strenuous exercise in healthy subjects. Am J Cardiol. 1988;61:875–9.
32. De Simone G, Devereux RB, Roman MJ, Ganau A, Saba PS, Alderman MH, et al. Assessment of left ventricular function by the midwall fractional shortening-systolic stress relation in human hypertension. J Am Coll Cardiol. 1994;23:1444–51.
33. Aurigemma GP, Silver KH, Priest MA, Gaash WH. Geometric changes allow normal ejection fraction despite depressed myocardial shortening in hypertensive left ventricular hypertrophy. J Am Coll Cardiol. 1995;26:195–202.
34. Palatini P, Visentin P, Nicolosi G, Mione V, Stritoni P, Michieletto P, et al. Endocardial versus midwall measurement of left ventricular function in mild hypertension: an insight from the Harvest study. J Hypertens. 1996;14:1011–7.
35. Palatini P, Frigo G, Visentin P, Mario L, Mormino P, Pessina AC. Left ventricular contractile performance in the early stage of hypertension in humans. Eur J Appl Physiol. 2001;85:118–24.
36. Astrand I. Aerobic work capacity in men and women with special reference to age. Acta Physiol Scand. 1960;169(Suppl):1–91.
37. Adams KF, Vincent LM, McAllister SM, El-Ashmawy H, Sheps DS, Hill C. The influence of age and gender on left ventricular response to supine exercise in asymptomatic normal subjects. Am Heart J. 1987;113:731–42.
38. Poliner LR, Dehmer GJ. Left ventricular performance in normal subjects. Circulation. 1980;62:528–34.
39. Steingart RM, Wexler J, Slagle S, Scheuer J. Radionuclide ventriculographic response to graded supine and upright exercise: critical role of the Frank-Starling mechanism at submaximal exercise. Am J Cardiol. 1984;53:1671–7.
40. Fisman EZ, Frank AG, Ben-Ari E, Kessler G, Pines A, Drory Y, et al. Altered left ventricular volume and ejection fraction responses to supine dynamic exercise in athletes. J Am Coll Cardiol. 1990;15:582–8.
41. Julius S, Amery A, Whitlock LS, Conway J. Influence of age on the hemodynamic response to exercise. Circulation. 1967;36:222–30.
42. Younis LT, Melin JA, Robert AR, Detry JM. Influence of age and sex on left ventricular volumes and ejection fraction during upright exercise in normal subjects. Eur Heart J. 1990;11:916–24.
43. Mann DL, Denenberg BS, Gash AK, Makler PT, Bove AA. Effects of age on ventricular performance during graded supine exercise. Am Heart J. 1986;111:108–15.
44. Bongiovi S, Palatini P, Visentin PA MF, Pessina AC. Age and blood pressure related changes in left ventricular diastolic filling. J Hypertens. 1992;10:25–30.

45. Ginzton LE, Contant R, Brizendine M, Laks MM. Effect of long-term high intensity aerobic training on left ventricular volume during maximal upright exercise. J Am Coll Cardiol. 1989;14:364–71.
46. Tomai F, Ciavolella M, Gaspardone A, De Fazio A, Basso EG, Giannitti C, et al. Peak exercise left ventricular performance in normal subjects and in athletes assessed by first-pass radionuclide angiography. Am J Cardiol. 1992;70:531–5.
47. Fagard R, Van Den Broeke C, Amery A. Left ventricular dynamics during exercise in elite marathon runners. J Am Coll Cardiol. 1989;14:112–8.
48. Tabau IF, Swlachcic J, Braun S, Marie EM. Impaired left ventricular functional reserve in hypertensive patients with left ventricular hypertrophy. Hypertension. 1989;14:1–8.
49. Upton MT, Rerych SK, Roeback JR Jr, Newman GE, Douglas JM Jr, Wallace AG, et al. Effect of brief and prolonged exercise on left ventricular function. Am J Cardiol. 1980;45:1154–60.
50. Bachmann K, Zenawy R, Riess PJ, Zoloch KA. Blutdrucktelemetrie:kontinuerliche, direkte blutdruckmessungen im altag und beim sport. Dtsch Med Wochenschr. 1970;14:741–7.
51. Palatini P, Mos L, Munari L, Mormino P, Del Torre M, Valle F, et al. Beats modulate blood pressure during running. Am J Hypertens. 1989;2:872–4.
52. Palatini P, Mos L, Mormino P, Di Marco A, Munari L, Fazio G, et al. Blood pressure changes during running in humans: the "beat" phenomenon. J Appl Physiol. 1989;67:52–9.
53. Rost R. Athletics and the heart. Chicago: Year Book Medical; 1987.
54. Kronig B. History of telemetric automatic long-term blood pressure recording. In: Meyer-Sabellek W, Anlauf M, Gotren R, Steinfeld L, editors. Blood pressure measurements. Darmstadt: Steinkopff Verlag; 1990. p. 95–110.
55. Fagard R, Aubert A, Staessen J, Eynde EV, Vanhees L, Amery A. Cardiac structure and function in cyclists and runners. Comparative echocardiographic study. Br Heart J. 1984;62:124–9.
56. Palatini P, Mormino P, Mos L, Di Marco A, Munari L, Del Torre M, et al. Blood pressure changes during physical exercise. J Hypertens. 1988;6(Suppl. 4):88–90.
57. Chaney RH, Arndt S. Predictability of blood pressure response to isometric stress. Am J Cardiol. 1983;51:787–90.
58. Jones RI, Lahiri A, Cashman PMM, Dore C, Raftery EB. Left ventricular function during isometric hand grip and cold stress in normal subjects. Br Heart J. 1986;55:246–52.
59. Sullivan J, Hanson P, Rahko PS, Folts ID. Continuous measurement of left ventricular performance during and after maximal isometric deadlift exercise. Circulation. 1992;85:1406–13.
60. Bezucha GR, Lenser MC, Hanson PG, Nagle FJ. Comparison of hemodynamic responses to static and dynamic exercise. J Appl Physiol. 1982;53:1589–93.
61. Seals DR, Hanson PG, Washburn RA, Painter PL, Ward A, Nagle FJ. Cardiovascular response to static contraction in borderline hypertension. Clin Cardiol. 1985;8:348–52.
62. Laird WP, Fixler DE, Huffines FD. Cardiovascular response to isometric exercise in normal adolescents. Circulation. 1979;59:651–61.
63. Grossman W, Mclaurin LPP, Saltz SB, Paraskos JA, Dalen JE, et al. Changes in the inotropic state on the left ventricle during isometric exercise. Br Heart J. 1973;35:697–704.
64. Helfant RH, deVilla MA, Meister SG. Effect of sustained isometric handgrip exercise on left ventricular performance. Circulation. 1971;44:982–93.
65. Kino M, Lance VQ, Shahamatpour A, Spodick DH. Effects of age in response to isometric exercise. Am Heart J. 1975;90:575–81.
66. Lind AR, McNicol GW. Muscular factors which determine the cardiovascular responses to sustained and rhythmic exercise. Can Med Assoc J. 1967;96:706–15.
67. Seals DR, Washburn RA, Hanson PG, Painter PL, Nagle FJ. Increased cardiovascular response to static contraction of larger muscle groups. J Appl Physiol. 1983;54:434–7.
68. McCloskey DI, Streatfield KA. Muscular reflex stimuli on the cardiovascular system during isometric contractions of muscle group of different mass. J Physiol. 1975;250:431–41.
69. Silke B, Watt SJ, Taylor SH. The circulatory response to lifting and carrying and its modification by beta-adrenoreceptor blockade. Int J Cardiol. 1984;6:527–36.
70. MacDougall ID, Tuxen D, Sale G, Moroz JR, Sutton JR. Arterial blood pressure response to heavy resistance exercise. J Appl Physiol. 1985;58:785–90.

71. Palatini P, Mos L, Munari L, Valle F, Del Torre M, Rossi A, et al. Blood pressure changes during heavy resistance exercise. J Hypertens. 1989;7:572–3.
72. Laporta D, Grassino A. Assessment of transdiaphragmatic pressure in humans. J Appl Physiol. 1985;58:1469–76.
73. Hamilton WF, Woodbury RA, Harper HT Jr. Arterial, cerebrospinal, and venous pressures in man during cough and strain. Am J Physiol. 1944;141:42–50.
74. Niebauer J, Börjesson M, Carre F, Caselli S, Palatini P, Quattrini F, et al. Recommendations for participation in competitive sports of athletes with arterial hypertension: a position statement from the sports cardiology section of the European Association of Preventive Cardiology (EAPC). Eur Heart J. 2018;39:3664–71.
75. Palatini P. Exaggerated blood pressure response to exercise: pathophysiologic mechanisms and clinical relevance. J Sports Med Phys Fitness. 1998;38:1–9.
76. Fagard RH. Athletes with systemic hypertension. Cardiol Clin. 2007;25:441–8.
77. Baglivo HP, Fabregues G, Burrieza H, Esper RC, Talarico M, Esper RJ. Effect of moderate physical training on left ventricular mass in mild hypertensive persons. Hypertension. 1990;15(suppl 1):I-153–6.
78. Kokkinos PF, Narayan P, Colleran JA, Pittares A, Notargiacomo A, Reda D. Effects of regular exercise on blood pressure and left ventricular hypertrophy in African-American men with severe hypertension. N Engl J Med. 1995;333:1462–7.
79. Zanettini R, Bettega D, Agostoni O, Ballestra B, del Rosso G, di Michele R, et al. Exercise training in mild hypertension: effects on blood pressure, left ventricular mass and coagulation factor VII and fibrinogen. Cardiology. 1997;88:468–73.
80. Palatini P, Visentin P, Dorigatti F, Guarnieri C, Santonastaso M, Cozzio S, et al. Regular physical activity prevents development of left ventricular hypertrophy in hypertension. Eur Heart J. 2009;30:225–32.
81. Boman K, Gerdts E, Wachtell K, Dahlöf B, Nieminen MS, Olofsson M, et al. Exercise and cardiovascular outcomes in hypertensive patients in relation to structure and function of left ventricular hypertrophy: the LIFE study. Eur J Cardiovasc Prev Rehabil. 2009;16:242–8.
82. Hinderliter A, Sherwood A, Gullette EC, Babyak M, Waugh R, Georgiades A, et al. Reduction of left ventricular hypertrophy after exercise and weight loss in overweight patients with mild hypertension. Arch Intern Med. 2002;162:1333–9.
83. Reid CM, Dart AM, Dewar EM, Jennings GL. Interactions between the effects of exercise and weight loss on risk factors, cardiovascular haemodynamics and left ventricular structure in overweight subjects. J Hypertens. 1994;12:291–301.
84. Cornelissen VA, Fagard RH. Effects of endurance training on blood pressure, blood pressure-regulating mechanisms, and cardiovascular risk factors. Hypertension. 2005;46:667–75.
85. Palatini P. Cardiovascular effects of exercise in young hypertensives. Int J Sports Med. 2012;33:683–90.
86. Rimmele U, Zellweger BC, Marti B, Seiler R, Mohiyeddini C, Ehlert U, et al. Trained men show lower cortisol, heart rate and psychological responses to psychosocial stress compared with untrained men. Psychoneuroendocrinology. 2007;32:627–35.
87. Palatini P, Bratti P, Palomba D, Saladini F, Zanatta N, Maraglino G. Regular physical activity attenuates the BP response to public speaking and delays the development of hypertension. J Hypertens. 2010;28:1186–93.
88. Laterza MC, de Matos LD, Trombetta IC, Braga AM, Roveda F, Alves MJ, et al. Exercise training restores baroreflex sensitivity in never-treated hypertensive patients. Hypertension. 2007;49:1298–306.

Effect of Physical Activity on Blood Pressure and Prevention of Hypertension

2

Véronique Cornelissen and Marina Bersaoui

2.1 Physical Activity (PA) and Hypertension: Data from Large Cohort Trials

2.1.1 PA in Daily Life and Incident Hypertension

Large epidemiological studies, which allowed for age and other confounding characteristics, have yielded consistent findings showing an inverse relation between the incidence of hypertension and habitual levels of physical activity (PA), assessed by means of questionnaires or sometimes an interview [1]. Huai et al. pooled 13 of these cohort studies [2] and found that among 136,846 adults with normal blood pressure (BP) at baseline, 11.4% developed hypertension after a median follow-up of 10 years. Engaging in high or moderate levels of leisure time PA (PA) was associated with decreased risk of hypertension (high versus low: RR, 0.81; 95% CI, 0.76–0.85; I^2 = 28% and moderate versus low: RR, 0.89; 95% CI, 0.85–0.94; I^2 = 0%) [2]. On the other hand, higher levels of commuting PA (*n* = 2 cohorts) and occupational PA (*n* = 6 cohorts) were not associated with a lower risk for hypertension [2]. More recently, Liu et al. [3] reported in a larger group of 330,222 adults (21 cohorts) who were initially free of hypertension a similar pooled relative risk for hypertension of 0.84 (95% CI, 0.78,0.90) in the most active individuals. As shown in Fig. 2.1, an inverse linear dose–response relation was established between the amount of leisure-time PA and incident hypertension, with no lower cutoff of benefit [3]. For each 10 metabolic equivalent of task (MET)-hours per week increment in leisure-time PA, which corresponds to meeting the recommended minimum PA level of 150 min per week (about 2 and a half hours), the risk of developing hypertension was found to fall by 6% [RR 0.94; 95%CI 0.92,0.96)]. When participants

V. Cornelissen (✉) · M. Bersaoui
O & N 4 Department of Rehabilitation Sciences, Leuven, Belgium
e-mail: veronique.cornelissen@kuleuven.be; Marina.bersaoui@kuleuven.be

P. Palatini et al. (eds.), *Exercise, Sports and Hypertension*, Updates in Hypertension and Cardiovascular Protection,
https://doi.org/10.1007/978-3-031-07958-0_2

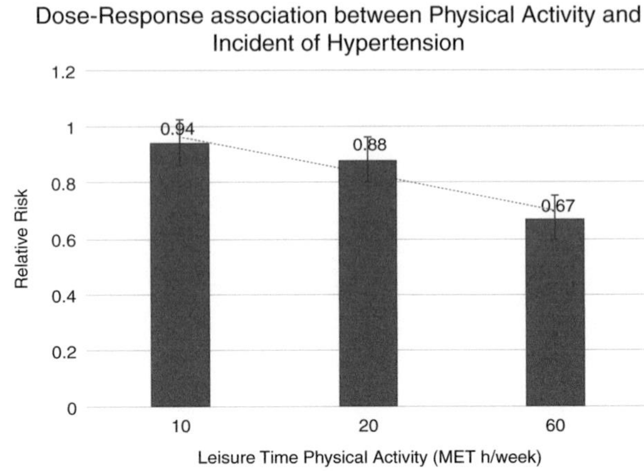

Fig. 2.1 Dose–response association between leisure-time PA (MET h/week) and incident hypertension predicted relative risk (RR) point estimates. (Adapted from Liu et al. [3])

performed twice this amount of activity, the risk was further reduced by 12% [RR 0.88; (95%CI 0.83,0.92)] [3].

Also changing behaviour toward a more physically active lifestyle has been associated with smaller increments in BP over time [4]. Williams et al. reported that a decrease of vigorous PA over a 7.4-year period of follow-up increased the odds of developing hypertension [4]. Moreover, it was shown that the odds of developing hypertension depended on the running distance at follow-up without relation to baseline activity [4]. This implies that uptake of a physically active lifestyle is not sufficient but that the adoption of a lifelong physically active life is crucial for sustained antihypertensive effects.

2.1.2 PA in Daily Life and Future CV Disease in Patients with Hypertension

In addition to its role in the prevention of hypertension, a physically active lifestyle is key in preventing the development and progression of cardiovascular (CV) diseases among those patients living with hypertension. Several cohort studies previously reported reduced overall and CV morbidity and mortality in active hypertensive patients compared to their inactive peers [5–8]. Two recent epidemiological studies [9, 10] added further evidence to the cardioprotective effect of a physically active lifestyle in patients with hypertension. The Copenhagen City Heart Study [9], including a random sample of 18,974 white men and women aged 20 to 98 years, examined the association between self-reported activity level in leisure-time assessed from the PA Questionnaire (level I: inactivity; II: light activity; and III: moderate/high-level activity) and overall mortality and CV morbidity. As shown in Table 2.1, an inverse association between higher levels of PA and all-cause mortality was found at all levels of BP. Additionally, they proved that this association was dose-dependent, regardless of BP level. Moreover, also CV outcome (admissions for acute myocardial infarction, heart failure, stroke, or death of same causes) was

Table 2.1 Association between levels of leisure time PA and overall mortality and CV events (Adapted from Joseph et al. [9])

		Overall mortality	CV events
Normal pressure	Inactivity	1.00 (reference)	1.00 (reference)
	Light activity	0.76 (0.64–0.91)**	0.73 (0.57–0.93)*
	Moderate/vigorous activity	0.68 (0.56–0.84)***	0.66 (0.51–0.86)**
Prehypertension	Inactivity	1.00 (reference)	1.00 (reference)
	Light activity	0.84 (0.77–0.93)**	0.81 (0.71–0.91)***
	Moderate/vigorous activity	0.76 (0.69–0.85)***	0.81 (0.71–0.93)**
Hypertension: stage 1	Inactivity	1.00 (reference)	1.00 (reference)
	Light activity	0.78 (0.72–0.84)***	0.77 (0.70–0.85)***
	Moderate/vigorous activity	0.69 (0.63–0.75)***	0.69 (0.62–0.77)***
Hypertension: stage 2	Inactivity	1.00 (reference)	1.00 (reference)
	Light activity	0.82 (0.75–0.89)***	0.74 (0.68–0.82)***
	Moderate/vigorous activity	0.72 (0.66–0.80)***	0.77 (0.69–0.86)***

Cox regression with time-dependent covariates showing hazard ratios and 95% CIs for all-cause mortality and CV events for each of the BP levels according to the level of PA. Hazard rates were adjusted for sex, age, calendar time, smoking status, BMI class, diabetes, previous CV disease, and education

*p<0.05; **p<0.01; ***p<0.001

significantly reduced by PA independent of the BP-level. Of interest is that reductions in all-cause mortality and CV events were already achieved at low levels of PA and that no interaction between the level of PA and BP groups was seen. This suggests that patients will already achieve important health benefits from just moving from an inactive lifestyle toward low volumes of physical activity. Additionally, the effect on outcome will be the same, irrespective of BP level [9]. Using data from 20,179 hypertensive individuals of a substudy of the China Kadoorie Biobank study, Zhou et al. examined the association between different domains of PA with the risk of CV disease at 10 years of follow-up [10]. In concordance with previous research, they found that being physically active was significantly associated with a reduced risk of CV disease among patients with hypertension: the hazard ratios for CV diseases were 0.87 (95%CI: 0.79–0.97), 0.73 (95%CI: 0.65–0.83) and 0.75 (95%CI: 0.65–0.85) for participants within 2, 3 and 4 quartiles of PA compared to the lowest active group [10]. Though, in contrast to the results of the Copenhagen City Heart Study [9], the association between PA level and CV disease risk was not linear, but U-shaped with the lower hazard rate observed at 35.4 MET-h/d, suggesting that an optimal PA level existed for prevention of CV disease among hypertensive patients [10]. Future research is needed to confirm or refute this U-shaped association.

2.2 Impact of Exercise Therapy on BP: Data from Meta-Analyses of Randomized Controlled Trials

Based on numerous meta-analyses, structured and planned PA, henceforward called exercise, is recognized by all guidelines as a key intervention (class IA recommendation) to lower BP in hypertensive patients [11–14]. This is supported by a recent network meta-analysis showing that exercise is at least equally effective in reducing BP of patients with hypertension as first-line antihypertensive medication [15]. In line with pharmacokinetics of drugs, it is also to be expected that the responses to exercise therapy will depend on particular characteristics of the intervention (i.e., type, frequency, duration and intensity, timing) and may vary among different patient populations (young versus old, men versus women, etc.). For this chapter, we will rely on meta-analyses published after 2000 that investigated the effect of the three main types of exercise: aerobic endurance training, dynamic resistance training and isometric resistance training and will briefly touch on the impact of each of the above-mentioned characteristics.

2.2.1 Blood Pressure Changes Following Dynamic Aerobic Endurance Exercise Therapy

Dynamic aerobic endurance exercise, defined as physical activities that involve large muscle groups in dynamic repetitive activities aiming to increase cardiorespiratory fitness, has unequivocally shown its efficacy in lowering BP and is therefore considered the exercise modality of choice when aiming to lower BP in hypertensive patients [11–13, 16–18]. A review by Hanssen et al. [17] summarizing data of 21 meta-analyses on the BP lowering potential of aerobic exercise found overall effects of −4.1 mmHg/−2.2 mmHg. Comparable reductions in daytime ambulatory BP [−3.2 mmHg, (−5.0 to −1.3)/(−2.7 mmHg, (−3.9 to −1.5)] observed by pooling data from 16 randomized controlled trials add further support to the BP lowering potential of aerobic exercise training [19]. Importantly, in the largest meta-analysis to date, including >4000 participants, Cornelissen and Smart [20] found BP decreases to be most pronounced in 26 study groups with hypertensive participants (−8.3 [−10.7 to −6.0]/−5.2 [−6.8 to −3.4] mmHg) than in the 50 groups of prehypertensive subjects (−2.1 [−3.3 to −0.83]/−1.7 [−2.7 to −0.68]) and 29 groups of subjects with normal BP levels (−0.75 [−2.2 to +0.69]/−1.1 [−2.2 to −0.068]). As efficacy of antihypertensive drug treatment is heterogeneous among ethnic groups, and exercise guidelines are based on trials involving Caucasian populations, Bersaoui et al. [21] aimed to assess the BP lowering effect of aerobic exercise among nonwhite populations. Trials among African descendants were scant with only 5 study groups that could be included. More trials (n = 13 study groups) were identified among Asian populations. Notably, aerobic exercise significantly reduced BP in each of these nonwhite ethnic groups [−7.2 (−10.6; −3.9)/−4.7 (−7.1; −2.2) mmHg in the Asian subgroup and − 12.4 (−17.9; −6.9) /−4.1 (−7.2; −1.1) mmHg in African descendants]. Subanalysis indicated a trend toward larger reductions in systolic BP in African descendants with hypertension compared to Asian hypertensives [21]. Earlier, Whelton et al. [22] also suggested that African descendants might have significantly larger reductions in systolic BP, and Asian participants significantly greater reductions in diastolic BP compared to white participants. With regard to sex, Cornelissen and Smart [20] found that BP decreases were twice as large in men, which was in contrast to Kelley et al. [23] and Igarashi et al. [24] who reported similar BP reductions among both sexes. Evidence to date seems to suggest that the BP-lowering effect of aerobic exercise can be expected both in young hypertensive individuals [25] as well as older patients [20]. However, it needs to be recognized that given the lack of adjustment for important confounders in all of these subgroup analyses and in particular the absence of direct comparison studies between men and women, young and old or participants of different ethnic origin, further research is required to establish whether differences in the BP response to aerobic exercise training according to important demographics exist, and if so why.

How to prescribe an aerobic exercise program that maximally lowers BP? In univariate weighted regression analysis [26] and subgroup analyses [20], weekly training frequency did not contribute significantly to explain the interstudy variance of the BP response to aerobic exercise training, that is, training frequencies between 3 and 7 days per week lowered BP [26]. However, comparative studies found that the fall in BP was significantly greater in 5 versus 3 days walking group [27] or 7 versus 1 days per week schedules [28] Today, for patients with hypertension, most guidelines endorse aerobic exercise on most, if not all days per week, because of the immediate reduction in BP seen following a single exercise session [14, 16]. This phenomenon of postexercise hypotension [29] is considered a viable tool in daily BP management by lowering a hypertensive patient's BP into more normal ranges for specific periods of the day. Regarding intensity, moderate intensity aerobic exercise (40–60% heart rate reserve) is recommended to prevent and treat high BP [11, 12, 16, 18]. However, many hypertensive patients with diverse comorbidities are older or limited in the level of PA they can undertake. In this context, it is of note that Cornelissen et al. [30] found equal reductions in office BP, BP during submaximal exercise and during recovery from exercise in older sedentary individuals following 10 weeks of aerobic exercise at 33% heart rate reserve versus 66% heart rate reserve. In agreement, a Cochrane meta-analysis including 73 trials found moderate-certainty evidence suggesting that walking reduces systolic BP (−4.1 mmHg, 95% CI -5.2 to −3.0), n = 5060) [31]. For diastolic BP, only low-certainty evidence was found [31]. Likewise, post exercise hypotension is already observed following low intensity aerobic exercise, though it should be acknowledged that more intense sessions induce larger and more sustained BP reductions [32]. Following here, we have witnessed a growing interest in the application of high intensity interval training (HIIT) in clinical populations. However, evidence to support HIIT for the purpose of BP lowering remains inconclusive and debatable, especially in hypertensive patients who are at higher CV risk. Meta-analytic research by Costa et al. [33] and Way et al. [34] found comparable reductions in office BP and ambulatory BP in adults with hypertension following HIIT and moderate intensity continuous training, though Leal et al. [35] reported larger reductions in office diastolic BP, but not for systolic BP in support of HIIT. On the other hand, a single session of high intensity exercise promoted a greater postexercise hypotension than a single session of moderate continuous exercise on ambulatory daytime BP [36].

2.2.2 Blood Pressure Changes Following Dynamic Resistance Exercise Therapy

Dynamic resistance training involves concentric and/or eccentric contractions of muscles while both the length and the tension of the muscles change and is usually performed to improve muscle strength. Despite initial scepticism about the BP lowering capability of dynamic resistance training, important advances in the last two decades resulted in a recognition of the value of dynamic resistance exercise in the management of hypertensive patients. Today, dynamic resistance exercise, 2–3 days per week, is endorsed by the guidelines as part of lifestyle intervention in patients with hypertension [11–13]. This is reinforced by meta-analytic data [37] showing that moderate intense dynamic resistance training provoked BP reductions that were comparable to those previously reported with aerobic endurance training, advising as such the potential of dynamic resistance training as a stand-alone antihypertensive therapy. Moreover, like for aerobic endurance exercise, hypertensive individuals seemed to benefit the most: that is, BP reduction of −6/−5 mmHg were seen in hypertensive patients versus 0/1 mmHg in patients with normal pressure [37]. Similarly, a single session of dynamic resistance training performed at 40–80% of 1RM elicit small but meaningful reductions in ambulatory BP, with hypertensive patients showing the best response [38]. Nonetheless, it needs to be recognized that data on the effectiveness of dynamic resistance exercise on ambulatory BP are still lacking, and no studies have been performed among African descendants. Therefore, more RCTs are needed to more definitively determine whether dynamic resistance training can act as an equal alternative to aerobic endurance training in hypertensive patients.

2.2.3 Blood Pressure Changes Following Isometric Resistance Exercise Therapy

Emerging evidence supporting the BP lowering effect of isometric resistance exercise has led to the revision of many hypertension guidelines with most of them now recommending low intensity isometric resistance training at least as an adjunct therapy in the management of hypertension [11–13, 18]. An isometric training regimen usually consists of several intermittent bouts of sustained handgrip or leg contractions at 10–30% maximal strength lasting 2 min each, interspersed with a short period of rest, for a total of 12 to 15 min per session. As such, this type of intervention which can be performed easily at any place and any time with minimal time investment makes it an accessible tool to every patient with hypertension. The meta-review by Hanssen et al. [17] found a mean BP-lowering effect of isometric resistance training ($n = 33$ trials) of −10.0/−5.8 mmHg. The individuals with normal BP (17 trials) obtained a BP reduction of −6.6/−3 mmHg while it was a little bit less in hypertensive individuals −4.3/−5.0 mmHg (CI: 95%). Earlier, an individual participant meta-analysis by Smart et al. [39], combining data from 12 studies involving 326 participants (52.7% medicated for hypertension, 191 assigned to IRT and 153 controls) found a BP-lowering effect of −6.2 (−7.75, −4.68)/−2.78(−3.92, −1.65) mmHg. Subanalyses detected no clinically significant effects in SBP and DBP based on sex, age (<45 years vs. >45 years) medication status, BMI category or hypertensive status (normotensives vs hypertensives) or extremity category (arm vs leg exercise). However, the unmedicated group (−10.18, CI 95%, −15.50 to −4.86 mmHg) showed a trend toward a greater reduction in SBP than the medicated (−5.86 (CI 95%, −9.19 to −2.54 mmHg) group [39]. Of note, the number of studies performed in females and patients with hypertension is still extremely small, making it difficult to quantify any sex-related and clinical status related differences about the antihypertensive effect of isometric resistance training and to generalize the results to the overall population. Moreover, results on the effect of isometric exercise on post exercise hypotension remain inconclusive [40–42]. As such, clearly, further research is still called for to explore the promising merits of low intensity isometric training as a BP lowering therapy.

2.3 Conclusion

PA and exercise are imperative in an effective BP management strategy. Aerobic endurance exercise remains the primary modality to recommend to patients with hypertension, though evidence is growing with regard to BP lowering potential of dynamic and isometric resistance training. To date, both are only considered as a second-line treatment in hypertension. Future research and stronger evidence are warranted to elucidate whether isometric resistance and dynamic resistance training can be recommended as a suitable alterative to aerobic exercise in hypertensive patients. Finally, there is a need for more research directly comparing the effectiveness of different exercise programs among sexes, ethnic groups, age-groups, and so on to allow for tailoring the exercise prescription to best meet the needs of each specific patient group.

References

1. Cornelissen V, Fagard R. Hypertension. In: Saxton J, editor. Exercise and chronic disease: an evidence-based approach. Abingdon: Routledge; 2011.
2. Huai P, Xun H, Reilly KH, Wang Y, Ma W, Xi B. Physical activity and risk of hypertension: a meta-analysis of prospective cohort studies. Hypertension. 2013;62(6):1021–6.
3. Liu X, Zhang D, Liu Y, Sun X, Han C, Wang B, et al. Dose-response association between physical activity and incident hypertension: a systematic review and meta-analysis of cohort studies. Hypertension. 2017;69(5):813–20.
4. Williams PT. A cohort study of incident hypertension in relation to changes in vigorous physical activity in men and women. J Hypertens. 2008;26(6):1085–93.
5. Vatten LJ, Nilsen TI, Holmen J. Combined effect of blood pressure and physical activity on cardiovascular mortality. J Hypertens. 2006;24(10):1939–46.
6. Fossum E, Gleim GW, Kjeldsen SE, Kizer JR, Julius S, Devereux RB, et al. The effect of baseline physical activity on cardiovascular outcomes and new-onset diabetes in patients treated for hypertension and left ventricular hypertrophy: the LIFE study. J Intern Med. 2007;262(4):439–48.

7. Fang J, Wylie-Rosett J, Alderman MH. Exercise and cardiovascular outcomes by hypertensive status: NHANES I epidemiological follow-up study, 1971–1992. Am J Hypertens. 2005;18(6):751–8.
8. Hu G, Jousilahti P, Antikainen R, Tuomilehto J. Occupational, commuting, and leisure-time physical activity in relation to cardiovascular mortality among finnish subjects with hypertension. Am J Hypertens. 2007;20(12):1242–50.
9. Joseph G, Marott JL, Torp-Pedersen C, Biering-Sørensen T, Nielsen G, Christensen AE, et al. Dose-response association between level of physical activity and mortality in normal, elevated, and high blood pressure. Hypertension. 2019;74(6):1307–15.
10. Zhou T, Su J, Tao R, Qin Y, Zhou J, Lu Y, et al. The association between daily total physical activity and risk of cardiovascular disease among hypertensive patients: a 10-year prospective cohort study in China. BMC Public Health. 2021;21(1):517.
11. Williams B, Mancia G, Spiering W, Agabiti Rosei E, Azizi M, Burnier M, et al. 2018 practice guidelines for the management of arterial hypertension of the European Society of Hypertension and the European Society of Cardiology: ESH/ESC task force for the Management of Arterial Hypertension. J Hypertens. 2018;36(12):2284–309.
12. Whelton PK, Carey RM, Aronow WS, Casey DE, Collins KJ, Dennison Himmelfarb C, et al. 2017 ACC/AHA/AAPA/ABC/ACPM/AGS/APhA/ASH/ASPC/NMA/PCNA guideline for the prevention, detection, evaluation, and Management of High Blood Pressure in adults: a report of the American College of Cardiology/American Heart Association task force on clinical practice guidelines. J Am Coll Cardiol. 2018;71(19):e127–248.
13. Unger T, Borghi C, Charchar F, Khan NA, Poulter NR, Prabhakaran D, et al. 2020 International Society of Hypertension Global Hypertension Practice Guidelines. Hypertension. 2020;75(6):1334–57.
14. Pescatello LS, MacDonald HV, Ash GI, Lamberti LM, Farquhar WB, Arena R, et al. Assessing the existing professional exercise recommendations for hypertension: a review and recommendations for future research priorities. Mayo Clin Proc. 2015;90(6):801–12.
15. Noone C, Leahy J, Morrissey EC, Newell J, Newell M, Dwyer CP, et al. Comparative efficacy of exercise and anti-hypertensive pharmacological interventions in reducing blood pressure in people with hypertension: a network meta-analysis. Eur J Prev Cardiol. 2020;27(3):247–55.
16. Pescatello LS, MacDonald HV, Lamberti L, Johnson BT. Exercise for hypertension: a prescription update integrating existing recommendations with emerging research. Curr Hypertens Rep. 2015;17(11):87.
17. Hanssen H, Boardman H, Deiseroth A, Moholdt T, Simonenko M, Kränkel N, et al. Personalized exercise prescription in the prevention and treatment of arterial hypertension: a consensus document from the European Association of Preventive Cardiology (EAPC) and the ESC Council on hypertension. Eur J Prev Cardiol. 2021;29:205–15.
18. Hansen D, Niebauer J, Cornelissen V, Barna O, Neunhäuserer D, Stettler C, et al. Exercise prescription in patients with different combinations of cardiovascular disease risk factors: a consensus statement from the EXPERT working group. Sports Med. 2018;48(8):1781–97.
19. Cornelissen VA, Buys R, Smart NA. Endurance exercise beneficially affects ambulatory blood pressure: a systematic review and meta-analysis. J Hypertens. 2013;31(4):639–48.
20. Cornelissen VA, Smart NA. Exercise training for blood pressure: a systematic review and meta-analysis. J Am Heart Assoc. 2013;2(1):e004473.
21. Bersaoui M, Baldew SM, Cornelis N, Toelsie J, Cornelissen VA. The effect of exercise training on blood pressure in African and Asian populations: a systematic review and meta-analysis of randomized controlled trials. Eur J Prev Cardiol. 2020;27(5):457–72.
22. Whelton SP, Chin A, Xin X, He J. Effect of aerobic exercise on blood pressure: a meta-analysis of randomized, controlled trials. Ann Intern Med. 2002;136(7):493–503.
23. Kelley GA, Kelley KA, Tran ZV. Aerobic exercise and resting blood pressure: a meta-analytic review of randomized, controlled trials. Prev Cardiol. 2001;4(2):73–80.
24. Igarashi Y, Akazawa N, Maeda S. Regular aerobic exercise and blood pressure in east Asians: a meta-analysis of randomized controlled trials. Clin Exp Hypertens. 2018;40(4):378–89.

25. Williamson W, Foster C, Reid H, Kelly P, Lewandowski AJ, Boardman H, et al. Will exercise advice be sufficient for treatment of young adults with prehypertension and hypertension? A systematic review and meta-analysis. Hypertension. 2016;68(1):78–87.
26. Cornelissen VA, Fagard RH. Effects of endurance training on blood pressure, blood pressure-regulating mechanisms, and cardiovascular risk factors. Hypertension. 2005;46(4):667–75.
27. Tully MA, Cupples ME, Hart ND, McEneny J, McGlade KJ, Chan WS, et al. Randomised controlled trial of home-based walking programmes at and below current recommended levels of exercise in sedentary adults. J Epidemiol Community Health. 2007;61(9):778–83.
28. Jennings G, Nelson L, Nestel P, Esler M, Korner P, Burton D, et al. The effects of changes in physical activity on major cardiovascular risk factors, hemodynamics, sympathetic function, and glucose utilization in man: a controlled study of four levels of activity. Circulation. 1986;73(1):30–40.
29. Kenney MJ, Seals DR. Postexercise hypotension. Key features, mechanisms, and clinical significance. Hypertension. 1993;22(5):653–64.
30. Cornelissen VA, Arnout J, Holvoet P, Fagard RH. Influence of exercise at lower and higher intensity on blood pressure and cardiovascular risk factors at older age. J Hypertens. 2009;27(4):753–62.
31. Lee LL, Mulvaney CA, Wong YKY, Chan ES, Watson MC, Lin HH. Walking for hypertension. Cochrane Database Syst Rev. 2021;2:CD008823.
32. Eicher JD, Maresh CM, Tsongalis GJ, Thompson PD, Pescatello LS. The additive blood pressure lowering effects of exercise intensity on post-exercise hypotension. Am Heart J. 2010;160(3):513–20.
33. Costa EC, Hay JL, Kehler DS, Boreskie KF, Arora RC, Umpierre D, et al. Effects of high-intensity interval training versus moderate-intensity continuous training on blood pressure in adults with pre- to established hypertension: a systematic review and meta-analysis of randomized trials. Sports Med. 2018;48(9):2127–42.
34. Way KL, Sultana RN, Sabag A, Baker MK, Johnson NA. The effect of high intensity interval training versus moderate intensity continuous training on arterial stiffness and 24h blood pressure responses: a systematic review and meta-analysis. J Sci Med Sport. 2019;22(4):385–91.
35. Leal JM, Galliano LM, Del Vecchio FB. Effectiveness of high-intensity interval training versus moderate-intensity continuous training in hypertensive patients: a systematic review and meta-analysis. Curr Hypertens Rep. 2020;22(3):26.
36. Marçal IR, Goessler KF, Buys R, Casonatto J, Ciolac EG, Cornelissen VA. Post-exercise hypotension following a single bout of high intensity interval exercise vs a single bout of moderate intensity continuous exercise in adults with or without hypertension: a systematic review and meta-analysis of randomized clinical trials. Front Physiol. 2021;12:675289.
37. MacDonald HV, Johnson BT, Huedo-Medina TB, Livingston J, Forsyth KC, Kraemer WJ, et al. Dynamic resistance training as stand-alone antihypertensive lifestyle therapy: a meta-analysis. J Am Heart Assoc. 2016;5(10):e003231.
38. Casonatto J, Goessler KF, Cornelissen VA, Cardoso JR, Polito MD. The blood pressure-lowering effect of a single bout of resistance exercise: a systematic review and meta-analysis of randomised controlled trials. Eur J Prev Cardiol. 2016;23(16):1700–14.
39. Smart NA, Way D, Carlson D, Millar P, McGowan C, Swaine I, et al. Effects of isometric resistance training on resting blood pressure: individual participant data meta-analysis. J Hypertens. 2019;37(10):1927–38.
40. Goessler K, Buys R, Cornelissen VA. Low-intensity isometric handgrip exercise has no transient effect on blood pressure in patients with coronary artery disease. J Am Soc Hypertens. 2016;10(8):633–9.
41. van Assche T, Buys R, de Jaeger M, Coeckelberghs E, Cornelissen VA. One single bout of low-intensity isometric handgrip exercise reduces blood pressure in healthy pre- and hypertensive individuals. J Sports Med Phys Fitness. 2017;57(4):469–75.
42. Olher RR, Bocalini DS, Bacurau RF, Rodriguez D, Figueira A, Pontes FL, et al. Isometric handgrip does not elicit cardiovascular overload or post-exercise hypotension in hypertensive older women. Clin Interv Aging. 2013;8:649–55.

Effect of Regular Exercise on Autonomic Nervous System Activity

3

Gino Seravalle and Guido Grassi

3.1 Physical Activity Versus Physical Inactivity

Lifestyle factors and physical inactivity are associated with cardiovascular (CV) disease development [1–3]. Physical activity is one of the main targeted areas in primary cardiovascular prevention [2]. Worldwide, 25% of adults and 75% adolescents currently do not meet the recommendations for physical activity set by the WHO [3]. On the contrary several evidences show that adults obtain important benefits and increase longevity by becoming more physically active, independently of established CV risk factors [4, 5]. In a recent systematic review it has been studied the different relationships between physical activity levels and patient outcomes [6]. The results have shown that (a) the associations of physical activity with beneficial health begin when adopting even very modest levels, (b) meeting the recommendations reduces mortality and cardiovascular risk to about 75% of the maximal benefit obtained by physical activity alone, and (c) physical activity levels beyond the guidelines' recommended levels reduce risk even more. Actually recommendations are not conclusive regarding advice on resistance training. A combination of aerobic physical activity and resistance training appears to be effective for people with diabetes and in preventing and managing cardiovascular disease [7–9]. This is due to the decrease in body weight, body mass index and abdominal visceral fat, and improvement in cardiorespiratory fitness and insulin sensitivity. Nevertheless there is insufficient evidence to support substituting aerobic exercise with resistance training [10]. On the contrary all the recommendations are in accord defining

G. Seravalle (✉)
Cardiology Department, IRCCS Istituto Auxologico Italiano, S. Luca Hospital, Milan, Italy

G. Grassi
Clinica Medica, University Milano-Bicocca, Monza, Italy
e-mail: Guido.Grassi@unimib.it

P. Palatini et al. (eds.), *Exercise, Sports and Hypertension*, Updates in Hypertension and Cardiovascular Protection,
https://doi.org/10.1007/978-3-031-07958-0_3

sedentary behavior an independent risk factor for cardiovascular morbidity and mortality and the reductions in total daily sitting should be recommended in public health guidelines [11].

3.2 Physiological Effects of Exercise

Regular physical exercise is a therapeutic lifestyle intervention for achieving optimal cardiovascular (CV) and overall health, as emphasized by several guidelines [12–15]. Physical activity triggers beneficial physiological effects on the entire body (Fig. 3.1) and can be a valuable tool for preventing and treating chronic diseases such as hypertension, coronary heart disease, heart failure, obesity and metabolic syndrome, and diabetes. Due to its beneficial effects on coronary flow reserve, myocardial capillary density, endothelial function, arterial blood pressure, heart rate, and lipid profile, regular physical activity represents the cornerstone of cardiological rehabilitative intervention [16].

When a subject exercises at progressively higher-power outputs, there is a linear increase in oxygen uptake to match the demand of the active skeletal muscles until the maximal oxygen consumptions (VO_{2max}) is reached. The VO_{2max} is an indicator of the system's ability to deliver oxygen to active muscles as well as a biomarker of health. The VO_{2max} can be twice in trained subjects and can be increased by approximately 15% with training. The determinants of oxygen consumption are

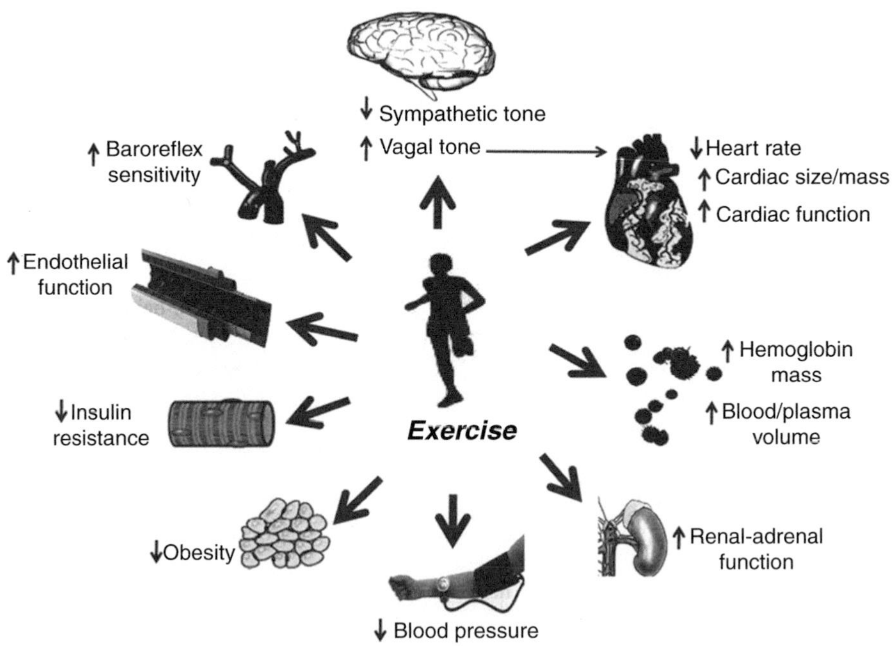

Fig. 3.1 Physiologic effects of regular physical exercise

Table 3.1 Hemodynamic and metabolic effects of exercise training

Variable	Effect
Stroke volume	↑
Arterial blood pressure	↓
Heart rate	↓
Capillary density	↑
Mitochondrial density	↑
Endothelial function	↑
Blood volume	↑
Blood viscosity	↓
HDL cholesterol	↑
LDL cholesterol	↓
Triglycerides	↓
Glucose	=↓
Insulin sensitivity	↑

HDL high-density lipoproteins, *LDL* low-density lipoproteins, = unchanged

summarized in the Fick equation: $VO_2 = CO \times (CaO_2 - CVO_2)$, where VO_2 is oxygen consumption, CO is cardiac output, and $CaO_2 - CVO_2$ is the arterial-venous blood O_2 difference. Cardiac output is the product of stroke volume and heart rate. It increases linearly with exercise intensity. This is the case also for the a-vO_2 difference [17, 18]. During exercise is possible to observe a progressive increase in systolic blood pressure while diastolic blood pressure remains relatively unchanged [19]. Differences may be observed when exercise is performed with the arms, where blood pressure may be 10% greater than when legs are used due to the greater resistance of the vascular bed in the upper side.

Several factors may affect exercise performance such as muscle buffering capacity, gender, age, genetics, chronic inactivity, medical conditions and drug therapies [18–22]. On the other hand exercise training is associated with significant adaptations. In particular endurance training elicits many adaptations in skeletal muscles and in the metabolic and cardiorespiratory system improving the ability to deliver and utilize oxygen for energy production, the capacity for prolonged exercise, sports performance, and daily life activities in absence of fatigue (Table 3.1) [23].

3.3 Physical Exercise Prescription

Usually exercise prescription should be in accord to relative intensity and it is intended to produce an approximately equivalent exercise stress in individuals with different absolute exercise capacities. The traditional approach has been to prescribe exercise intensity as a percentage of maximal oxygen uptake (VO_{2max}) or maximum heart rate (HR_{max}) and these methods remain commonly used. Due to the differences in the metabolic thresholds for the same $\%VO_{2max}$ or $\%HR_{max}$, someone recommends that exercise intensity should be prescribed relative to oxygen consumption reserve (VO_2R), to heart rate reserve (HRR), to the aerobic

Table 3.2 Practical physical activity recommendations in different pathophysiological conditions (adapted from [12–15]

Obesity	Volume exercise >250 min (or >1500 kcal)/week
	Moderate-intensity exercise (40–60% HRR)
	Involving large muscle groups (walking, stepping, cross training)
	3–5 days/week
Hypertension	Moderate-intensity exercise (40–60% HRR)
	Endurance exercise
	30–45 min per day
	3–5 days/week
Dyslipidemia	Caloric expenditure >900 kcal/week
	Moderate–high intensity (40–60% HRR)
	>40 min/session
	>4 days/week
T2DM	Energy expenditure 1000–2000 kcal/week
	Moderate-intensity exercise (40–60% HRR)
	>150 min/week

(Aer) or anaerobic (An) threshold (T) [24]. While for athletes it is common to "individualize" training programs according to their specific characteristics, the sport differences, the pre-game or post-game period, for healthy nonathletes or subjects affected by pathophysiological conditions this is usually more generalized and included in recommendations made by several scientific societies (Table 3.2) [3–6, 12–15].

3.4 The Autonomic Nervous System: How to Measure and Quantify

3.4.1 Heart Rate and Heart Rate Variability

Resting heart rate is really easy to assess and is worldwide used as a main parameter associated to blood pressure values and breathing to evaluate the healthy status of a subject. The wide diffusion of wearable systems also allows to evaluate changes during physical activity or sleeping period and also to detect the appearance of an arrhythmia. Resting heart rate is a sensitive indicator of the autonomic nervous system activity and an increase in this parameter has been associated with increased risk of cardiovascular disease and total mortality [25, 26]. Exercise training is accompanied by a decrease in resting heart rate due to an increase in parasympathetic activity and a reduction in sympathetic activity [27, 28]. Changes in resting heart rate and in responses to physical activities are quite easy to observe just after few weeks of training and help to understand whether hemodynamic adaptations are activated [29].

The heart rate is under the influence of the autonomic nervous system by acetylcholine and norepinephrine release [30]. Sympathetic and parasympathetic fibers are not homogeneously distributed with a prevalence action of right fibers and a greatly rapid response of parasympathetic fibers due to the rapid release and removal of acetylcholine. Heart rate is under control of anterior part of the brain, thalamus and hypothalamus, which receive information by peripheral receptors located in aortic arch and in carotid sinus (sensible to changes in arterial pressure) or in the lungs and atria (sensible to respiratory activity, intrathoracic pressure and stretching of the atria) [31].

Two other parameters have been found to have physiological importance. The baroreflex sensitivity, that is the quantification of changes in heart rate in response to defined pressure changes, which represent an indirect measure of central modulation of the heart [31]. A reduction in baroreflex sensitivity is present in several pathophysiological conditions with a consequent sympathovagal imbalance toward an adrenergic preponderance [32].

The second parameter is represented by the analysis of its oscillatory components that allows to quantify the interactions between autonomic neural activity, blood pressure and respiratory control systems and is called heart rate variability (HRV) [33, 34]. A decrease in the HRV can be observed during an hyperadrenergic tone and is correlated with an increased risk of cardiac mortality and is a predictive risk factor for cardiovascular events [33]. It can be measured through prolonged EKG recordings that can accurately measure RR intervals and is calculated using time domain indexes, frequency indexes and nonlinear indexes [35]. Usually it is used to assess cardiac vagal tone [35, 36].

3.4.2 The Sympathetic Nervous System

Several methods either invasive or noninvasive are available to measure the adrenergic tone. The more sensible and reproducible are the invasive ones which are mainly used for clinical research; the indirect methods are less sensible and reproducible and are frequently used in routine clinical examinations.

3.4.2.1 Microneurography

Microneurography is the only method available for direct recordings of postganglionic sympathetic traffic in humans. This method is minimally invasive (insertion of a thin needle of tungsten usually in the peroneal nerve fascicle) and allows to record the sympathetic nerve traffic both to the skin and the muscle. The analysis consists in the use of an integrated signal of multiple nerve fibers to report sympathetic nerve activity as burst frequency (count of the number of bursts occurring in a minute), burst incidence (the number of bursts occurring per 100 heart beats) or measurement of the total nerve activity (mean burst amplitude or area × number of bursts in 1 min) [28, 32, 37–42]. Although it represents the gold standard, it has several limitations. First, it is minimally invasive and restricted to an expert laboratory. Second, it needs limb relaxed and immobile. Third, it can be not applied to internal organs although simultaneous recordings with different methodologies have shown that microneurography is a good marker of sympathetic responses in several internal organs [43, 44]. Fourth, it needs a skilled technician.

3.4.2.2 Norepinephrine Spillover

The radiotracer-derived measurement is a method based on the measurement of norepinephrine outflow to the circulation. Tritiated I-norepinephrine is infused in the patient's circulation, allowing to measure organ-specific norepinephrine spill over to plasma by isotope dilution [43–45]. Obviously this is an invasive method (catheterism) that needs availability and disposal of radiotracer thus limiting its use. On the contrary, it allows to measure the spill over at the level of different organs (heart, kidney, brain or total body) [43, 44] allowing a precise differentiation of activity of the sympathetic nervous system in different pathophysiological conditions. Its use is limited to specialized centers.

3.4.2.3 Catecholamines

Plasmatic and urinary catecholamines or their products are frequently used in daily clinical activity due to the wide availability of the methodology and labs for analysis. Their use is limited to the assessment of secondary forms of hypertension [46]. Due to the reduced specificity and reproducibility [47] their use is now reduced in research sets.

3.5 Sympathetic Neural Adaptation to Exercise

The literature on this topic is full of articles making use of different types of physical activity which makes a general conclusion difficult. If the question is the reflex control of muscle sympathetic nerve activity (MSNA), usually exercise involves small muscle groups of the forearm or of the legs, while when investigation involves the effects on resting MSNA usually exercise involves the use of whole-body and large muscle mass. Several other factors may complicate the situation: (a) the training intensity, frequency and duration; (b) age and gender; (c) the population enrolled (healthy subjects or patients affected by pathophysiological conditions).

We will briefly examine the microneurographic studies performed during acute exercise, the long-term effects of exercise training and the post-exercise effects.

3.5.1 Acute Effects

Due to technical limitations these studies are performed during static or dynamic (rhythmic) exercise performed by upper or lower part of the body while MSNA recording were performed in the lower or upper part respectively. These studies have shown that MSNA increases during sustained handgrip exercise [48–54] and this increase is proportional to exercise intensity [55] (Fig. 3.2). It has been also shown that exercise in the lower limb needs both more intensity and duration to induce an increase in adrenergic tone. At low intensity leg cycling is accompanied by a MSNA inhibition due to loading of cardiopulmonary baroreceptors which is induced by a muscle pump-induced increase in venous return and central blood volume [56, 57]. The gradual increase in workload (40% VO_{2peak}) for more than

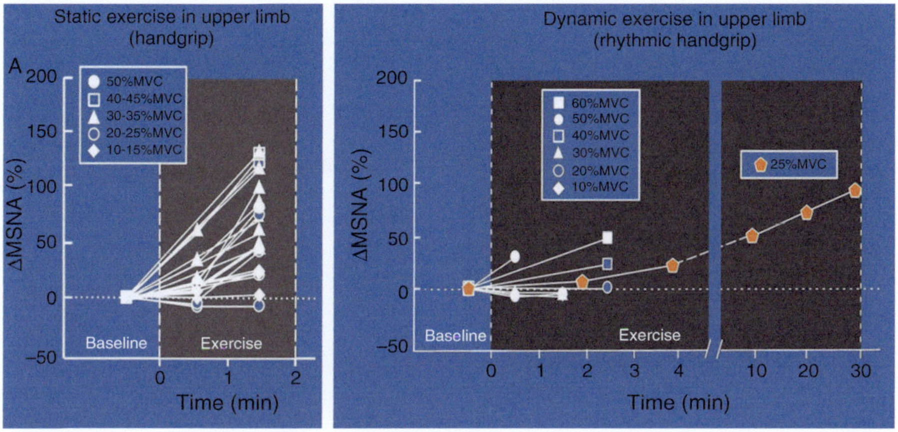

Fig. 3.2 Changes in muscle sympathetic nerve activity (MSNA) during static exercise (left panel) and dynamic exercise (right panel) at different % of maximal voluntary contraction (MVC). (Modified from [55], with permission)

30 min is accompanied by an increase in MSNA [58] and is related to a cardiovascular drift: reduction in stroke volume and arterial blood pressure and parallel increase in heart rate due to progressive increases in cutaneous blood flow and cutaneous vasodilation with the mediation of central reflex command [59, 60].

3.5.2 Long-Term Effects

Different is the influence of endurance training on sympathetic tone in healthy humans. In a study by Grassi and coworkers [28] 10 weeks of endurance training (2 h/day for 5 days/week) capable of increasing maximum oxygen consumption from 34.8 ± 2.1 to 40.4 ± 1.8 mL/kg per min, was accompanied by significant hemodynamic and autonomic changes. The study showed a significant reduction in systolic and diastolic blood pressure (136.3 ± 2.9/83.5 ± 2.0 vs. 124.8 ± 3.1/75.4 ± 2.7 mmHg, $p < 0.05$), a reduction in heart rate, and a significant reduction in MSNA (from 21.2 ± 2.3 to 14.0 ± 1.8 bursts per min, $p < 0.02$) (Fig. 3.3). In this study the use of vasoactive drug infusions allowed to investigate the effects of endurance training on the baroreceptor control of MSNA. The results showed that physical training was able to improve baroreceptor control of systemic circulation via the sympathetic nervous system (Fig. 3.3) and that this effect was less evident for the baroreceptor control of cardiac sympathetic activity. Similar results have also been shown in hypertensive subjects [61]. In a randomized control trial employing heart rate variability to investigate the effect of combined aerobic and resistance training (50–80% of HR_{max}, 5 times/week for 4 weeks) in sedentary hypertensive women, Masroor and coworkers [62] have shown a significant reduction in systolic (−13.4%) and diastolic (−8.51%) blood pressure values and a significant decrease in low frequency/high frequency ratio (LF/HF ratio) as index of sympathovagal balance.

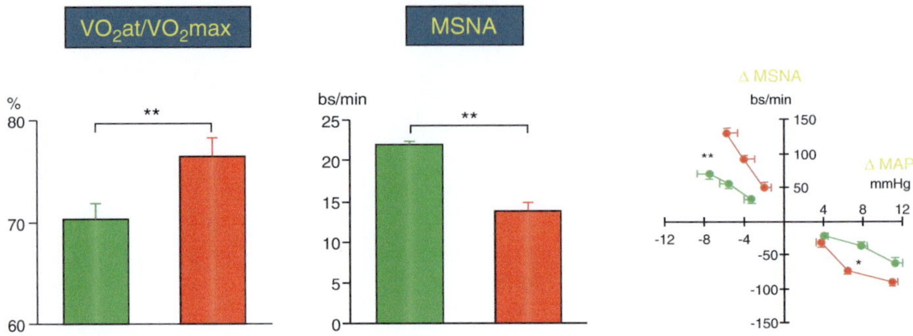

Fig. 3.3 Changes in oxygen consumption at anaerobic threshold (VO_{2at}) and maximal oxygen consumption (VO_{2max}) ratio and muscle sympathetic nerve activity (MSNA) after 10 weeks of physical training (red histograms). On the right, baroreflex MSNA responses to vasoactive drug infusion before (green line) and after (red line) 10 weeks of physical training. Asterisks ($*p < 0.05$, $**p < 0.01$) refer to statistical significance between mean values obtained before and at the end of the endurance training program. (Modified from [28], with permission)

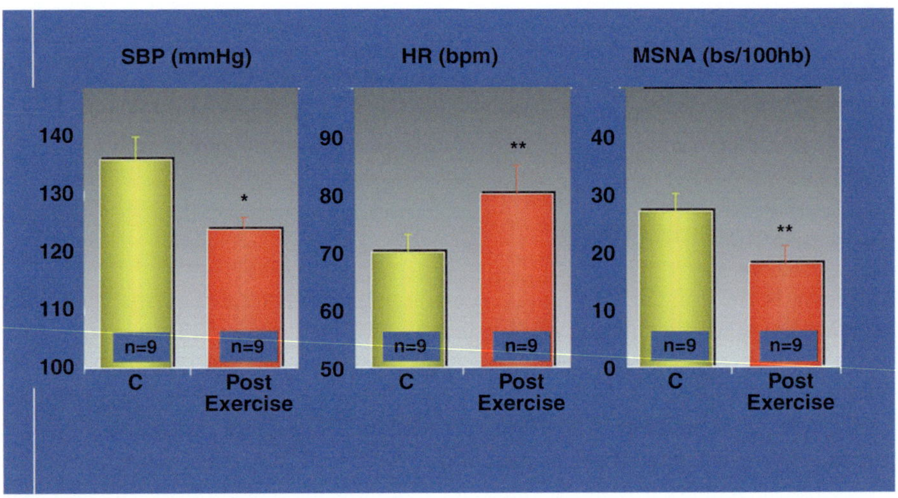

Fig. 3.4 Mean values of systolic blood pressure (SBP), heart rate (HR), and muscle sympathetic nerve activity (MSNA) measured at rest and 60 min after exercise in 9 men with borderline hypertension. Asterisks ($*p < 0.05$, $**p < 0.005$) refer to statistical significance vs. resting condition. (Modified from [63], with permission)

3.5.3 Post-Exercise Effects

The period following a single bout of exercise is characterized by a reduction in systolic and diastolic blood pressure, a decrease in total peripheral, forearm, and hand vascular resistance and a decrease in plasma catecholamines and sympathetic outflow [63–65] (Fig. 3.4). Other studies have also suggested the involvement of other important mechanisms like activations of opioid and serotoninergic systems which are known to inhibit sympathetic outflow [66, 67]. On the contrary some studies, with not superimposable amount of physical activity, have shown an increase in the adrenergic tone associated with a stimulation of the renin-angiotensin-aldosterone system [64, 68]. More recently, animal studies have clearly shown that dynamic exercise resulted in a post-exercise reduction in MAP associated with a significant reduction in total peripheral resistance, a significant elevation in cardiac output and a significant decrease in sympathetic nerve activity [69]. Taken in conjunction with findings that cardiac afferents blockade inhibits post-exercise hypotension and increases renal sympathetic activity [70], this could suggest that cardiac afferents affect sympathetic post-exercise outflow.

References

1. Yusuf S, Hawken S, Ounpuu S, Dans T, Avezum A, Lanas F, McQueen M, Budaj A, Pais P, Varigos J, Lisheng L, INTERHART Study Investigators. Effect of potentially modifiable risk factors associated with myocardial infarction in 52 countries (the INTERHEART study): case-control study. Lancet. 2004;364:937–52.
2. Stewart J, Manmathan G, Wilkinson P. Primary prevention of cardiovascular disease: a review of contemporary guidance and literature. JRSM Cardiovasc Dis. 2017;6:2048004016687211.
3. World Health Organization. Global action plan on physical activity 2018–2030: more active people for a healthier world. Geneva: WHO; 2018.
4. Mok A, Khaw KT, Luben R, Wareham N, Brage S. Physical activity trajectories and mortality: population based cohort study. BMJ. 2019;365:I2323.
5. Aerts N, Le Goff D, Odorico M, Le Reste JY, Van Bogaert P, Peremans L, Musinguzi G, Van Royen P, Bastiaens H. Systematic review of international clinical guidelines for the promotion of physical activity for the primary prevention of cardiovascular diseases. BMC Fam Pract. 2021;22:97.
6. Kraus WE, Powell KE, Haskell WL, Janz KF, Campbell WW, Jakicic JM. Physical activity, all-cause and cardiovascular mortality, and cardiovascular disease. Med Sci Sports Exerc. 2019;51:1270–81.
7. Davidson LE, Hudson R, Kilpatrick K, Kuk JL, McMillan K, Janiszewski PM. Effects of exercise modality on insulin resistance and functional limitation in older adults: a randomized controlled trial. Arch Intern Med. 2009;169:122–31.
8. Taggart J, Williams A, Dennis S, Newall A, Shortus T, Zwar N. A systematic review of interventions in primary care to improve health literacy for chronic disease behavioral risk factors. BMC Fam Pract. 2012;13:49.
9. Sigal RJ, Kenny GP, Boule NG, Wells GA, Prud'homme D, Fortier M. Effects of aerobic training, resistance training, or both on glycemic control in type 2 diabetes: a randomized trial. Ann Intern Med. 2007;147:357–69.
10. Saeidifard F, Medina-Inojosa JR, West CP, Olson TP, Somers VK, Bonikowske AR. The association of resistance training with mortality: a systematic review and meta-analysis. Eur J Prev Cardiol. 2019;26:1647–65.
11. De Rezende LF, Rodrigues Lopes M, Rey-Lopez JP, Matsudo VK, Luiz OC. Sedentary behavior and health outcomes: an overview of systematic review. PLoS One. 2014;9:e105620.
12. Mancia G, et al. ESH/ESC guidelines for management of arterial hypertension. The task force for the management of arterial hypertension of the European Society of Hypertension/ European Society of Cardiology. J Hypertens. 2013;31:1281–357.
13. Haskell WL, et al. Am Coll sports med/AHA members. Physical activity and public health: updated recommendation for adults from the American College of Sports Medicine and the American Heart Association. Circulation. 2007;116:1081–93.

14. Zinman B, et al. Physical activity/exercise and diabetes. Diabetes Care. 2004;27:S58–62.
15. Kushner RF, Ryan DH. Assessment of lifestyle management of patients with obesity: clinical recommendations from systematic reviews. JAMA. 2014;312:943–52.
16. Lavie CJ, Thomas RJ, Squires RW, Allison TG, Milani RV. Exercise training and cardiac rehabilitation in primary and secondary prevention of coronary heart disease. Mayo Clin Proc. 2009;84:373–83.
17. McArdle WD, Katch FI, Katch VL. Essentials of exercise physiology. 3rd ed. Philadelphia, PA: Lippincott, Williams & Wilkins; 2005.
18. Laughlin MH. Cardiovascular response to exercise. Am J Physiol. 1999;277:S244–59.
19. MacDougall JD. Blood pressure responses to resistive, static, and dynamic exercise. In: Fletcher GF, editor. Cardiovascular response to exercise. New York, NY: American Heart Association; 1994. p. 155–73.
20. Jackson AS, Wier LT, Ayers GW, Beard EF, Stuteville JE, Blair SN. Changes in aerobic power of women, ages 20-64 yr. Med Sci Sports Exerc. 1996;28:884–91.
21. Trappe SW, Costill DL, Vukovich MD, Jones J, Melham T. Aging among elite distance runners: a 22-yr longitudinal study. J Appl Physiol. 1996;80:285–90.
22. Bouchard C, Dionne FT, Simoneau JA, Boulay MR. Genetics of aerobic and anaerobic performances. Exerc Sport Sci Rev. 1992;20:27–58.
23. Seravalle G, Grassi G, Mancia G. Trained athletes. In: Gussak IB, Kostis JB, editors. Iatrogenicity. New Brunswick, NJ: Rutgers University Press; 2018. p. 309–17.
24. Mann T, Lamberts RP, Lambert MI. Methods of prescribing relative exercise intensity: physiological and practical considerations. Sports Med. 2013;43:613–25.
25. Bohm M, Reil JC, Deedwania P, Kim JB, Borer JS. Resting heart rate: risk indicator and emerging risk factor in cardiovascular disease. Am J Med. 2015;128:219–28.
26. Seravalle G, Quarti Trevano F, Grassi G. Heart rate as a predictor of cardiovascular risk. Minerva Med. 2021;112:130–43.
27. Carter JB, Banister EW, Blaber AP. Effect of endurance exercise on autonomic control of heart rate. Sports Med. 2003;33:33–46.
28. Grassi G, Seravalle G, Calhoun D, Mancia G. Physical training and baroreceptor control of sympathetic nerve activity in humans. Hypertension. 1994;23:294–301.
29. Bellenger CR, Fuller JT, Thomson RL, Davison K, Robertson EY, Buckely JD. Monitoring athletic training status through autonomic heart rate regulation: a systematic review and meta-analysis. Sports Med. 2016;46:1461–86.
30. Levy MN. Autonomic interactions in cardiac control. Cardiovasc Res. 1970;4:160–7.
31. Mancia G, Mark AL. Arterial baroreflexes in humans. In: Shepherd JT, Abboud FM, editors. Handbook of physiology, section 2: the cardiovascular system. Bethesda, MD: American Physiological Society; 1983. p. 755–93.
32. Grassi G, Seravalle G, Mancia G. Sympathetic activation in cardiovascular disease: evidence, clinical impact and therapeutic implications. Eur J Clin Invest. 2015;45:1367–75.
33. Nunan D, Sandercock GR, Brodie DA. A quantitative systematic review of normal values for short-term heart rate variability in health adults. Pacing Clin Electrophysiol. 2010;33:1407–17.
34. Shaffer F, McCraty R, Zerr CL. A healthy heart is not a metronome: an integrative review of the heart's anatomy and heart rate variability. Front Psychol. 2014;5:1040. https://doi.org/10.3389/fpsyg.2014-01040.
35. Kleiger RE, Stein PK, Bigger JT Jr. Heart rate variability: measurement and clinical utility. Ann Noninvasive Electrocardiol. 2005;10:88–101.
36. Bernardi L, Spallone V, Stevens M, Hilsted J, Frontoni S, Pop-Busui R, Ziegler D, Kempler P, Freeman R, Low P, Tesfaye S, Valensi P. Toronto consensus panel on diabetic neuropathy. Methods of investigation for cardiac autonomic dysfunction in human research studies: investigations methods for cardiac autonomic function. Diabetes Metab Res Rev. 2011;27:654–64.
37. Vallbo AB, Hagbarth KE, Torebjork HE, Wallin BG. Somatosensory, proprioceptive, and sympathetic activity in human peripheral nerves. Physiol Rev. 1979;59:919–57.

38. Wallin BG, Fagius J. Peripheral sympathetic neural activity in conscious humans. Circ Res. 1985;57:461–9.
39. Grassi G. Assessment of sympathetic cardiovascular drive in human hypertension: achievements and perspectives. Hypertension. 2009;54:690–7.
40. Grassi G, Mark AL, Esler M. The sympathetic nervous system alterations in human hypertension. Circ Res. 2015;116:976–90.
41. Macefield V. Sympathetic microneurography. Handb Clin Neurol. 2013;117:353–64.
42. Greaney J, Kenney W. Measuring and quantifying skin sympathetic nervous system activity in humans. J Neurophysiol. 2017;118:2181–93.
43. Wallin BG, Esler M, Dorward P, Eisenhofer G, Ferrier C, Westerman R, Jennings G. Simultaneous measurements of cardiac noradrenaline spillover and sympathetic outflow to skeletal muscle in humans. J Physiol. 1992;453:45–58.
44. Wallin BG, Thompson JM, Jennings GL, Esler MD. Renal noradrenaline spillover correlates with muscle sympathetic activity in humans. J Physiol. 1996;491:881–7.
45. Esler M, Leonard P, O'Dea K, Jackman G, Jennings G, Korner P. Biochemical quantification of sympathetic nervous activity in humans using radiotracer methodology: fallibility of plasma noradrenaline measurements. J Cardiovasc Pharmacol. 1982;4(suppl 1):S152–7.
46. Därr R, Kuhn M, Bode C, Bornstein SR, Pacak K, Lenders JWM, Eisenhofer G. Accuracy of recommended sampling and assay methods for the determination of plasma-free and urinary fractionated metanephrines in the diagnosis of pheochromocytoma and paraganglioma: a systematic review. Endocrine. 2017;56:495–503.
47. Grassi G, Bolla G, Seravalle G, Turri C, Lanfranchi A, Mancia G. Comparison between reproducibility and sensitivity of muscle sympathetic nerve traffic and plasma noradrenaline in man. Clin Sci (Lond). 1997;92:285–9.
48. Mark AL, Victor RG, Nehred C, Wallin BG. Microneurographic studies of the mechanisms of sympathetic nerve responses to static exercise in humans. Circ Res. 1985;57:461–9.
49. Saito M, Mano T, Abe H, Iwase S. Responses in muscle sympathetic nerve activity to sustained had-grips of different tensions in humans. Eur J Appl Physiol Occup Physiol. 1986;55:493–8.
50. Seals DR, Chase PB, Taylor JA. Autonomic mediation of the pressor responses to isometric exercise in humans. J Appl Physiol. 1988;64:2190–6.
51. Seals DR. Influence of muscle mass on sympathetic neural activation during isometric exercise. J Appl Physiol. 1989;67:1801–6.
52. Victor RG, Pryor SL, Secher NH, Mitchell JH. Effects of partial neuromuscular blockade on sympathetic nerve responses to static exercise in humans. Circ Res. 1989;65:468–76.
53. Saito M. Differences in muscle sympathetic nerve response to isometric exercise in different muscle groups. Eur J Appl Physiol Occup Physiol. 1995;70:26–35.
54. Katayama K, Kaur J, Young BE, Barbosa TC, Ogoh S, Fadel PJ. High-intensity muscle metaboreflex activation attenuates cardiopulmonary baroreflex-mediated inhibition of muscle sympathetic nerve activity. J Appl Physiol. 2018;125:812–9.
55. Katayama K, Saito M. Muscle sympathetic nerve activity during exercise. J Physiol Sci. 2019;69:589–98. https://doi.org/10.1007/s12576-019-00669-6.
56. Mack G, Nose H, Nadel ER. Role of cardiopulmonary baroreflexes during dynamic exercise. J Appl Physiol. 1988;65:1827–32.
57. Katayama K, Ishida K, Saito M, Loike T, Hirasawa A, Ogoh S. Enhanced muscle pump during mild dynamic leg exercise inhibits sympathetic vasomotor outflow. Physiol Rep. 2014;2:e12070.
58. Saito M, Sone R, Ikeda M, Mano T. Sympathetic outflow to the skeletal muscle in humans increases during prolonged light exercise. J Appl Physiol. 1997;82:1237–43.
59. Coyle EF, Gonzalez-Alonso J. Cardiovascular drift during prolonged exercise: new perspectives. Exerc Sport Sci Rev. 2001;29:88–92.
60. Rowell LB. Control of regional blood flow during dynamic exercise. In: Rowell LB, editor. Human cardiovascular control. Oxford University Press: New York; 1993. p. 204–54.

61. Laterza MC, de Matos LDNJ, Trombetta IC, Braga AMW, Roveda F, Alves MJNN, Krieger EM, Negrao CE, Rondon MUPB. Exercise training restores baroreflex sensitivity in never-treated hypertensive patients. Hypertension. 2007;49:1298–306.
62. Masroor S, Bhati P, Verma S, Khan M, Hussain ME. Heart rate variability following combined aerobic and resistance training in sedentary hypertensive women: a randomized control trial. Indian Heart J. 2018;70:S28–35.
63. Floras JS, Sinkey CA, Aylward PE, Seals DR, Thoren PN, Mark AL. Postexercise hypotension and sympathoinhibition in borderline hypertensive men. Hypertension. 1989;14:28–35.
64. Halliwell JR, Taylor JA, Hartwig TD, Eckberg DL. Augmented baroreflex heart rate gain after moderate-intensity, dynamic exercise. Am J Physiol. 1996;270:R420–6.
65. Cleroux J, Kouname N, Nadeau A, Coulombe D, Lacourciere Y. After effects of exercise on regional and systemic hemodynamics in hypertension. Hypertension. 1992;19:183–91.
66. Hara K, Floras JS. Influence of naloxone on muscle sympathetic nerve activity, systemic and calf hemodynamics and ambulatory blood pressure after exercise in mild essential hypertension. J Hypertens. 1995;13:447–61.
67. Yao T, Andersson S, Thoren P. Long-lasting cardiovascular depression induced by acupuncture-like stimulation of the sciatic nerve in unanaesthetized spontaneously hypertensive rats. Rain res. 1982;240:77–85.
68. Piepoli M, Coats AJS, Adamopoulos S, Bernardi L, Feng YH, Conway J, Sleight P. Persistent peripheral vasodilatation and sympathetic activity in hypotension after maximal exercise. J Appl Physiol. 1993;75:1807–14.
69. Kulics JM, Collins HL, DiCarlo SE. Postexercise hypotension is mediated by reductions in sympathetic nerve activity. Am J Physiol. 1999;276:H27–32.
70. Collins HL, DiCarlo SE. Attenuation of postexercise hypotension by cardiac afferent blockade. Am J Physiol. 1993;265:H1179–83.

Endothelial Function and Physical Exercise: A Key to Cardiovascular Protection?

4

Martina Chiriacò, Stefano Masi, Agostino Virdis, and Stefano Taddei

Abbreviations

3-NT	3-Nitrotyrosine
8-OHdG	8-Hydroxy-2-deoxyguanosine
AP-1	Activator protein 1
AT-II	Angiotensin II
CAD	Coronary artery disease
EDHF	Endothelium derived hyperpolarizing factor
ET-1	Endothelin-1
FBF	Forearm blood flow
FGF-β	Fibroblast growth factor β
FMD	Flow-mediated dilation
GTN	Glyceryl trinitrate
HF	Heart failure
HIIT	High intensity interval training
IL-1	Interleukin-1
IL-6	Interleukin-6
IMT	Intima–media thickness
MCP-1	Monocyte chemoattractant protein-1
MDA-LDL	Malondialdehyde-modified LDL
mtROS	Mithochondrial reactive oxygen species
NADPH	Nicotinamide adenine dinucleotide phosphate
NO	Nitric oxide

M. Chiriacò (✉) · S. Masi · A. Virdis · S. Taddei
Department of Clinical and Experimental Medicine, Santa Chiara Hospital, Università degli Studi di Pisa, Pisa, Italy
e-mail: martina.chiriaco@spec-med.unipi.it; stefano.masi@unipi.it; agostino.virdis@med.unipi.it; stefano.taddei@med.unipi.it

P. Palatini et al. (eds.), *Exercise, Sports and Hypertension*, Updates in Hypertension and Cardiovascular Protection,
https://doi.org/10.1007/978-3-031-07958-0_4

PBF	Peripheral blood flow
PDGF	Platelet-derived growth factor
RAAS	Renin–angiotensin–aldosterone system
ROS	Reactive oxygen species
TGF-β	Transforming growth factor beta
TNF-α	Tumor necrosis factor α
TOSC	Total oxyradical scavenging capacity
VCAM-1	Vascular cell adhesion molecule 1

4.1 Endothelial Function and Its Mediators

Endothelial cells play an important role in the local regulation of vascular tone through the production and release of vasodilator and vasoconstrictor mediators in response to chemical and mechanical stimuli.

The main vasodilator substances involved in the regulation of vascular tone are nitric oxide (NO), prostacyclin (PGI_2) and endothelium-derived hyperpolarizing factor (EDHF). The endothelium also synthesizes and secretes vasoconstrictor substances: among these, the most notable are endothelin-1 (ET-1), prostaglandin H and COX-derived thromboxane [1].

Endothelial dysfunction is defined as the alteration of endothelium function resulting from the activation of endothelial cells, involving a more predominant secretion of vasocontrictor mediators. The condition is characterized by the presence of a pro-inflammatory and pro-thrombotic state and by a reduced NO bioavailability, which result in an increased vascular tone [2, 3].

Endothelial dysfunction affects all vascular beds and is determined by many complex interacting mechanisms; among these, the most important ones involve an increased production of reactive oxygen species (ROS), inflammation and increased leukocyte cell adhesion [4]. In their dysfunctional phenotype, endothelial cells produce oxidative stress, recruit inflammatory cells promoting their migration through the vascular wall and favor smooth muscle cell proliferation as a result of reduced NO availability [5, 6]. Many factors can influence endothelial function, causing a shift in endothelial cell phenotype to their pro-atherosclerotic dysfunctional state and leading to vascular remodeling, inflammation and progression of atherosclerosis.

Among these, shear stress is an important physical factor in the regulation of endothelial cell function. The inconstant force exerted on vascular walls by turbulent blood flow, associated with low shear stress, stimulates the migration of endothelial cells and the altered production of vasoactive molecules [7, 8]. By contrast, high shear stress favors vasodilation by improving NO bioavailability [9, 10].

Shear stress also modulates the expression of cellular adhesion molecules on endothelial cells like vascular cell adhesion molecule 1 (VCAM-1) and selectins, which, in turn, can lead to the adhesion of leukocytes to the endothelium surface, promoting their migration into the subendothelial space and the formation of atherosclerotic lesions [11, 12]. Hemodynamic forces can also affect the production of pro-inflammatory cytokines and endothelial growth factors. Imbalances in the expression of platelet-derived growth factor (PDGF), fibroblast growth factor β (FGF- β), transforming growth factor beta (TGF-β), interleukin-6 (IL-6), and interleukin-1 (IL-1) can stimulate the activation and migration of inflammatory cells, creating a pro-inflammatory environment that leads to the progression of vascular disease and the proliferation of smooth muscle cells, ultimately resulting in vascular remodelling and atherosclerosis [13].

The other main factor contributing to reduced NO availability and endothelial dysfunction is oxidative stress. ROS, in fact, are highly unstable molecules that react and damage cellular macroelements, including proteins, lipids, and nucleic acids. In normal conditions, the constant shear stress promotes the activation of transcription factors, which increase the expression of antioxidant molecules and contrast oxidative stress [14]. In contrast, in conditions of low shear stress, as in turbulent flow, there is an activation of nicotinamide adenine dinucleotide phosphate (NADPH) oxidase and an increased ROS production in endothelial cells. In this state there is also an upregulation of the expression of the transcription factors NFkB and activator protein 1 (AP-1), which stimulate ROS production and the expression of leukocytes adhesion and chemotactic molecules, favoring the progression of atherosclerotic disease [14].

ROS can also interact with proteins, oxidizing cysteine and tyrosine residues and altering their structure and function. Under normal oxidative conditions, vascular smooth muscle cells exhibit very low proliferation rates, in pathological conditions such as hypertension, increased levels of ROS induce post-translational modifications of proteins involved in the control of the cellular cycle, stimulating cell proliferation, de-differentiation and migration [15]. This proliferative phenotype leads to the thickening of the media, a reduced size of the lumen and an increased wall stiffness which are typical of the parietal hypertrophic remodeling observed in hypertension.

Hypertension is characterized by an hyperactivation of the renin–angiotensin–aldosterone system (RAAS) [16]. Angiotensin II (AT-II) activates many signaling pathways involved in the genesis of both endothelial dysfunction and vascular remodeling. In particular, it stimulates the production of ROS through AT1-mediated NADPH oxidase activation, increases leukocytes adhesion in resistance arteries, stimulates the NFkB-mediated expression of VCAM-1, induces the expression of pro-inflammatory molecules such as IL-6, monocyte chemoattractant protein-1 (MCP-1) and tumor necrosis factor α (TNF-α) and directly causes endothelial cell damage by inhibiting cell regeneration [17, 18].

4.2 Clinical Significance of Endothelial Dysfunction in Cardiovascular Disease

Endothelial dysfunction can be observed in different conditions characterized by high cardiovascular risk such as hypertension, dyslipidemia, diabetes, and smoking. The correlation between endothelial dysfunction and cardiovascular disease such as atherosclerosis, coronary disease, acute coronary syndromes, and heart failure has been extensively studied in the last decades [19–23].

The pathophysiological mechanisms underlying the relationship between endothelial dysfunction and atherosclerosis are complex. The most notable ones involve inflammation, oxidative stress, leukocyte activation and have been described in the previous section. Indeed, endothelial dysfunction is linked to vascular remodeling which is considered a markers of atherosclerotic damage [24–26].

There is extensive evidence on the association between endothelial dysfunction and cardiovascular disease. In patients with previous acute coronary syndrome, for example, impaired endothelium-dependent vasodilation correlates with cardiovascular event rates while the restoration of endothelial function is associated with improvement of event-free survival [27].

In addition, impaired endothelial function, assessed by flow-mediated dilation (FMD), independently predicts the occurrence of in-stent restenosis in patients undergoing percutaneous coronary intervention [28].

In a long-term follow-up of women with angina, reversible myocardial perfusion defects on nuclear imaging and absence of coronary disease, the presence of coronary endothelial dysfunction was associated with the development of coronary disease at follow-up [29].

Moreover, in a large-scale study involving more than 2109 healthy young adults, the number of cardiovascular risk factors was correlated with increased carotid intima–media thickness (IMT), a marker of vascular damage that has been shown to predict cardiovascular events [30]. This finding was evident only in subjects with endothelial dysfunction, suggesting that the status of systemic endothelial function may modify the association between risk factors and atherosclerosis [31].

The role of endothelial dysfunction in heart failure (HF) has been proven in various studies showing a worse prognosis in patients with HF which may depend on the decreased NO availability found in endothelial dysfunction [32–34] and possibly from increased oxidative stress which also appears to be reversible after HF recompensation, indicating that endothelial dysfunction may be involved in the occurrence of acute HF [33, 35].

4.3 Physical Activity and Endothelial Function in the Elderly

During the years, pharmacological, nonpharmacological and nutraceutical approaches have been studied for the improvement of endothelial function; among these, physical exercise, which is known to reduce cardiovascular morbidity and mortality in the general population [36], has been shown to be one of the most effective nonpharmacological interventions to at least partially prevent age-related endothelial dysfunction.

Besides evidence in animal models showing that continuous exercise improves endothelium-dependent vasodilation evoked by the vasodilator acetylcholine (ACh) in dogs and rats [37, 38], several studies conducted in human subjects have shown similar results in different clinical settings.

In particular, the effect of physical training on endothelial function has been extensively studied in elderly subjects, given that ageing is an independent risk factor for the development of atherosclerotic disease and is associated with a progressive decline in endothelium-dependent vasodilation, most likely due to both increased oxidative stress and reduction in NO bioavailability [39].

A clinical study by Taddei et al. [1] involving 49 healthy subjects, of whom 12 were elderly (over 60 years old) sedentary people, 14 elderly athletes (triathletes, runners, and cyclists), 12 young sedentary subjects and 11 young athletes, investigated forearm blood flow (FBF) modifications with strain-gauge plethysmography induced by the infusion of vasoactive substances.

ACh-induced increase in FBF, through its endothelium-dependent vasodilator activity, was blunted in elderly individuals as compared to young subjects, both in the sedentary and active groups. Interestingly, while the response to ACh was similar in young sedentary and athletic subjects, in the elderly group athletes showed a greater response to ACh compared to their sedentary counterpart.

Moreover, the inhibition of the vasodilator response to acetylcholine induced by the NO-synthase inhibitor L-NMMA was significantly greater in elderly athletes compared to elderly sedentary control subjects. While in elderly sedentary control subjects, the infusion of vitamin C, an antioxidant, increased the vasodilation induced by ACh and restored the inhibiting ability of L-NMMA on the response to the vasodilator agonist, this was not seen in young subjects or elderly athletes.

These results confirm the presence of endothelial dysfunction associated with advancing age and suggest that physical activity has positive effects on endothelial response to vasodilator stimuli only in elderly individuals, in whom it can prevent the reduction in NO availability that is characteristic of impaired endothelium-dependent vasodilation in elderly individuals.

The results of that study also showed that sedentary elderly subjects exhibit age-related endothelial dysfunction caused by oxidative stress–induced reduction in NO availability, confirmed by the different response to L-NMMA and vitamin C. Long-term physical training appears to reverse this alteration by preventing oxidative stress and preserving NO availability.

On the basis of the previous study, Franzoni et al. [39] sought to investigate the characteristics of conduit artery endothelial function and its relationship with antioxidant status in young and older athletes (mean age 63.6 years) and in matched healthy sedentary subjects. Endothelial function was assessed through FMD, a non-invasive technique consisting in the measurement of changes in arterial diameter of superficial arteries (brachial, radial, or femoral vessels) through ultrasonographic technique. Flow-mediated changes in conduit artery diameter are caused by the generation of endothelial-derived vasoactive mediators induced by shear stress. Shear stress is increased by inducing reactive hyperaemia after the inflation and deflation of a sphygmomanometer cuff around the forearm, distally to the diameter measuring point. Vasodilation can also be induced by the systemic administration of vasodilating substances such as glyceryl trinitrate (GTN), that allows the assessment of endothelium-independent dilation. The athletes enrolled in the study were mainly long-distance runners who engaged in vigorous endurance exercise at least 5 times a week and participated in competitive races. Older sedentary subjects showed lower vasodilation at FMD than their athletic counterparts and both young subgroups, confirming the presence of endothelial dysfunction in the elderly.

There were no differences in endothelium-independent dilation in response to GTN administration. The study also analyzed the plasmatic antioxidant capacity through total oxyradical scavenging capacity (TOSC), finding that older sedentary subjects had lower antioxidant capacity compared to the other groups, while older athletes had TOSC comparable to young sedentary subjects. In addition, FMD was not dependent on age in the athletic subjects but it was greater in patients with higher TOSC. Franzoni et al. therefore showed that endothelium-dependent vasodilation decreases with age, along with plasma antioxidant capacity. Notably, FMD and antioxidant capacity are preserved in older trained subjects. Moreover, the study also assessed individual maximum oxygen consumption (VO_2 max), which predicted vasodilation better than age, highlighting the role of exercise training in endothelial function, independently from biological ageing.

4.4 Does Age Matter?

While the previous studies comparatively evaluated the effects of physical exercise on elderly and young subjects, Goto et al. [40] sought to determine the effects of different exercise intensities on endothelium-dependent vasodilation in healthy young subjects, in order to assess the short-term effects of physical training at different maximum oxygen consumption (VO_{2max}) in previously untrained individuals. Vasodilation was evaluated through the measurement of forearm blood flow (FBF) responses to acetylcholine. After a training period of 12 weeks of different intensities, defined by the value of VO_{2max} reached during exercise, which consisted in 30 min of bicycle ergometer 5 to 7 times per week, plethysmographic measurements of FBF after acetylcholine (Ach) infusion showed an increase in FBF only for the moderate intensity exercise group. In addition, the authors also studied the effect of exercise on oxidative stress, evaluating levels of serum malondialdehyde-modified LDL (MDA-LDL) and 8-hydroxy-2-deoxyguanosine (8-OHdG), which are circulating markers of oxidative stress, finding that high-intensity exercise increased plasma 8-OHdG and serum MDA-LDL levels while moderate exercise showed a trend to a non significant decrease for both markers. This finding is in contrast with the notion that long-term exercise reduces oxidative stress in patients with ischemic heart disease [41] and healthy subjects [42]; but it is in line with the observation that short-term bouts of exercise are linked to oxidative stress with an increase in LDL susceptibility to oxidation and consequent higher risk of atherosclerosis [43].

Hallmark et al. [44] studied the short-term effects of moderate or high-intensity exercise (30 min of cycling) on healthy young inactive obese (BMI > 30 kg/m^2) and lean subjects by assessing FMD at 1, 2 and 4 h after exercise and comparing it with measurements obtained on a day when exercise tests were not performed (control day). The study showed that only high-intensity exercise acutely improves endothelial function in lean subjects, and that the increase in FMD in obese subjects was blunted compared to lean patients as FMD did not increase significantly from baseline values at any exercise intensity in obese subjects.

The effect of a particular type of physical activity, high intensity interval training (HIIT), on oxidative stress and endothelial function has been studied in an indirect way by Streese and colleagues [45] who assessed the effects of a 12 weeks HIIT program (vs. standard physical activity) on retinal arteriolar and venular diameters, that represent an accessible vascular bed to investigate microvascular phenotype and vascular remodelling. Oxidative stress was measured through plasma levels of the marker 3-nitrotyrosine (3-NT), and through assessment of gene expression of the protein p66Shc and DNA methylation. The protein p66Shc, forms multimeric complexes in the cytoplasm and in the mithochondrial matrix and, in conditions of cellular stress, migrates in the intermembranous mithochondrial space leading to an increased production of mithochondrial ROS (mtROS). Regulation of p66Shc might be a possible target to reduce the vascular damage mediated by mtROS [26]. Besides improving metabolic parameters, HIIT reversed the retinal phenotype inducing an increase in retinal arteriolar diameters and a decrease in venular diameters when compared with the control group. In addition, the training program reduced the expression of p66Shc, and induced restoration of DNA methylation status of p66Shc promoter and 3-NT plasma levels.

4.5 Physical Activity Can Improve Impaired Endothelium-Dependent Vasodilation in Patients with Cardiovascular Risk Factors or Disease

Physical activity does not have beneficial effects on endothelial function only in healthy subjects as described before; in fact, several studies have found a beneficial effect also in several cardiovascular and metabolic pathologies (Fig. 4.1).

For example, endothelial dysfunction is an established characteristic of HF and contribute to the state of peripheral vasoconstriction associated with neurohormonal activation typical of HF [46].

The notion that physical activity, and in particular endurance training, is beneficial in HF, increasing exercise tolerance and decreasing peripheral vascular resistance has led to investigate the mechanisms responsible for the observed improvements.

Hambrecht and colleagues [47] sought to assess the alterations induced by a long-term exercise training program consisting of 40 min of ciclying, 5 days per week for 6 months (vs. controls) on endothelial function in lower limb skeletal muscle of HF patients with reduced ejection fraction (HFrEF) and their relationship with maximal exercise tolerance. Endothelial function was assessed invasively through measurement of PBF in the left femoral artery after administration of ACh, L-NMMA, or bolus injection of nitroglycerin. PBF was calculated from average peak velocity and arterial cross-sectional area determined through angiography. After the exercise training program, PBF improved significantly in response to acetylcholine administration and the decrease in PBF determined by NO-synthase

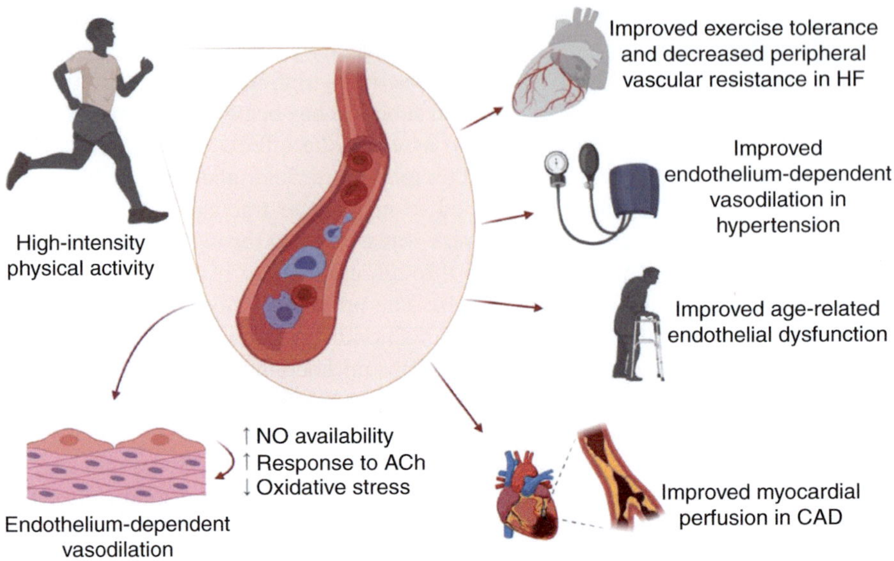

Fig. 4.1 High-intensity physical activity improves endothelial function by increasing NO bioavailability, reducing oxidative stress and increasing endothelial response to vasodilator stimuli such as ACh. Improved endothelium-dependent vasodilation is associated with better outcomes in conditions at high cardiovascular risk, heart failure, *CAD* hypertension, and aging. *ACh* acetylcholine, *CAD* coronary artery disease, *HF* heart failure, *NO* nitric oxide

inhibitory action of L-NMMA was significantly higher in HF patients after training, suggesting that the improvement in endothelial function caused by training is determined at least in part by an increase in NO production.

Hambrect et al. [48] also studied the effects of physical exercise in patients with coronary artery disease (CAD). In these patients, exercise training has been shown to improve myocardial perfusion without modification of coronary lesions. Among the possible explanations for this observation is the recruitment of collateral vessels with exercise, but this hypothesis is not supported by angiographic findings in resting patients [49–51]. Hambrect and colleagues therefore conducted a trial on patients with CAD and coronary endothelial dysfunction and without other confounding cardiovascular risk factors, to assess whether an improvement in endothelial function induced by exercise may be correlated with improved coronary flow reserve.

The enrolled patients had coronary disease of two vessels of which one hemodinamically significant and requiring revascularization and the other non critical that responded abnormally to intra-arterial ACh infusion (no response or vasoconstriction), documenting endothelial dysfunction.

The patients were assigned to an exercise-training group or a control group. After 4 weeks of high intensity endurance training the vasoconstrictive responses to ACh were significantly attenuated compared to baseline measurement. In addition, coronary blood-flow velocity, measured by doppler velocitometry and coronary blood-flow reserve were both increased. The endothelium-independent vasodilation assessed by nitroglycerin infusion did not change after exercise. These results indicate that exercise training improves endothelium-dependent vasodilation of epicardial vessels in patients with CAD and may explain the improved myocardial blood flow induced by high-intensity physical training.

Endothelial dysfunction has been extensively studied in subjects with hypertension and several pharmacological and nonpharmacological interventions have been used to test endothelium-dependent vasodilation. Among these, physical training has been investigated by Higashi et al. [52], who tested the effects of long-term (12 weeks) aerobic exercise on endothelial function in patients with essential hypertension through FBF measurement by plethysmography.

Hypertensive patients had lower vasodilatory response to ACh than nonhypertensive subjects, after the 12 weeks program of training. The response to ACh improved significantly in the active group of hypertensive patients while it did not in the control group. The infusion of L-NMMA inhibited the exercise-induced enhancement of forearm vasodilatory response to ACh in the exercising group. Besides hypertensive subjects, long-term aerobic exercise augmented ACh-induced NO release also in the normotensive group, highlighted by the abolishment of the enhanced response of forearm vasodilation to ACh after exercising.

These findings confirm that long-term physical exercise improves endothelium-dependent function through an increase in the NO production in both hypertensive and normotensive subjects.

4.6 Future Perspectives

The available evidence is highly suggestive of a central role of endothelium-dependent vasodilation in determining the better outcomes observed in the studies on the effects of physical activity in high cardiovascular risk conditions and in ageing. Nevertheless, there is still a need for direct evidence of a mediation role of improved endothelial function in the association between physical exercise and improved cardiovascular outcomes and exercise tolerance. Clinical studies measuring endothelial function changes during exercise may provide additional insight into the possible direct association between physical training and vascular changes; in addition, long-term follow-up periods may provide more reliable data on the reduction of risk for cardiovascular diseases in patients with physical activity-induced endothelial function improvement.

4.7 Conclusions

Physical training is linked to enhanced exercise tolerance, better cardiovascular outcomes and overall improved quality of life. One of the physiological mechanisms responsible for the beneficial effects of physical activity may depend on the improved endothelial function seen in both healthy subjects and in patients at high cardiovascular risk who exercise regularly. Generally, the effects of physical activity seem to be maximal for high-intensity prolonged training regimens and are mainly dependent on the improvement of endothelium-dependent vasodilation, involving a higher NO bioavailability and an improved response to vasodilator stimuli. The notion that endothelial dysfunction, which is a pathological trait seen in several high cardiovascular risk conditions, can be improved through exercise, is of great interest both in clinical research and practice. In fact, monitoring the effects of physical exercise through its action on endothelial function may be useful in routine clinical practice, particularly through the use of noninvasive methodological assessments such as FMD, to improve adherence to exercise and lifestyle modifications.

References

1. Taddei S. Endothelium-dependent vasodilation in hypertensive patients. Endothelium. 1996;4:1–9.
2. Rajendran P, et al. The vascular endothelium and human diseases. Int J Biol Sci. 2013;9:1057–69.
3. Ghiadoni L, Taddei S, Virdis A. Hypertension and endothelial dysfunction: therapeutic approach. Curr Vasc Pharmacol. 2011;10:42–60.
4. Granger DN, Rodrigues SF, Yildirim A, Senchenkova EY. Microvascular responses to cardiovascular risk factors. Microcirculation. 2010;17:192–205.
5. Guzik TJ, Touyz RM. Oxidative stress, inflammation, and vascular aging in hypertension. Hypertension. 2017;70:660–7.
6. Xu S, Touyz RM. Reactive oxygen species and vascular remodelling in hypertension: still alive. Can J Cardiol. 2006;22:947–51.
7. Davies PF, Remuzzi A, Gordon EJ, Dewey CF, Gimbrone MA. Turbulent fluid shear stress induces vascular endothelial cell turnover in vitro. Proc Natl Acad Sci U S A. 1986;83:2114–7.
8. Von Offenberg Sweeney N, et al. Cyclic strain-mediated regulation of vascular endothelial cell migration and tube formation. Biochem Biophys Res Commun. 2005;329:573–82.
9. Kuchan MJ, Frangos JA. Shear stress regulates endothelin-1 release via protein kinase C and cGMP in cultured endothelial cells. Am J Physiol Heart Circ Physiol. 1993;264:H150.
10. Hendrickson RJ, et al. Sustained pulsatile flow regulates endothelial nitric oxide synthase and cyclooxygenase expression in co-cultured vascular endothelial and smooth muscle cells. J Mol Cell Cardiol. 1999;31:619–29.
11. Gerszten RE, et al. Adhesion of monocytes to vascular cell adhesion molecule-1-transduced human endothelial cells: implications for atherogenesis. Circ Res. 1998;82:871–8.
12. Merten M, Chow T, Hellums JD, Thiagarajan P. A new role for P-selectin in shear-induced platelet aggregation. Circulation. 2000;102:2045–50.
13. Cahill PA, Redmond EM. Vascular endothelium—gatekeeper of vessel health. Atherosclerosis. 2016;248:97–109.
14. Hsich HJ, Liu CA, Huang B, Tseng AH, Wang DL. Shear-induced endothelial mechanotransduction: the interplay between reactive oxygen species (ROS) and nitric oxide (NO) and the pathophysiological implications. J Biomed Sci. 2014;21:3.
15. Rao GN, Berk BC. Active oxygen species stimulate vascular smooth muscle cell growth and proto-oncogene expression. Circ Res. 1992;70:593–9.
16. Ferrari R. RAAS inhibition and mortality in hypertension. Glob Cardiol Sci Prac. 2013;2013:269–78.
17. Osborn JW, Fink GD. Region-specific changes in sympathetic nerve activity in angiotensin II-salt hypertension in the rat. Exp Physiol. 2010;95:61–8.
18. Rajagopalan S, et al. Angiotensin II-mediated hypertension in the rat increases vascular superoxide production via membrane NADH/NADPH oxidase activation: contribution to alterations of vasomotor tone. J Clin Investig. 1996;97:1916–23.

19. Celermajer DS, et al. Passive smoking and impaired endothelium-dependent arterial dilatation in healthy young adults. N Engl J Med. 1996;334:150–5.
20. Ghiadoni L, et al. Effect of acute blood pressure reduction on endothelial function in the brachial artery of patients with essential hypertension. J Hypertens. 2001;19:547–51.
21. Goodfellow J, et al. Endothelium and inelastic arteries: an early marker of vascular dysfunction in non-insulin dependent diabetes. Br Med J. 1996;312:744–5.
22. Landmesser U, Drexler H. The clinical significance of endothelial dysfunction. Curr Opin Cardiol. 2005;20:547–51.
23. Celermajer DS, et al. Non-invasive detection of endothelial dysfunction in children and adults at risk of atherosclerosis. Lancet. 1992;340:1111–5.
24. Masi S, et al. The importance of endothelial dysfunction in resistance artery remodelling and cardiovascular risk. Cardiovasc Res. 2020;116:429–37.
25. Kosmopoulos M, et al. The relationship between telomere length and putative markers of vascular ageing: a systematic review and meta-analysis. Mech Ageing Dev. 2021;201:111604.
26. Chiriacò M, et al. Inflammation and vascular ageing: from telomeres to novel emerging mechanisms. High Blood Press Cardiovasc Prev. 2019;26:321–9.
27. Fichtlscherer S, Breuer S, Zeiher AM. Prognostic value of systemic endothelial dysfunction in patients with acute coronary syndromes: further evidence for the existence of the 'vulnerable' patient. Circulation. 2004;110:1926–32.
28. Patti G, et al. Impaired flow-mediated dilation and risk of restenosis in patients undergoing coronary stent implantation. Circulation. 2005;111:70–5.
29. Bugiardini R, Manfrini O, Pizzi C, Fontana F, Morgagni G. Endothelial function predicts future development of coronary artery disease: a study of women with chest pain and normal coronary angiograms. Circulation. 2004;109:2518–23.
30. Lorenz MW, Markus HS, Bots ML, Rosvall M, Sitzer M. Prediction of clinical cardiovascular events with carotid intima-media thickness: a systematic review and meta-analysis. Circulation. 2007;115:459–67.
31. Juonala M, et al. Interrelations between brachial endothelial function and carotid intima-media thickness in young adults: the cardiovascular risk in young Finns study. Circulation. 2004;110:2918–23.
32. Heitzer T, Baldus S, Von Kodolitsch Y, Rudolph V, Meinertz T. Systemic endothelial dysfunction as an early predictor of adverse outcome in heart failure. Arterioscler Thromb Vasc Biol. 2005;25:1174–9.
33. Fischer D, et al. Endothelial dysfunction in patients with chronic heart failure is independently associated with increased incidence of hospitalization, cardiac transplantation, or death. Eur Heart J. 2005;26:65–9.
34. Katz SD, et al. Vascular endothelial dysfunction and mortality risk in patients with chronic heart failure. Circulation. 2005;111:310–4.
35. Colombo PC, et al. Endothelial cell activation in patients with decompensated heart failure. Circulation. 2005;111:58–62.
36. Roccella EJ. The sixth report of the joint National Committee on prevention, detection, evaluation, and treatment of high blood pressure. Arch Intern Med. 1997;157:2413–46.
37. Delp MD, McAllister RM, Laughlin MH. Exercise training alters endothelium-dependent vasoreactivity of rat abdominal aorta. J Appl Physiol. 1993;75:1354–63.
38. Wang J, Wolin MS, Hintze TH. Chronic exercise enhances endothelium-mediated dilation of epicardial coronary artery in conscious dogs. Circ Res. 1993;73:829–38.
39. Franzoni F, et al. Physical activity, plasma antioxidant capacity, and endothelium-dependent vasodilation in young and older men. Am J Hypertens. 2005;18:510–6.
40. Goto C, et al. Effect of different intensities of exercise on endothelium-dependent vasodilation in humans: role of endothelium-dependent nitric oxide and oxidative stress. Circulation. 2003;108:530–5.
41. Leaf DA, Kleinman MT, Hamilton M, Deitrick RW. The exercise-induced oxidative stress paradox: the effects of physical exercise training. Am J Med Sci. 1999;317:295.
42. Ji LL. Exercise-induced modulation of antioxidant defense. Ann NY Acad Sci. 2002;959:82–92.

43. Ji LL. Antioxidants and oxidative stress in exercise. In: Proceedings of the Society for Experimental Biology and Medicine, vol. 222. Oxford: Blackwell; 1999. p. 283–92.
44. Hallmark R, et al. The effect of exercise intensity on endothelial function in physically inactive lean and obese adults. PLoS One. 2014;9:e85450.
45. Streese L, et al. High-intensity interval training modulates retinal microvascular phenotype and DNA methylation of p66Shc gene: a randomized controlled trial (EXAMIN AGE). Eur Heart J. 2020;41:1514–9.
46. Kubo SH, Rector TS, Bank AJ, Williams RE, Heifetz SM. Endothelium-dependent vasodilation is attenuated in patients with heart failure. Circulation. 1991;84:1589–96.
47. Hambrecht R, et al. Regular physical exercise corrects endothelial dysfunction and improves exercise capacity in patients with chronic heart failure. Circulation. 1998;98:2709–15.
48. Hambrecht R, et al. Effect of exercise on coronary endothelial function in patients with coronary artery disease. N Engl J Med. 2000;342:454–60.
49. Niebauer J, et al. Impact of intensive physical exercise and low-fat diet on collateral vessel formation in stable angina pectoris and angiographically confirmed coronary artery disease. Am J Cardiol. 1995;76:771–5.
50. Schuler G, et al. Regular physical exercise and low-fat diet effects on progression of coronary artery disease. Circulation. 1992;86:1–11.
51. Ferguson RJ, et al. Effect of physical training on treadmill exercise capacity, collateral circulation and progression of coronary disease. Am J Cardiol. 1974;34:764–9.
52. Higashi Y, et al. Regular aerobic exercise augments endothelium-dependent vascular relaxation in normotensive as well as hypertensive subjects: role of endothelium-derived nitric oxide. Circulation. 1999;100:1194–202.

Exercise and Microcirculation in Hypertension

5

Damiano Rizzoni, Claudia Agabiti-Rosei, and Carolina de Ciuceis

5.1 Introduction

Microcirculation, which includes the small resistance arteries (lumen diameters of 100–350 μm), arterioles (lumen diameters <100 μm), capillaries (<7 μm), and venules, represents the part of the vascular system that is responsible for regulation of nutrient and oxygen supply within the tissue according to change in demand. Because their composition, small arteries and arterioles, and much less capillaries, determine the vascular peripheral resistance. Indeed, compared to large arteries, tunica media of small arteries contains fewer elastic fibers and more smooth muscle with relatively thick walls which are capable of great vasoconstriction/vasodilatation to adjust rate of blood flow. Similarly, arterioles monitor blood flow into capillary through precapillary sphincter and they are regulated by sympathetic innervation and local chemical mediators that can alter diameter and thus resistance. Capillaries are the smallest blood vessels connecting arterial outflow and venous return, they are made of one layer of endothelial cells and basement membrane, and their primary function is exchange between blood and interstitial fluid and the delivery of nutrients and oxygen to tissues.

Therefore, their role is important especially for tissues undergoing great variations in flow and metabolic requirement such as skeletal muscle.

D. Rizzoni (✉)
Division of Medicine, Spedali Civili of Brescia, Montichiari, Brescia, Italy

Department of Medical and Surgical Sciences, University of Brescia, Brescia, Italy

Clinica Medica, Department of Clinical and Experimental Sciences, University of Brescia, Brescia, Italy
e-mail: damiano.rizzoni@unibs.it

C. Agabiti-Rosei · C. de Ciuceis
Department of Medical and Surgical Sciences, University of Brescia, Brescia, Italy
e-mail: claudia.agabitirosei@unibs.it; carolina.deciuceis@unibs.it

P. Palatini et al. (eds.), *Exercise, Sports and Hypertension*, Updates in Hypertension and Cardiovascular Protection,
https://doi.org/10.1007/978-3-031-07958-0_5

Increasing pressure in the microvascular network leads to vasoconstriction and alterations in the morphology of the small arteries and arterioles in order to maintain a constant flow at the level of the capillaries, thus avoiding pressure and flow fluctuations [1].

The presence of an optimal capacity for endothelium to respond to mechanical and chemical stimuli and to produce vasoactive substances together with the ability of smooth muscle cells to achieve a required contractile state by continuously integration of vasodilator and vasoconstrictor signals are crucial in order to allow an effective regulation of vascular tone in healthy conditions.

Several cardiovascular diseases, such as arterial hypertension and type 2 diabetes, may be associated to impairment of both microvascular structure and function which contribute to enhanced peripheral vascular resistance and further increase in blood pressure. In experimental model of hypertension as well as in patients with essential hypertension, a remodeling process of small resistance arteries occurs responsible for an increased media to lumen ratio of small resistance arteries which is the hallmark of hypertension disease. Similarly, retinal arterioles from hypertensive patients show increased wall-to-lumen ratio. Capillary rarefaction is another morphological change observed in hypertensive animals and patients which contributes to increased vascular resistance.

In addition to structural alterations, endothelial cells may be dysfunctional in hypertension leading to a reduced ability to regulate the amount of blood and oxygen supplied to the tissue and an impairment of vascular tone. An alteration in endothelial phenotype and function is also an early sign of reduced cardiovascular health and may have important impact for regulation of skeletal muscle vascular tone especially during physical exercise.

The importance of microcirculation is supported by the evidence that structural damage of small vessels is a predictor of later cardiovascular events and may have prognostic implications [2–4].

Recently, development of noninvasive technique to evaluate microvascular endothelial function allow to demonstrate that retinal arteriolar endothelial dysfunction is an independent predictor of long-term major adverse cardiovascular prognosis in patients with coronary artery disease or cardiovascular risk factors [5].

One of the main consequences of microvascular alterations in these patients is demodulation of blood flow regulation to contracting skeletal muscle which may lead to tissue ischemia and fatigue.

Several pharmacological compounds have been reported to be effective in improving or regressing structural and functional alterations in microvessels related to hypertension including renin angiotensin system inhibitors or calcium antagonists [6].

Exercise training has been also extensively demonstrated to lower blood pressure in hypertensive patients [7, 8], and is therefore considered one of the main nonpharmacological approaches in the prevention and treatment of hypertension [9, 10]. Among mechanisms by which physical exercise positively affects hypertensive disease may regard an improvement or regression of structural and functional microvascular damage in the skeletal muscle. Indeed, exercise training has been reported to regress microvascular remodeling [11–13], normalize capillary density in hypertensive animals [13] and humans [14], and to improve endothelial function in different microvascular districts, thus representing an important tool in the management of hypertension or other cardiovascular diseases.

5.2 Regulation of Blood Flow and Vascular Tone in Skeletal Muscle

Skeletal muscle blood flow is important for skeletal muscle peripheral resistance and blood pressure regulation in resting condition and especially during physical exercise. Muscle blood flow is closely related to the oxygen demand of the exercising muscles and it directly increases with tissue oxygen requests [15]. During exercise such as conventional cycle ergometry, O_2 extraction increases hyperbolically with maximum work rate, thus achieving values of about 80–90% at peak O_2 uptake (VO_2). Skeletal muscle blood flow rapidly rises at the onset of exercise reaching up to almost 100-fold at maximal exercise [15], and this increase is more evident in well-trained individuals compared to untrained ones [15]. Together with changes in hemodynamics and higher cardiac output, adaptation in microcirculation is important mostly for maintaining optimal perfusion in contracting skeletal muscle during exercise.

Indeed, several mechanisms such as mechanical and chemical factors, local and erythrocyte metabolic and endothelium-derived substances, as well as the sympathetic nervous system activity have been suggested to be involved in regulating vascular resistance and skeletal muscle blood flow both in resting condition and during physical exercise [16].

In this respect, activation of sympathetic nervous system represents the most important feature. It induces increase in cardiac output and peripheral vasoconstrictor signaling in order to maintain adequate mean arterial pressure during great metabolic vasodilatation which occurs during exercise. This process is mediated primarily by noradrenaline which is released from sympathetic nerve endings and binds to α-adrenoceptors on smooth muscle cells in small resistance arteries. However, specific signaling at the level of contracting skeletal muscle do not produce vasoconstriction but results in blunting of the vasoconstrictor response in order to appropriately regulate flow for tissue oxygen delivery. This suggests the presence of a different and unique regulation in the skeletal muscle which is commonly referred to as "functional sympatholysis" [17]. Therefore, sympathetic nervous system activity acts by inducing constriction of resistance vessels to counteract vasodilation occurring in the active muscle group during high-intensity exercise.

Moreover, sympathetic activity may be mediated by a number of local vasoactive substances which are produced in different cells (such as erythrocytes, endothelial cells, and skeletal muscle cells) and properly integrate with neural vasoconstrictor signals within contracting skeletal muscles in order to modulate blood flow control during exercise.

Among vasoactive substances, of particular importance for muscle blood flow regulation are nitric oxide (NO) and prostacyclin. These two vasodilators are both stimulated by several compounds (e.g., adenosine, ATP, acetylcholine, and bradykinin) and are affected by mechanically induced signals, such as shear stress. It was previously demonstrated that infusion of prostanoids into the brachial artery increased blood flow and that prostacyclin and prostaglandin E2 concentrations were increased during muscle contraction in the forearm and leg, respectively, suggesting that prostanoids are involved in muscle blood flow regulation [18]. Inhibition of cyclooxygenase (COX), which initiates the conversion of arachidonic acid to PGI2, has shown no effect on blood flow at rest or during exercise in the human forearm or leg [19, 20].

NO, which is derived by both neuronal NO synthase (nNOS) [21] and endothelial NO synthase (eNOS), may regulate skeletal muscle blood flow by inducing vasodilation by acting on the smooth muscle cells in the arterioles. Vallance and coworkers showed a 50% reduction in forearm blood flow after blocking NO synthase (NOS) by infusion of NG-monomethyl-L-arginine (L-NMMA) [22] but this effect was not confirmed during exercise [23]. Interestingly, the simultaneous inhibition of both prostanoid and NO has demonstrated a clear reduction in leg blood flow during exercise [24, 25] therefore suggesting the presence of a compensatory and redundant vasodilator mechanism regulating adequate blood flow in the skeletal muscle (Fig. 5.1) [26].

In addition, adenosine triphosphate (ATP) plays a crucial role in regulating skeletal muscle blood flow. ATP secreted by muscle cells during contraction may induce vasodilation by inducing production of NO and prostacyclin or through its conversion into adenosine [16]. ATP and adenosine are present in both plasma and muscle interstitial fluid and mediate vasodilation by acting on endothelial or skeletal muscle cell receptors, thus causing the production of NO and prostacyclin [25, 27].

ATP and NO have been suggested to act also as sympatholytic compounds able to modulate the effect of sympathetic activity [17] and contribute vasodilator mechanism in the skeletal muscle during exercise by optimizing blood flow to the contracting muscles. ATP has been shown to elicit sympatholytic effects in humans [28] mainly through a desensitization of the adrenergic receptor, whereas NO has been found to induce sympatholysis only in rodents [29].

In addition, some evidence in both in vitro models and in humans suggests that when the erythrocytes travel through the microvessels in skeletal muscle they can release the vasodilators ATP and NO in response to off-loading of oxygen to ensure increased blood flow and oxygen, albeit studies investigating this topic are still limited [16].

Shear stress, the frictional force applied from blood flow onto the endothelial cells lining the lumen of all blood vessels, represents another factor playing a role in the acute regulation of arteriolar diameter and thus blood flow. Increase in shear stress leads to production of NO from eNOS in the arteriolar wall leading to vasodilation [30], although its role in large flow increase occurring during exercise seems limited.

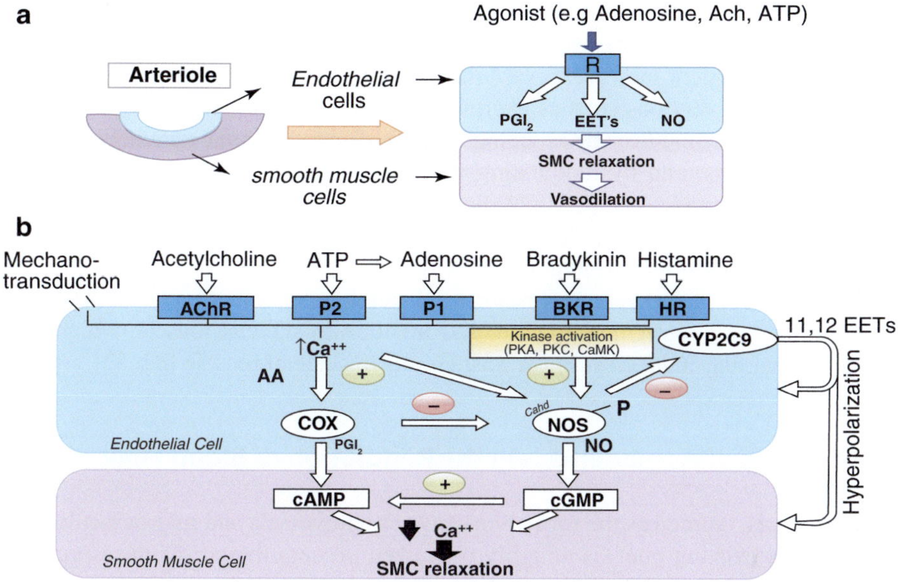

Fig. 5.1 Schematic illustration of vasodilator interactions in skeletal muscle arterioles. (**a**) Illustration of a simplified view of endothelium-dependent induction of vasodilatation. Vasodilator agonists, such as adenosine or acetylcholine (ACh), act on specific receptors on endothelial cells lining the luminal side of an arteriole. The receptor activation leads to the formation of compounds which cause relaxation of smooth muscle cells adjacent to the endothelial cells resulting in vasodilatation of the arteriole. (**b**) Detailed illustration of how vasodilator systems in the vascular wall can be activated and of proposed interactions between vasodilator systems. In vascular endothelial cells, several compounds, including acetylcholine, ATP, adenosine, and bradykinin, as well as mechanical signals including shear stress, activate both endothelial NO synthase (eNOS) and the arachidonic acid pathway leading to formation of prostacyclin (PGI2) and eicosatrienoic acids (EETs). Activation of NOS and the arachidonic acid pathway occurs via an increase in intracellular calcium but eNOS activity is also regulated by protein phosphorylation at different sites. Redundancy exists between the NO and the prostacyclin systems where one described mechanism is inhibition of NOS by prostacyclin. Redundancy also exists between the NO system and cytochrome P450 2C9 (CYP 2C9), which produces 11,12-eicosatrienoic acid (11,12-EET) that can induce smooth muscle cell (SMC) relaxation by hyperpolarization. During normal conditions, NO exerts an inhibitory effect on CYP 2C9 but when NO formation is inhibited, the activity of CYP 2C9 increases. In the smooth muscle cell cyclic guanosine monophosphate (cGMP) can promote cyclic adenosine monophosphate (cAMP) levels by inhibiting phosphodiesterase III, which degrades cAMP. *AChR* acetylcholine receptor, *AA* arachidonic acid, *ATP* adenosine 5-triphosphate, *BKR* bradykinin receptor, *11, 12 EETs* 11, 12 eicosatrienoic acid, *CaM* calmodulin, *CaMK* calmodulin kinase, *cAMP* cyclic adenosine monophosphate, *cGMP* cyclic guanosine monophosphate, *COX* cyclooxygenase, *CYP 2C9* cytochrome P450 2C9, *HR* histamine receptor, *PGI2* prostacyclin, *PKA* protein kinase A; *PKC* protein kinase C, *P1* purinergic receptor 1, *P2* purinergic receptor 2, *SMC* smooth muscle cell. (*Hellsten Y, Nyberg M, Jensen LG, Mortensen SP. Vasodilator interactions in skeletal muscle blood flow regulation. J Physiol 2012: 590 (Pt 24): 6297–6305*)

In addition, skeletal muscle blood flow may be affected by changes in microvascular structure or function which occur in pathological conditions such as hypertension with subsequent increase in vascular resistance as discussed below. Similarly, therapeutic interventions such as exercise training may elicit beneficial effects on skeletal muscle blood flow by inducing favorable microvascular remodeling, capillary angiogenesis, and by modulating vasomotor reactivity of small arteries and arterioles. In particular, activation of the angiogenic process, with increase in capillary network, seems to have the major influence in ameliorating local blood flow in several tissues including skeletal muscle [31].

Furthermore, phenotypic expression of skeletal muscle fiber type also has powerful influences on vascular structure and function in skeletal muscle, which may influence training-induced vascular adaptations in skeletal muscle [32, 33].

5.2.1 Role of Angiogenesis in the Regulation of Blood Flow

Angiogenesis, defined as the formation of new microvessels and microvascular networks from existing ones, is a highly organized process that arises in response to hypoxia and other stimuli and that relieves tissue ischemia. A large number of pro- and antiangiogenic or angiostatic factors are involved in regulating angiogenesis where the balance between them seems to determine the resulting growth, maintenance or regression of capillaries in a tissue [34] (Fig. 5.2).

VEGF and VEGFR-2 are thought to be the most important promoters of capillary growth in most tissues, including skeletal muscle [35], while TIMP-1 and TSP-1 represent important angiostatic factors which limit and inhibit angiogenic process [34].

In skeletal muscle, VEGF is present in endothelial cells as well as within skeletal muscle cells and, upon contraction [36], a fraction of the VEGF is secreted into the extracellular fluid where it binds VEGF receptor 2 on capillary endothelial cells.

In adult skeletal muscle, upregulation of VEGF and other factors such as Flk-1, angiopoietin-2, and platelet/endothelial cell adhesion molecule-1 (PECAM-1) represent a common angiogenic response of endothelial cells. These angiogenic signals from growth factors can be influenced by the local microenvironment resulting in differing forms of capillary growth (sprouting and splitting) to produce a coordinated expansion of the vascular bed. Muscle overload induces changes in expression levels in genes associated with extracellular matrix remodeling, such as matrix metalloproteinase-2 (MMP-2), tissue inhibitor of metalloproteinases (TIMP), and thrombospondin, resulting in sprouting angiogenesis, whereas changes in neuropilin, midkine, and restin levels are observed during splitting angiogenesis. All these factors may be differently modulated in physiological or pathological conditions. Indeed, VEGF is involved in several angiogenic steps, and influences endothelial activation, proliferation, and migration, and capillary sprouting and splitting or intussusception and has a great impact on exercise-induced angiogenesis [34].

Similarly, eNOS is a proangiogenic factor with the ability to modulate VEGF expression, thus influencing capillary growth [37].

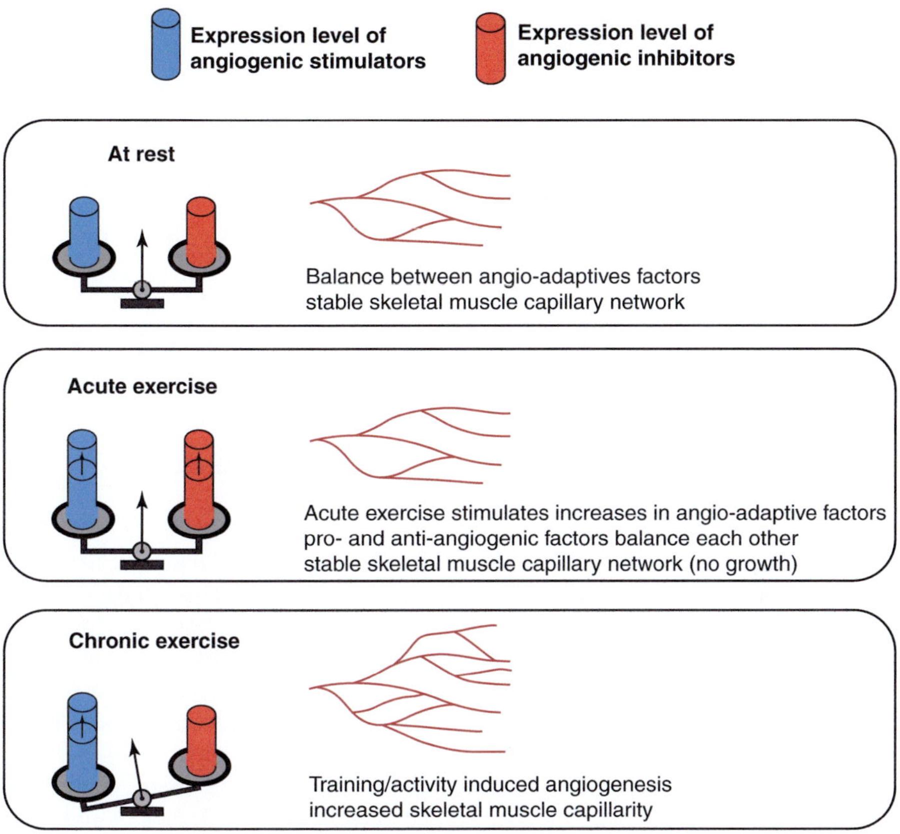

Fig. 5.2 Regulation of angiogenesis at rest and after physical exercise. Under basal conditions (at rest), angiogenic stimulators and inhibitors are in functional balance with each other resulting in a stabilized and quiescent microvascular network in skeletal muscle. Acute exercise stimulates upregulation of both angiogenic stimulators and inhibitors such that balance between these opposing factors remains unaltered and thus a single bout of exercise is not sufficient to elicit microvascular growth. In contrast, repeated or chronic exercise stimulus leads to sustained activation of angiogenic stimulators while the responsiveness of angiogenic inhibitors to individual bouts of exercise is gradually reduced, resulting in a net balance that favors an angiogenic response and the resulting expansion of skeletal muscle microvascular network. VEGF-A, fibroblast growth factor-2, or angiopoietins are some examples of angiogenic stimulators, whereas angiostatin, endostatin, vasohibin, and tissue inhibitors of metalloproteinases are examples of angiogenic inhibitors (note that these factors are mentioned as illustrative examples only and do not represent the exhaustive list of those potentially involved during skeletal muscle angio-adaptation). (*Olfert, I.M. & Birot, O. 2011. Importance of anti-angiogenic factors in the regulation of skeletal muscle angiogenesis. Microcirculation 18, 316–330*)

Other proangiogenic factors are matrix metalloproteinases (MMPs) and angiopoietin-2, which are essential for the degradation of the extracellular matrix and capillary destabilization during sprouting angiogenesis [34].

Antiangiogenic factors include angiopoietin-1 (Ang1) which is important for stabilization of the newly formed capillary and competes with Ang2 for the angiopoietin receptor-2 (Tie2). Tissue inhibitor matrix metalloproteinases (TIMPs) inhibit MMPs and thereby limit the extent of extracellular matrix degradation [34]. Thrombospondin-1 (TSP-1) is a multifunctional protein with binding sites specific for cell-to-cell and cell-to-matrix interactions with the ability to inhibit migration and proliferation and promote apoptosis of endothelial cells, thus reducing the VEGF effects [34]. Deletion of TSP-1 in mice has been shown to increase capillarization in cardiac and skeletal muscles providing evidence for an important role for TSP-1 in restricting capillary growth [38]. Moreover, soluble VEGF receptor-1 (sVEGFR-1) binds and inactivates VEGF and has been proposed to be an important regulator of VEGF signaling [34].

Different factors may interfere with VEGF and TSP-1 such as aging [39] and lifestyle-related disease [14], which may blunt the angiogenic process.

5.2.2 Role of Skeletal Muscle Composition in Regulation of Blood Flow

Several evidences demonstrated that also composition in skeletal muscle fiber type is involved in blood flow regulation. Skeletal muscle fibers are characterized by different properties in oxidative capacity, vascularization, and mechanisms of vascular control, with subsequent differences in regional blood flow distribution as well as in fiber recruitment among muscles during exercise. Therefore, a change in skeletal muscle fiber composition may be associated to alteration in microvascular blood flow in contracting muscle with important functional consequences.

Skeletal muscle is a complex tissue composed of connective tissue, nerves and muscle fibers. Based on their biochemical characteristics, which include oxidative capacity, constitutive proteins, capillary density, myoglobin density, and the type of muscular myosin heavy chain (MHC) [40], three classical fiber types may be distinguished: type I (oxidative slow-twitch), type IIa (oxidative fast-twitch), and type IIb (glycolytic fast-twitch) fibers in rodent, which are equivalent to type IIx (glycolytic fast-twitch) fibers in humans [40]. Type 1 fibers have slower myosin heavy chain (MyHC) isoforms and are rich in mitochondria, thus making them fatigue resistant and capable to support sustained contraction [41, 42]. These fibers also possess high oxidative capacity and low glycolytic capacity, and have more fatty acid oxidation and triglyceride accumulation compared to type 2 fibers, whereas type 2 fibers have faster MyHC isoforms and less mitochondria [42]. Type 1 fibers are typically recruited in endurance and tonic contractile activities such as long-distance running and maintaining posture [43], whereas type 2 fibers are more sensitive to fatigue and support fast, intense contractile activities of short duration, such as sprinting [42, 43]. Indeed, muscles composed predominantly of type I slow-twitch fibers have increased capillarization, arteriolar density, oxidative capacity, and endothelium-dependent dilation when compared with muscle composed mainly of type II fast-twitch fibers.

Interestingly, type 1 fibers also show greater insulin sensitivity and insulin responsiveness than type 2 fibers, thus suggesting that change from type 1 to type 2 fibers may alter insulin sensitivity contributing to skeletal muscle dysfunction, exercise intolerance, and poor glucose control.

Therefore, variability in the proportion of skeletal-muscle fiber types may explain marked differences in aspects of certain chronic disease states including obesity, insulin resistance, and hypertension.

5.3 Microvascular Alterations in Essential Hypertension

Hypertension is characterized by abnormal regulation of the vasomotor tone, enhanced vasoconstriction, reduced vasodilation, structural alterations of vessels and microvascular networks. These functional and structural alterations in the microcirculation may compromise an optimal skeletal muscle blood flow in response to physical exercise resulting in reduced oxygen availability during exercise, tissue ischemia, and impaired tolerance to physical activity.

5.3.1 Structural Changes of the Vasculature

Morphological alterations in hypertension involve small resistance arteries, arterioles, and capillaries. A reduced internal diameter together with a greater media thickness has been observed in mesenteric arteries from experimental model of hypertension as well in subcutaneous resistance arteries from essential hypertensive patients, which results in increased media-to-lumen ratio without net cell growth (no change in media cross-sectional area), a process defined inward eutrophic remodeling [44].

On the other hand, in some forms of secondary hypertension (renovascular hypertension) [45] as well as in other cardiovascular diseases, such as diabetes mellitus or obesity, in spite of the presence of hypertension [46–48], hypertrophic remodeling has been reported with increased both media to lumen ratio and media cross-sectional area, thus indicating that a cellular hypertrophy (cell volume increase) or hyperplasia (cell number increase) occur [45]. It has been suggested that hypertrophic remodeling may be more disadvantageous in terms of future cardiovascular events [49].

Remodeling process may represent the most prevalent and earliest form of arterial damage in hypertension [50] and may represent a generalized phenomenon which may be observed is different vascular districts. Accordingly, an increased wall-to-lumen ratio of retinal arterioles, assessed with different noninvasive techniques, has been demonstrated in patients with essential hypertension [51, 52]. From a physiological point of view, the main consequence of remodeling consists of changes in distensibility [53] with subsequent reduction in flow reserve at the level of subcutaneous tissues and, more clinically important, in the coronary [54] and cerebral microcirculation [55]. In the skeletal muscle, this change may compromise the increase in blood flow during physical exercise.

Furthermore, a rarefaction of arterioles and capillaries affecting the microvascular network has been observed in hypertension first, it seems to be a functional change due to increase vascular tone and vasoconstriction upstream at arteriolar level in basal condition, and then it becomes structural or anatomical, when total capillary number is reduced at full dilated condition after venous congestion and the nonperfused vessels disappear. These factors may contribute differently in each vascular bed, and may vary between models of hypertension.

Capillary rarefaction was observed in gracilis, myocardium [12], temporalis, and kidney [13] in SHR, when compared to WKY, and it has been also demonstrated in various tissues of hypertensive patients [56–59] including skeletal muscle [14, 60].

Henrich et al. demonstrated more than 30 years ago that hypertensive patients present a rarefaction in both the quadriceps muscle (by about 37%) and in the pectoralis major muscle (by about 51%) which may cause a reduction in the transcapillary fluid exchange [60]. Similarly, it has been observed that hypertensive patients show decreased capillary density along with lower levels of VEGF protein in muscle homogenates compared to controls, suggesting an impairment of angiogenesis in these patients [14]. In the same study, capillary–fiber ratio was not different between the two groups probably resulting in reduced capacity for oxygenation of the muscle fibers because of a longer diffusion distance for oxygen. Interestingly, microvascular rarefaction has also been detected in offspring of hypertensives suggesting that blood pressure alone does not affect angiogenesis [61].

Despite the evidence of a reduction of microvascular network in hypertension [14, 55, 56, 58, 60], the underlying cellular mechanisms remain uncertain. An impairment of different angiogenetic factors, such as vascular endothelial growth factor (VEGF), VEGF receptor VEGFR-2, TIMP-1, and thrombospondin-1 (TSP-1) [38], has been suggested. However, there are some discrepancies among studies [57, 62].

No concordant data are present about circulating TIMP-1 levels which were found to be reduced in skeletal muscles from hypertensive patients compared to normotensive subjects possibly resulting in an increased matrix remodeling and capillary basement membrane thickening. Nevertheless, reduction of capillary thickness did not parallel the increase in TIMP-1 levels [62].

In addition, animal models lacking TSP-1 by genetic modulation express increased capillarization compared to control animals [38]; however, its role in capillary rarefaction in hypertension is not clear.

Among the factors implicated in angiogenesis, the angiotensin system seems to be involved, which has a large impact on the cardiovascular system and which is a contributing factor in essential hypertension [63].

Moreover, a part from capillary number reduction, the function of capillaries may also be affected by change in their composition. Indeed, capillaries lack tunica media and their wall is characterized by an endothelial cell layer together with a basement membrane. In some studies, patients with mild essential hypertension showed a thickening of the capillary wall (probably of basement membrane). In addition, a decreased capillary lumen diameter was observed using electron microscopy without change in skeletal muscle capillary density as confirmed by a similar capillary fiber ratio when compared to normotensive subjects [57, 62]. However, the underlying mechanism for the thickening of the basement membrane in hypertension is not known.

Taken together, these alterations in the microvascular network are expected to negatively affect the conditions for oxygen supply and delivery in skeletal muscles and may result in limited diffusion through the capillaries.

5.3.2 Functional Alterations of the Vasculature

Endothelial dysfunction is a pathological condition associated with an impaired ability to regulate vascular tone mainly characterized by an imbalance between substances with vasodilating, antimitogenic and antithrombogenic properties (endothelium-derived relaxing factors) and substances with vasoconstricting, prothrombotic, and proliferative characteristics (endothelium-derived contracting factors) [64].

Endothelial dysfunction may be detected in essential hypertension as demonstrated by increased peripheral resistance and decreased maximal vasodilatation after intrabrachial infusion of acetylcholine, an endothelium-dependent vasodilator, evaluated as forearm blood flow during strain gauge plethysmography which can be restored by an antioxidant such as vitamin C [65].

Indeed, endothelial dysfunction may be caused by an impairment of NO availability [65], secondary to oxidative stress, mainly caused by both the increased reactive oxygen species production (ROS) that scavenges NO and antioxidant capacity reduction [65–67]. In addition, an altered function of the prostanoid system, such as prostaglandins and thromboxane A2 [68] and increased cyclooxygenase derived contractile products may also play a role [66]. Other sources of ROS include uncoupling of endothelial nitric oxide synthase (eNOS) which increases superoxide formation [67].

ROS have been demonstrated to be involved in microvascular dysfunction related to physical inactivity. Data derived from animal studies indicate that physical inactivity attenuates endothelium-dependent vasodilation, reduces the expression of endothelial NO synthase (eNOS) [69] and increases formation of ROS through NADPH oxidase and a reduction in important antioxidant enzymes, such as superoxide dismutase 2 [67].

The presence of functional alterations could affect the vasodilator capacity necessary for increasing local blood flow and oxygen delivery in the skeletal muscle during exercise in hypertension ultimately resulting in tissue ischemia and impaired tolerance to physical activity.

Indeed, hypertensive subjects performing 8 weeks of aerobic high-intensity training (knee extensor exercise by cycling ergometer two to three times a week) showed lower leg blood flow and oxygen delivery to contracting leg muscles when compared to normotensive subjects [70]. However, this blunted exercise response was not associated with altered vasodilator response to the NO- and prostanoid-dependent vasodilators acetylcholine [70] and adenosine [25, 68] and the two groups also had similar muscle protein levels and phosphorylation status of enzymes catalyzing NO formation [70]. Accordingly, a similar reduction in blood flow was observed during pharmacological inhibition of NO and prostanoid formation by infusion of L-NMMA and indomethacin in hypertensive patients compared to a normotensive group, suggesting that the capacity to produce NO and vasodilator prostanoids during leg exercise and the effect of NO and vasodilator prostanoids on the regulation of exercise hyperemia at the local muscular level are not affected in essential hypertension [70]. These data suggest that the mechanisms underlying the reduction in exercise induced blood flow in hypertension are not completely clear and seem to involve factors other than NO and prostanoids.

Among vascular constrictor factors, ET-1 appears to play an important role for impaired vasodilator response to forearm exercise in hypertensive subjects [71]. In accordance with that, ETA receptor inhibition, which mediates the vasoconstrictor effect of endothelin-1, has been demonstrated to increase blood flow to the exercising leg in aged individuals [72]. This suggests that endogenous ET-1 may limit exercise hyperemia in presence of enhanced ET-1-mediated vasoconstrictor tone, such as in essential hypertension [73]. In fact, skeletal muscle and plasma endothelin-1 levels were higher in hypertensive than normotensive individuals and higher plasma ET-1 levels were associated to a lower blood flow to the exercising leg of hypertensive subjects [70, 74].

Alternatively, it is possible that alterations in the blunting of sympathetic outflow, normally observed in contracting muscles of healthy animals and humans, may result in lower blood flow to contracting skeletal muscle [28]. Indeed, sympathetic outflow has been shown to be impaired in rat models of hypertension [75] as well as in the forearm of human hypertensive subjects [76].

Similarly, an altered influence of sympathetic activity on the vasculature and thus the degree of vasoconstrictor tone may also be involved in changes in microvascular function related to physical inactivity. Exercise training can reduce noradrenaline responsiveness [77] and therefore may elicit beneficial effects also in hypertension.

5.3.3 Alterations in Skeletal Muscle

Changes in the structure and function of different organs, including vasculature, in hypertension and other cardiovascular disease, such as obesity or hyperglycemia, are often associated with lipid accumulation, oxidative stress and inflammation [67, 78], which can also impact upon the physiology of skeletal muscle.

Skeletal muscle is the most abundant insulin-sensitive tissue, comprising 40%–50% of body mass, and it is responsible for approximately 20%–30% of resting oxygen consumption and handles 75%–95% of all insulin mediated glucose disposal [79]. Therefore, maintaining sensitivity to insulin is essential for maintaining and utilizing energy stores.

Hypertension is one of the key factors of the metabolic syndrome which may also have detrimental effects on the skeletal muscle as it may alter fiber composition, glucose uptake and insulin sensitivity of skeletal muscle, thereby causing inflammation and oxidative stress.

Decreased expression of insulin receptors and glucose transporter type 4 (GLUT4) protein (which regulates glucose uptake) in skeletal muscle has been found in patients with metabolic syndrome [80] and in experimental models of hypertension [81]. Furthermore, the skeletal muscle of hypertensive patients has a diminished insulin-stimulated glucose uptake [82], which may be ameliorated by antihypertensive treatment [83].

These changes contribute to increased glycolytic capacity and reduced oxidative capacity, and may exacerbate the underlying pathology by promoting muscle weakness and sedentary behavior.

Interestingly, NO mediates insulin induced stimulation of skeletal muscle perfusion and nutrient delivery [84]. In this regard, a reduction in NO, commonly observed during hypertension, may contribute to skeletal muscle dysfunction in metabolic syndrome.

Skeletal muscle fiber distribution also seems to be important in mediating insulin effects since insulin action is consistently less in type I fibers compared to type 2 fibers [80]. Lower proportion of type I fibers in metabolic syndrome muscle correlated with the severity of insulin resistance. In light of this, it is therefore important to promote the transformation of glycolytic fibers into oxidative muscle fibers.

In addition, Han et al. have demonstrated that patients with hypertension, independently of the treatment, show the presence of sarcopenia with higher body fat lower skeletal muscle mass compared with normotensive individuals [85]. The precise mechanisms linking sarcopenia with hypertension has not been clarified yet.

Indeed, loss of muscle mass promotes insulin resistance, which is an established risk factor for hypertension, it may enhance both inflammatory and oxidative pathways and increase arterial stiffness, which may mediate both sarcopenia and hypertension. Loss of muscle mass may also elevate blood pressure potentially by reducing myokines which are muscle contraction-induced factors with anti-inflammatory effects [85].

Variations in skeletal muscle fiber composition may represent another underlying mechanism for the alterations in sarcopenia, muscle strength, and contractility. Muscle fiber-type composition is determined by both genotype and environment where genetic component is about 40–50% for the observed variability in the proportion of type I fibers (slow-twitch) in human muscles [86].

Fiber-type composition and transformation of skeletal muscle fiber type may be determined by several polymorphisms of genes many of which have been associated with physical performance and athlete status, as well as metabolic and cardiovascular diseases. Several of these gene variants are involved in different biochemical and metabolic pathways which may interfere with muscle oxidative phenotype such as the calcineurin–NFAT pathway, mitochondrial biogenesis, glucose and lipid metabolism, cytoskeletal function, as well as in hypoxia and angiogenesis.

In an experimental model of hypertension, type IIA-fibers were present at a higher proportion in the soleus muscle of SHR compared to Wistar Kyoto rats (WKY) in all stages of hypertension [87].

Similarly, it has been demonstrated that skeletal muscles of patients with hypertension contain a higher percentage of type II fast-twitch, glycolytic fibers compared with normotensive controls [88].

5.4 Effect of Exercise in Healthy Subjects

Exercise training may induce cardiovascular changes that contribute to increase blood flow in skeletal muscles which is the result of a combination of structural and functional vascular adaptations. Exercise training can induce increases in blood flow capacity (BFC) by structural remodeling of the vascular tree (capillary bed and arterial tree) and by altered vasomotor reactivity of arteries and arterioles which control vascular resistance.

One of the primary adaptive responses of the skeletal muscle to aerobic exercise training is angiogenesis, which contributes to the improvement in muscular aerobic capacity, hence resulting in better oxygen transportation, delivery, and extraction.

Previous reports in normotensive individuals provided evidence that training may induce significant increases in the capillary bed of the skeletal muscle and myocardium [89]. Accordingly, 4 weeks of exercise training increased BFC as measured by reactive hyperemic responses to occlusion of blood flow to the forearm in human subjects [90] and induced capillarization in young men [91].

Exercise training [92, 93] has been suggested to counteract an antiangiogenic state condition in skeletal muscle and induce angiogenesis.

Previous studies reported that the level of VEGF mRNA in skeletal muscle [36, 94] as well as the level of VEGF protein in the skeletal muscle interstitium [36] were enhanced after an acute bout of exercise in normotensive individuals as well as within the first hours after exercise [39, 94]. Otherwise, both a decrease and an increase in VEGF protein levels within the muscle have been reported after dynamic exercise [94]. In fact, studies from Hoeier et al. demonstrated that acute exercise may induce only a transient increase in the mRNA level of several pro- as well as antiangiogenic factors. However, no differences in mRNA levels or VEGF protein in skeletal muscle were observed before and after a period of training despite enhanced capillarization [31]. These findings suggested that antiangiogenic factors increase after exercise and limit capillary growth for a well-controlled angiogenic process, whereas the existing VEGF stores in the muscle may be sufficiently large and an increase is not necessary for the angiogenic response, at least in young healthy individuals.

Moreover, exercise training induces nonuniform increases in capillarity and arteriolar density [95]. Indeed, data from animal models demonstrated that increases in skeletal muscle capillary density and mitochondrial content vary with mode of training (endurance or interval sprint training) and are greatest in the muscle tissue with the greatest increased oxidative capacity and fiber activity during training bouts [96].

Similarly, increased arteriolar density (increased number and/or size of arterioles) may contribute to increase BFC by increased maximal vascular conductance [96].

Moreover, endurance training improves oxygen extraction and lowers blood flow during submaximal exercise possibly because of an increase in shear stress. Indeed, the vasodilator terazosin, an α-adrenergic receptor blocker, induced capillary growth in human skeletal muscle, resulting in an increased fractional O_2 extraction, and a lower blood flow [97].

Exercise training also induces nonuniform increase in endothelial function in the skeletal muscle vasculature. This effect appears to be more pronounced in the muscles recruited during exercise training, although considerable inhomogeneities can be seen even within the same vasculature [95, 98, 99].

Furthermore, it is likely that changes in vascular smooth muscle reactivity contribute to the observed increased blood flow capacity after exercise training which involved sympathetic activity, vasodilator substance such as adenosine, and myogenic tone. For example, cyclic stretch of the vessel wall, which is acutely altered during an exercise bout, can lead to pronounced modifications in VSMC phenotype [100].

Interestingly, adult skeletal muscle undergoes conversion between these fiber types in response to exercise [101]. In particular, endurance training induces the transition from fast-twitch muscle fiber to slow-twitch muscle fiber, whereas strength training has an opposite effect. Muscle fiber transition is regulated by many factors, such as myogenic regulatory factors (MyoD and myogenin), peroxisome proliferator-activated receptor (PPAR)-gamma coactivator-1alpha (PGC-1alpha) and Ca2-dependent transcription factor, and the nuclear factor of activated T cells, cytoplasmic 1 (NFATc1) [101].

5.5 Effects of Exercise in Essential Hypertension

Benefits of physical exercise have been extensively established in experimental models and in humans with cardiovascular disease and they involve also the microcirculation. Structural and functional alterations of microcirculation associated with cardiovascular fitness and performance may contribute to reduction of blood pressure. Hypertension is associated with hemodynamic changes which result in reduced blood flow and oxygen delivery to contracting skeletal muscle. These factors could represent one important mechanism underlying the impaired exercise tolerance in this condition [16].

5.5.1 Effect on Microvascular Structure

Exercise mediates structural and mechanical changes and can correct capillary rarefaction in hypertension. However, contrasting results have been observed in experimental hypertension with respect to regression of microvascular remodeling [12, 13, 16].

In one study, training reduced resting blood pressure and caused normalization of both relative hindlimb vascular resistance and gracilis arterioles wall-to-lumen ratio in SHR, when compared to WKY [12].

Similarly, arteriole wall/lumen ratio from sedentary SHR was equally reduced (approximately 30%) and normalized by training in locomotor (soleus, gastrocnemius, gracilis) and nonlocomotor skeletal muscles (temporalis), in the myocardium and diaphragm, without changes in the renal cortex [13] suggesting that the vascular remodeling induced by exercise training may be dependent also on the vascular bed studied. Indeed, regression of arteriole remodeling may represent tissue-specific (skeletal muscle) and group-specific (SHR) adjustments to training to reduce local resistance and augment physical capacity of circulation, thus contributing to training-induced pressure-lowering effect.

In another study [16], 12 weeks of aerobic treadmill exercise did not affect lumen diameter, wall thickness, and wall–lumen ratio but was able to reduce vascular stiffness of both mesenteric resistance and small coronary arteries in SHR. Indeed, parallel changes in the extracellular matrix were observed such as reduction in collagen deposition and normalization of altered internal elastic lamina organization and expression of MMP-9 in mesenteric arteries from SHR. This was also related to better endothelial function in coronary and small mesenteric arteries and the concomitant decrease of oxidative stress and increase of NO bioavailability [16].

Exercise training may interfere with anatomical rarefaction and normalize capillary density, leading to capillary growth possibly by inducing angiogenesis. Training increased significantly both capillary density and capillary–fiber ratio in the gracilis and myocardium of WKY and SHR groups, causing a complete reversal of capillary rarefaction in trained SHR [12]. Indeed, capillarization after training was always larger in trained versus sedentary animals supporting the presence of angiogenic processes. The greater capillary supply of skeletal muscles and myocardium of trained SHR and WKY may reflect mainly the increased oxygen uptake of exercise-activated muscles, being an adaptive response to augmented local flow during exercise. Moreover, a period of low-intensity training also increased venule density (≈ twofold) only in locomotor and nonlocomotor muscles of SHR compared to WKY, whereas capillary density was similarly increased in all exercised muscles of both groups, with no change in temporalis and kidneys [13].

An increase in capillary-to-fiber ratio has been reported also in humans [14, 62]. The training intervention generally leads to increased capillary-to-fiber ratio in both normotensive [89] and hypertensive patients [14] albeit in some studies increased capillary-to-fiber ratio was observed after a period of training in the hypertensive subjects only [62] despite of equal training compliance and intensity compared to normotensive groups.

The resulting capillarization induced by exercise training may reflect the increase in proangiogenic stimuli such as VEGF. In healthy subjects, no differences in mRNA levels or VEGF protein in skeletal muscle were observed before and after a period of training despite enhanced capillarization [31]. However, this finding is in contrast with results from individuals with mild-to-moderate hypertension where 4-month period with combined endurance and strength training led to a 40%

increase in the skeletal muscle levels of VEGF [14]. The enhanced angiogenic potential with training in the hypertensive individuals was associated to a lowered blood pressure and an increased capillary-to-fiber ratio but unaltered capillary density. The discrepancy suggests that training mainly affects VEGF protein levels positively in individuals with reduced VEGF protein levels, for example, in cardiovascular disease [14]. In accordance with that, VEGF protein levels have been found to increase after endurance training of patients with cardiovascular disease [14] and in one study, increased VEGF levels were reported after only several training sessions [93]. Interestingly, in individuals with essential hypertension, eNOS protein levels were increased, whereas VEGF protein levels remained unaltered after acute exercise supporting the hypothesis that several factors other than NO may interfere with angiogenesis.

Moreover, data from humans show a capillary ultrastructure adaptation to training which consists of an increase in capillary and lumen area and a concomitant reduction of capillary basement membrane thickness in hypertensive patients to levels similar to the normotensive subjects [62]. This suggests that exercise training in essential hypertension is effective in improving diffusion conditions and hence oxygen extraction and exchange of metabolites in the skeletal muscle capillary network.

5.5.2 Effect on Microvascular Function

Exercise training, mainly endurance training, represents a nonpharmacological approach able to improve blood pressure control through a reduction in vascular resistance as well as vascular alterations and endothelial function in hypertensive patients as well as in animal models of hypertension [16, 102].

Regular physical activity can improve vascular function by ameliorating the balance between vasodilator and vasoconstrictor systems, thus contributing in the matching of blood flow and oxygen utilization in contracting skeletal muscles. Accordingly, an improvement of endothelial function after continuous aerobic exercise training has been reported in mesenteric resistance arteries and in small coronary arteries from SHR [16]. Similarly, exercise training significantly improved the responses to acetylcholine and flow-mediated dilation in in gastrocnemius muscle small arteries from hypertensive rats with chronic NO synthase inhibition in parallel with a decrease in blood pressure [103] suggesting that both an increase in vasodilator formation and a reduction in the levels of vasoconstrictors and ROS may be involved.

These data have been confirmed in human hypertension. Indeed, regular aerobic exercise (30 min of brisk walking 5 to 7 times weekly for 12 weeks) augments endothelium-dependent vascular relaxation measured as the forearm blood flow by strain-gauge plethysmography [104, 105] in patients with mild essential hypertension compared to untrained subjects supporting the hypothesis that long-term aerobic exercise augmented acetylcholine-stimulated nitric oxide release. In the same studies, compared to hypertensive patients, normotensive subjects showed higher responses of forearm vasculature to acetylcholine and in blood flow before exercise which did not change after training [104]. In addition, after training, a reduction of leg blood flow was observed in normotensive subjects during exercise, whereas exercise blood flow remained unaltered in hypertensive patients [70] indicating the presence of an insufficient blood flow and hence oxygen delivery before training in essential hypertension.

Furthermore, short term (8 weeks) resistance or endurance training improves endothelial function of resistance arteries and oxidant/antioxidant balance also in young patients with prehypertension [106]. Beneficial effects on endothelium-dependent vasodilation induced by exercise training in hypertension seem to be associated with an increase in the release of nitric oxide [104] and a reduction in oxidative stress [13].

However, in other studies, the regulation of exercise hyperemia at the local muscular level does not seem to affect NO and vasodilator prostanoids in essential hypertension since the vasodilator response to acetylcholine was found to be equally increased in hypertensive patients and normotensive subjects [25, 70]. However, these compounds appear to be involved in the lowering of systemic blood pressure and vascular tone induced by training since the effect of training on blood pressure was abolished when these systems were inhibited [70].

A part from an increased NO bioavailability [70, 104], other mechanisms underlying the beneficial effect of exercise training have been proposed such as improved balance between prostacyclin and thromboxane levels in skeletal muscle [26], improved balance between ROS formation and antioxidant systems [102], and lower circulating levels of ET-1 [74].

In addition, essential hypertension is linked to an increased sympathetic vasoconstrictor activity and reduced tissue perfusion, and an impaired functional sympatholysis is therefore likely to have a greater consequence for tissue perfusion in hypertensive than in normotensive individuals with a similar impairment in functional sympatholysis. However, Mortessen et al. [77] demonstrated that 8 weeks of aerobic training (3–4 times per week) improves functional sympatholysis during leg exercise and the α-adrenergic responsiveness independently of the presence of hypertension at least in middle-aged individuals.

5.5.3 Role of MicroRNAs

A body of evidence indicates that aerobic exercise training (ET) improves endothelial function, counteracts microvascular rarefaction and decreases blood pressure in hypertension [12, 107, 108]. However, the mechanisms underlying the association between ET and these effects in hypertension are not completely understood. In this context, a new class of gene expression regulators, known as microRNAs (miRNAs), seem to be an important factor in the gene regulation of hypertension and they represent possible therapeutic target for tackling capillary rarefaction and defective angiogenesis in this disease [109].

The miRNAs are noncoding short RNA molecules (approximately 17–25 nucleotides in length) which regulate gene expression on the posttranscriptional level. ET

Some miRNAs associated with hypertension that have potential for being regulated by exercise training.

miRNAS	Targets	miRNA function
miRNA-16	VEGF	Control of angiogenesis and vascular integrity
miRNA-21	PTEN; Bcl-2	Involved in nitric oxide production; apoptosis
miRNA-24	Trb-3	Mediator of contractile phenotype in VSMC
miRNA-126	VCAM-1; PI3KR2; Spred1	Suppress cell adhesion molecule; Proangiogenic
miRNA-146a	TRAF6; KLF4	Involved in inflammatory response
miRNA-155	eNOS; AT1R	eNOS expression and NO production

Fig. 5.3 Some miRNAs associated with hypertension that have potential for being regulated by exercise training. *VEGF* vascular endothelial growth factor, *PTEN* phosphatase and tensin homolog, *Bcl-2* B-cell CLL/lymphoma 2, Trb-3, Tribbles-like protein-3, *NO* Nitric oxide, *VECAM1* vascular cell adhesion molecule 1, *PI3KR2* Phosphatidyl-inositol 3-kinase regulatory subunit beta, *Spred1* Sprouty-related, *EVH1* Domain-containing protein-1, *TRAF6* TNF receptor associated factor 6, *KLF4* Krüppel-like factor 4, *AT1R* Type 1 receptor of angiotensin II. See text for details. (*Vander José das Neves, Tiago Fernandes, Fernanda Roberta Roque, Ursula Paula Renó Soci, Stéphano Freitas Soares Melo, Edilamar Menezes de Oliveira. Exercise training in hypertension: Role of microRNAs. World J Cardiol 2014 August 26; 6* (8)*: 713–727 (modified)*)

seems to be able to modulate miRNAs associated with neovascularization and vascular remodeling in hypertension explaining the relationship between ET and miRNAs in the pathogenesis of this disease (Fig. 5.3). The complexity of miRNAs-dependent gene expression is further due to the fact that a single miRNA can regulate hundreds of targets and more than one miRNA can cooperatively regulate a single miRNA [110]. In an even more complex manner the miRNA function might be controlled by differential processing mechanisms [111]. The miRNAs are involved in all biological processes, including cellular proliferation, differentiation, cellular migration and apoptosis, cardiogenesis, such as cardiomyocyte growth, remodeling, interstitial fibrosis, skeletal muscle proliferation and differentiation, brain morphogenesis, oncogenesis, and hematopoietic lineage differentiation [112–115]; thus, their deregulation often results in the development of cardiovascular diseases.

The miRNAs-155 is expressed in macrophages and it seems to be a key mediator of cardiac injury in hypertensive heart disease, promoting cardiac inflammation, hypertrophy, and failing in response to pressure overload [116]. Moreover miRNAs-155 targets endothelial nitric oxide synthase (eNOS) and the type 1 receptor of Angiotensin II (AT1R) which regulate the tonus of vascular smooth muscle cells (VSMC) [116]. About ET, it has been demonstrated that ET is able to decrease cardiac miRNA-208a level, which regulate expression of slow myosin, in healthy wistar and obese Zucker rats and improves the balance between the ß-myosin heavy chain (ßMHC) and αMHC gene expression [117, 118]. Thus, miRNA-155 is an example of pathological miRNA naturally reversed by ET and its downregulation is able to improve the contractile efficiency of the heart.

Regarding microcirculation, it is well known that the impaired NO availability play a key role in microvascular alterations, mainly due to oxidative stress with increased of reactive oxygen species and reduced antioxidant capacity. The microvascular rarefaction may be responsible for most hypertension associated organ damage [119]. It has been demonstrated that continuous aerobic ET exerts beneficial effects on the endothelial function of small arteries of gastrocnemius muscle from rats with chronic inhibition of NO synthase [103], in mesenteric resistance arteries and small coronary arteries from SHR [11] and in resistance arteries from young prehypertensive patients [106].

However, the beneficial effects of ET on miRNAs of the small and large vasculature is poorly understood. We have above mentioned that miRNAs play a key role in the development of endothelial dysfunction, vascular remodeling and reduce angiogenic capacity that are involved in the pathogenesis of hypertension [109]. In particular it has been demonstrated a correlation between hypertension, alterations in miRNAs and changes in renin-angiotensin-aldosterone system (RAAS) and in the phenotypes of VSMC, endothelial cells as well as in the inflammatory activation of macrophages [109, 120, 121]. The role of ET in this context has not been clarified as yet.

Considering atherosclerosis, Wu et al. studied the effects of treadmill ET for a period of 12 weeks, 5 times per week, 60 min/day, on the aorta of male ApoE null C57BL/6 J mice with atherosclerosis, which were fed a high-fat diet [122]. They showed that aerobic exercise is able to decrease angiotensin II and endothelin 1 levels, to decrease expression of miRNA-155 and to increase expression of miRNA-146a and miRNA-126 in the aorta of trained mice, in particular in the group treated with simvastatin.

As mentioned before the target of miRNA-155 is eNOS and its expression reduction is an essential factor for increasing eNOS expression and NO production [123]. The miRNA-155 binds to the eNOS mRNA 3′-UTR and destabilizes eNOS mRNA, resulting in decreased eNOS and NO production. In atherosclerosis, miRNA-155 is drastically upregulated [123]. However, anti-miRNA-155, statins (3-hydroxy-3-methylglutaryl coenzyme A reductase inhibitors), and other Rho kinase inhibitors prevent the increase in miRNA-155 [124]. To our knowledge, it is not clear if, in hypertension, ET diminishes miRNA-155 expression in vessels, but it is demonstrated that exercise can modulate the miRNA-155 expression in atherosclerotic vessels.

Another important miRNA involved in vascular integrity is miRNA-126, which acts by blocking regulators of the VEGF pathway [125–127]. It has been demonstrated that miRNA-126 could interfere with adhesion of leucocytes to the endothelium, enhancing angiogenesis through deletion of the cell adhesion molecule expression and negative regulation of the endothelial receptor of α4β1 integrin [128]. Harris et al. demonstrated that miRNA-126 is one of the most abundant miRNAs expressed in endothelial cells but not in VSMC [122, 128]. Phosphoinositol-3 kinase regulatory subunit 2 (PI3KR2), a negative regulator of the VEGF signaling, is an important target of miRNA-126, [127, 129, 130]. Fernandes et al. were the first to observe that hypertension could be associated with a reduction of miRNA-126 expression and an increase of PI3KR2 expression which could be the cause of impaired the VEGF angiogenic signaling pathways seen in this study in SHRs [131]. The study of Wu et al. showed that ET was able to increase miRNA-126 expression in the aorta of mice [122]. Thus, miRNA-126 might be an important modulator of vascular disease and vessel remodeling.

VEGF and antiapoptotic protein Bcl-2 were identified and validated as target of miRNA-16. In the study of Dejean et al., it has been observed that miRNA-16 directly interacts with VEGF mRNA and that the increase of miRNA-16 was able to reduce angiogenesis and tumor growth [132]. The overexpression of miRNA-16 resulted in reduced proliferation, migration, and cord formation of endothelial cells in vitro and reduced capacity of endothelial cells to form blood vessels in vivo [133].

Another miRNA involved in endothelial biology is miRNA-21 which acts by modulating apoptosis by bcl-2 and eNOS activity [134, 135]. The miRNA-21 is involved in vascular remodeling that affects VSMC and endothelial cells. Thus, miRNA-21 represents a critical miRNA for angiogenesis and its overexpression is able to induce a synthetic VSMC as seen after vascular injury [109, 120]. A higher miRNA-16 and miRNA-21 peripheral expression associated with a decrease in EGF and bcl-2 expression has been observed in a model of 12-week-old male spontaneously hypertensive rats (SHRs) [131]. In the soleus muscle of this model of SHRs, alterations in fiber type distribution were observed with higher percentage of type II fibers, decrease in slow-twitch fibers and reduced capillary/fiber ratio with small decrease in citrate synthase activity. In this study 10-week ET was able to reduce 21% of the blood pressure in SHRs, to normalize capillary rarefaction in the skeletal muscle of SHRs and to increase the capillary/fiber ratio in the skeletal muscle of control Wister Kyoto rats. The main novel finding of this study was the demonstration of the ability of ET to restore miRNA-16,-21 and -126 associated with revascularization in hypertension suggesting a potential mechanism by which ET ameliorates capillary rarefaction and defective angiogenesis in hypertension [125]. In addition it has been shown that ET is able to normalize VEGF, eNOS and PI3KR2 levels, the proapoptotic (Bad) and anti-apoptotic (Bcl-2, Bcl-x) mediators, indicating that ET may improve the balance between proapoptotic and antiapoptotic factors present in vascular disease, leading to regression of microvascular alterations in hypertension [131]. Therefore, these miRNAs may be potential therapeutic targets for pathological conditions characterized by capillary rarefaction such as hypertension.

Another miRNA that deserves to be remembered is the miRNA-34a. The target of this miRNA is sirtuin 1 (SIRT1) in the endothelial cells that is involved in the effect of aging on the vasculature [136]. In support of this mechanism is the demonstration that overexpression of miRNA-34a has been associated with senescence of endothelial cells. The hypothesis is that this miRNA is involved in development or progression of atherosclerosis in hypertension since it has been hypothesized that SIRT1 impairs the eNOS metabolism in the endothelial cells via SIRT1/eNOS pathway [137]. Nevertheless, other studies are needed in order to explain the possible association between miRNA-34a, vascular cells and ET in the pathogenesis of hypertension and vascular disease.

In summary, the above findings indicate that several miRNAs are involved in vascular integrity and angiogenesis and that they may be a potential new target for treatment. ET probably causes alterations in many of the miRNAs that are deregulated in the vascular system and this may explain the beneficial effects of exercise in hypertension.

5.5.4 Effect of MicroRNAs on the Skeletal Muscle

The role of ET in the prevention and treatment of hypertension and cardiovascular disease is well established but the vascular mechanism and the muscle changes are not fully understood. As mentioned above, the analysis of miRNAs could explain the correlation between ET and cardiovascular prevention. A better knowledge of miRNA pathways could be of help for identifying new strategies for prevention and treatment. Recent studies have revealed that myogenic transcription factors involved in differentiation and muscle contraction also activate the expression of a set of miRNAs with the function of "adjusting" the output of the transcription network, resulting in precise cellular responses to signals of development, physiology, and pathology (Fig. 5.4).

The miRNAs-1, -133a-b, -206, and -208 are muscle-specific and provide up to 25% of miRNAs expression in skeletal muscle; it has been demonstrated that they are involved in the growth, differentiation, and contractility of muscle [138, 139].

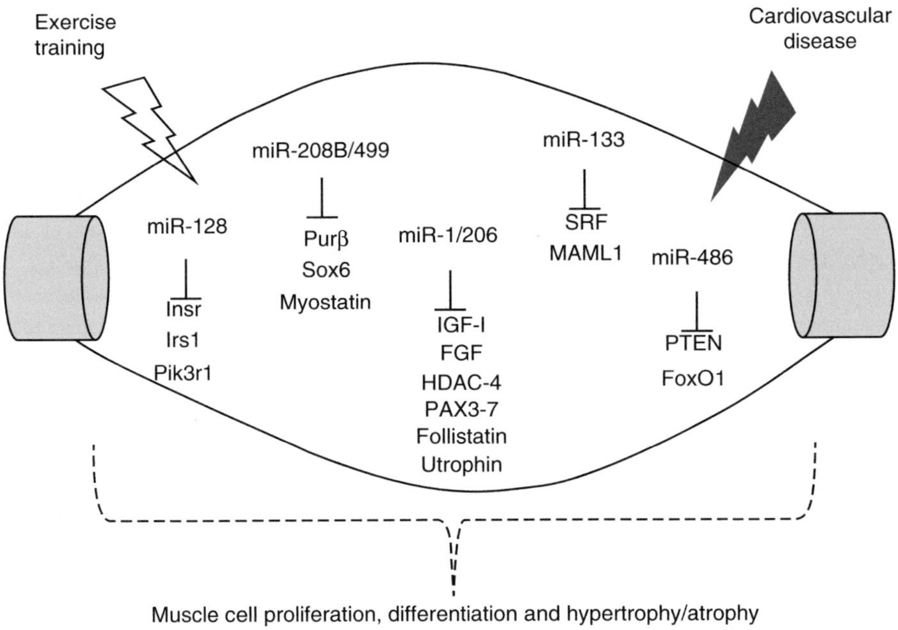

Fig. 5.4 Skeletal muscle miRNAs and selected target genes regulating cell proliferation, differentiation, and hypertrophy/atrophy by exercise training and cardiovascular diseases. The relationship between miRNAs and the mRNAs that encode proteins is shown. *Insr* Insulin receptor, *Irs1* Insulin receptor substrate 1, *Pik3r1* Phosphatidylinositol 3-kinases, regulatory 1; *Purβ* Purine-rich element binding protein B, *HDAC4* Histone deacetylase 4, *IGF-1* Insulin-like growth factor 1, *FGF* Fibroblast growth factor, *SRF* Serum response factor, *MAML1* Mastermind 1, *PTEN* Phosphatase and tensin homolog, *FoxO1* Forkhead box protein O1. (*Vander José das Neves, Tiago Fernandes, Fernanda Roberta Roque, Ursula Paula Renó Soci, Stéphano Freitas Soares Melo, Edilamar Menezes de Oliveira. Exercise training in hypertension: Role of microRNAs. World J Cardiol 2014 August 26; 6 (8): 713–727*)

Other miRSNAs responsible of myoblast proliferation or differentiation are miRNAs-24, -26a, -27b, -125b, -148a, -181, -214, and -489 [140].

Safdar et al. [141] observed an increase expression of miRNA-1 in skeletal muscle of mice after 3 h of a single session of aerobic ET. The chronic effect of exercise led to a decrease in the expression of miRNA-1 with consequent expression of important genes in muscle growth, such as c-Met, hepatocyte growth factor, and insulin-like growth factor 1 (IGF-1), and secondary muscle hypertrophy.

In the study of van Rooij and colleagues [142] it has been demonstrated the presence of two miRNAs in MHC genes: the miRNA-208b, encoded by the gene β *MHC*, and miRNA-499, encoded by the gene *Myh7b*, a little studied myosin that shares extensive homology with the β *MHC* gene. Both miRNAs, with feature of type I fibers, are expressed in skeletal muscles and are associated with oxidative profile. Indeed, it has been shown that in double knockout animals (dKO) for miRNAs-208b and − 499 there was a substantial loss of type I muscle myofibers in the soleus muscle of dKO with consequent loss of slow myofibers. This finding was confirmed by the reduction in protein and gene expression of βMHC and concomitant increase in the expression of type IIa and type b-IIx faster myosin isoforms [142]. The overexpression of miRNA-499 was able to reverse all myofibers from soleus fast into slow fibers, type I profile. Moreover, transgenic expression of miRNA-499 in the heart of miR-208a−/− mice, which is necessary to increase β *MHC (Myh7)* in the heart of adult animals in response to stress and hypothyroidism [143], was sufficient to restore the expression of βMHC and miR-208b to normal levels in the presence of propylthiouracil (PTU) [142]. In addition, it has been demonstrated that animals with overexpression of miRNA-499 ran 50% more than wild type during exercise tolerance test on the treadmill, suggesting that higher aerobic endurance is a consequence of modification in muscle fibers with predominance of slow type I fibers with oxidative metabolism.

In spite of these findings, the association of these miRNAs and the secondary changes in fiber type with CVD or hypertension is still unknown. It is likely that miRNA-208b and miRNA-499 are involved in the changes in muscle fiber profile which have been observed in hypertension and CVD. ET would play a key role for the standardization of these parameters because it is well known that ET improves oxidative stress associated with a predominance of type I fibers.

5.6 Conclusion

Skeletal muscle blood flow may be affected by changes in microvascular structure or function which occur in pathological conditions such as hypertension with subsequent increase in vascular resistance. ET may elicit beneficial effects on skeletal muscle blood flow by inducing favorable microvascular remodeling, capillary angiogenesis, and modulating vasomotor reactivity of small arteries and arterioles. In particular, activation of angiogenic processes with increase in capillary network seems to have a major influence in ameliorating local blood flow in several tissues including skeletal muscle. Furthermore, phenotypic expression of skeletal muscle fiber type also has powerful influences on vascular structure and function which may influence training-induced vascular adaptations in skeletal muscle. miRNAs, a new class of gene expression regulators, are involved in vascular integrity and angiogenesis and could explain the link between hypertension and the beneficial effects of exercise. In this context, miRNAs may be a potential new target for prevention and treatment of hypertension and cardiovascular disease.

References

1. Levy BI, Ambrosio G, Pries AR, Struijker-Boudier HA. Microcirculation in hypertension: a new target for treatment? Circulation. 2001;104:735–40.
2. Rizzoni D, Porteri E, Boari GE, De Ciuceis C, Sleiman I, Muiesan ML, Castellano M, Miclini M, Agabiti-Rosei E. Prognostic significance of small-artery structure in hypertension. Circulation. 2003;108:2230–5.
3. De Ciuceis C, Porteri E, Rizzoni D, Rizzardi N, Paiardi S, Boari GEM, Miclini M, Zani F, Muiesan ML, Donato F, Salvetti M, Castellano M, Tiberio GAM, Giulini SM, Rosei EA. Structural alterations of subcutaneous small-resistance arteries may predict major cardiovascular events in patients with hypertension. Am J Hypertens. 2007;20(8):846–52.
4. Mathiassen ON, Buus NH, Sihm I, Thybo NK, Mørn B, Schroeder AP, Thygesen K, Aalkjaer C, Lederballe O, Mulvany MJ, Christensen KL. Small artery structure is an independent predictor of cardiovascular events in essential hypertension. J Hypertens. 2007;25(5):1021–6.
5. Theuerle JD, et al. Impaired retinal microvascular function predicts long-term adverse events in patients with cardiovascular disease. Cardiovasc Res. 2021;117:1949–57.
6. Agabiti Rosei E, Heagerty AM, Rizzoni D. Effects of antihypertensive treatment on small artery remodelling. J Hypertens. 2009;27(6):1107–14.
7. Rogers MW, Probst MM, Gruber JJ, Berger R, Boone JB. Differential effects of exercise training intensity on blood pressure and cardiovascular responses to stress in borderline hypertensive humans. J Hypertens. 1996;14:1369–75.
8. Fagard RH, Cornelissen VA. Effect of exercise on blood pressure control in hypertensive patients. Eur J Cardiovasc Prev Rehabil. 2007;14(1):12–7.
9. Cornelissen VA, Fagard RH. Effects of endurance training on blood pressure, blood pressure-regulating mechanisms, and cardiovascular risk factors. Hypertension. 2005;46:667–75.
10. Visseren FLJ, Mach F, Smulders YM, Carballo D, Koskinas KC, Bäck M, Benetos A, Biffi A, Boavida JM, Capodanno D, Cosyns B, Crawford C, Davos CH, Desormais I, Di Angelantonio E, Franco OH, Halvorsen S, Hobbs FDR, Hollander M, Jankowska EA, Michal M, Sacco S, Sattar N, Tok-gozoglu L, Tonstad S, Tsioufis KP, van Dis I, van Gelder IC, Wanner C, Williams B, ESC Scientific Document Group. ESC Scientific Document Group. 2021 ESC guidelines on cardiovascular disease prevention in clinical practice. Eur Heart J. 2021;42(34):3227–337.
11. Roque FR, Briones AM, García-Redondo AB, Galán M, Martínez-Revelles S, Avendaño MS, Cachofeiro V, Fernandes T, Vassallo DV, Oliveira EM, Salaices M. Aerobic exercise reduces oxidative stress and improves vascular changes of small mesenteric and coronary arteries in hypertension. Br J Pharmacol. 2013;168(3):686–703.
12. Amaral SL, Zorn TM, Michelini LC. Exercise training normalizes wall-to-lumen ratio of the gracilis muscle arterioles and reduces pressure in spontaneously hypertensive rats. J Hypertens. 2000;18:1563–72.
13. Melo RM, Martinho E, Michelini LC. Training induced, pressure-lowering effect in SHR: wide effects on circulatory profile of exercised and non-exercised muscles. Hypertension. 2003;42:851–7.

14. Hansen AH, Nielsen JJ, Saltin B, Hellsten Y. Exercise training normalizes skeletal muscle vascular endothelial growth factor levels in patients with essential hypertension. J Hypertens. 2010;28:1176–85.
15. Andersen P, Saltin B. Maximal perfusion of skeletal muscle in man. J Physiol. 1985;366:233–49.
16. Nyberg M, Gliemann L, Hellsten Y. Vascular function in health, hypertension, and diabetes: effect of physical activity on skeletal muscle microcirculation. Scand J Med Sci Sports. 2015;25(Suppl 4):60–73.
17. Remensnyder JP, Mitchell JH, Sarnoff SJ. Functional sympatholysis during muscular activity. Observations on influence of carotid sinus on oxygen uptake. Circ Res. 1962;11:370–80.
18. Wilson JR, Kapoor SC. Contribution of prostaglandins to exercise-induced vasodilation in humans. Am J Physiol. 1993;265(1 Pt 2):H171–5.
19. Shoemaker JK, Naylor HL, Pozeg ZI, Hughson RL. Failure of prostaglandins to modulate the time course of blood flow during dynamic forearm exercise in humans. J Appl Physiol. 1996;81:1516–21.
20. Mortensen SP, Gonzalez-Alonso J, Damsgaard R, Saltin B, Hellsten Y. Inhibition of nitric oxide and prostaglandins, but not endothelial-derived hyperpolarizing factors, reduces blood flow and aerobic energy turnover in the exercising human leg. J Physiol. 2007;581:853–61.
21. Balon TW, Nadler JL. Nitric oxide release is present from incubated skeletal muscle preparations. J Appl Physiol. 1994;77(6):2519–21.
22. Vallance P, Collier J, Moncada S. Effects of endothelium-derived nitric oxide on peripheral arteriolar tone in man. Lancet. 1989;2(8670):997–1000.
23. Radegran G, Saltin B. Nitric oxide in the regulation of vasomo-tor tone in human skeletal muscle. Am J Physiol Heart Circ Physiol. 1999;276:H1951–60.
24. Boushel R, Langberg H, Gemmer C, Olesen J, Crameri R, Scheede C, Sander M, Kjaer M. Combined inhibition of nitric oxide and prostaglandins reduces human skeletal muscle blood flow during exercise. J Physiol. 2002;543:691–8.
25. Mortensen SP, Nyberg M, Thaning P, Saltin B, Hellsten Y. Adenosine contributes to blood flow regulation in the exercising human leg by increasing prostaglandin and nitric oxide formation. Hypertension. 2009;53:993–9.
26. Hellsten Y, Nyberg M, Jensen LG, Mortensen SP. Vasodilator interactions in skeletal muscle blood flow regulation. J Physiol. 2012;590(Pt 24):6297–305.
27. Rongen GA, Smits P, Thien T. Characterization of ATP-induced vasodilation in the human forearm vascular bed. Circulation. 1994;90(4):1891–8.
28. Rosenmeier JB, Hansen J, Gonzalez-Alonso J. Circulating ATP-induced vasodilatation overrides sympathetic vasoconstrictor activity in human skeletal muscle. J Physiol. 2004;558(Pt 1):351–65.
29. Jendzjowsky NG, DeLorey DS. Shortterm exercise training enhances functional sympatholysis through a nitric oxide-dependent mechanism. J Physiol. 2013;591(Pt 6):1535–49.
30. Pohl U, Holtz J, Busse R, Bassenge E. Crucial role of endothelium in the vasodilator response to increased flow in vivo. Hypertension. 1986;8(1):37–44.
31. Hoier B, Nordsborg N, Andersen S, Jensen L, Nybo L, Bangsbo J, Hellsten Y. Pro- and anti-angiogenic factors in human skeletal muscle in response to acute exercise and training. J Physiol. 2012;590(Pt 3):595–606.
32. Laughlin MH, Woodman CR, Schrage WG, Gute D, Price EM. Interval sprint training enhances endothelial function and eNOS content in some arteries that perfuse white gastrocnemius muscle. J Appl Physiol. 2004;96:233–44.
33. Armstrong RB, Laughlin MH. Exercise blood flow patterns within and among rat muscles after training. Am J Physiol Heart Circ Physiol. 1984;246:H59–68.
34. Olfert IM, Birot O. Importance of anti-angiogenic factors in the regulation of skeletal muscle angiogenesis. Microcirculation. 2011;18:316–30.
35. Millauer B, Wizigmann-Voos S, Schnürch H, Martinez R, Møller NP, Risau W, Ullrich A. High affinity VEGF binding and developmental expression suggest Flk-1 as a major regulator of vasculogenesis and angiogenesis. Cell. 1993;72:835–46.

36. Hoffner L, Nielsen JJ, Langberg H, Hellsten Y. Exercise but not prostanoids enhance levels of vascular endothelial growth factor and other proliferative agents in human skeletal muscle interstitium. J Physiol. 2003;550(Pt 1):217–25.
37. Tsurumi Y, Murohara T, Krasinski K, Chen D, Witzenbichler B, Kearney M, Couffinhal T, Isner JM. Reciprocal relation between VEGF and NO in the regulation of endothelial integrity. Nat Med. 1997;3:879–86.
38. Malek MH, Olfert IM. Global deletion of thrombospondin-1 increases cardiac and skeletal muscle capillarity and exercise capacity in mice. Exp Physiol. 2009;94:749–60.
39. Ryan NA, Zwetsloot KA, Westerkamp LM, Hickner RC, Pofahl WE, Gavin TP. Lower skeletal muscle capillarization and VEGF expression in aged vs. young men. J Appl Physiol. 2006;100(1):178–85.
40. Schiaffino S, Reggiani C. Fiber types in mammalian skeletal muscles. Physiol Rev. 2011;91:1447–531.
41. Smerdu V, Karsch-Mizrachi I, Campione M, Leinwand L, Schiaffino S. Type IIx myosin heavy chain transcripts are expressed in type IIb fibers of human skeletal muscle. Am J Physiol. 1994;267:C1723–8.
42. Hagiwara N. Genetic dissection of the physiological role of skeletal muscle in metabolic syndrome. New J Sci. 2014;2014:1e21.
43. Mizunoya W, Iwamoto Y, Shirouchi B, Sato M, Komiya Y, Razin FR, et al. Dietary fat influences the expression of contractile and metabolic genes in rat skeletal muscle. PLoS One. 2013;8(11):e80152–65.
44. Rizzoni D, Porteri E, Castellano M, Bettoni G, Muiesan ML, Muiesan P, Giulini SM, Agabiti-Rosei E. Vascular hypertrophy and remodeling in secondary hypertension. Hypertension. 1996;28(5):785–90.
45. Rizzoni D, Porteri E, Guefi D, Piccoli A, Castellano M, Pasini G, Muiesan ML, Mulvany MJ, Rosei EA. Cellular hypertrophy in subcutaneous small arteries of patients with renovascular hypertension. Hypertension. 2000;35(4):931–5.
46. Rizzoni D, Porteri E, Guelfi D, Muiesan ML, Valentini U, Cimino A, Girelli A, Rodella L, Bianchi R, Sleiman I, Rosei EA. Structural alterations in subcutaneous small arteries of normotensive and hypertensive patients with non-insulin-dependent diabetes mellitus. Circulation. 2001;103(9):1238–44.
47. De Ciuceis C, Porteri E, Rizzoni D, Corbellini C, La Boria E, Boari GEM, Pilu A, Mittempergher F, Di Betta E, Casella C, Nascimbeni R, Rosei CA, Ruggeri G, Caimi L, Rosei EA. Effects of weight loss on structural and functional alterations of subcutaneous small arteries in obese patients. Hypertension. 2011;58(1):29–36.
48. Grassi G, Seravalle G, Scopelliti F, Dell'Oro R, Fattori L, Quarti-Trevano F, Brambilla G, Schiffrin EL, Mancia G. Structural and functional alterations of subcutaneous small resistance arteries in severe human obesity. Obesity (Silver Spring). 2010;18(1):92–8.
49. Izzard AS, Rizzoni D, Agabiti Rosei E, Haegerty AM. Small artery structure and hypertension: adaptive changes and target organ damage. J Hypertens. 2005;23(2):247–50.
50. Park JB, Schiffrin EL. Small artery remodeling is the most prevalent (earliest?) form of target organ damage in mild essential hypertension. J Hypertens. 2001;19(5):921–30.
51. Ritt M, et al. Analysis of retinal arteriolar structure in never-treated patients with essential hypertension. J Hypertens. 2008;26:1427–34.
52. Kock E, et al. Morphometric analysis of small arteries in the human retina using adaptive optics imaging: relationship with blood pressure and focal vascular changes. J Hypertens. 2014;32(4):890–8.
53. Laurent S, Boutouyrie P. The structural factor of hypertension: large and small artery alterations. Circ Res. 2015;116(6):1007–21.
54. Rizzoni D, Palombo C, Porteri E, Muiesan ML, Kozàkovà M, La Canna G, Nardi M, Guelfi D, Salvetti M, Morizzo C, Vittone F, Rosei EA. Relationships between coronary flow vasodilator capacity and small artery remodelling in hypertensive patients. J Hypertens. 2003;21(3):625–31.

55. Rizzoni D, De Ciuceis C, Porteri E, Paiardi S, Boari GE, Mortini P, Cornali C, Cenzato M, Rodella LF, Borsani E, Rizzardi N, Platto C, Rezzani R, Rosei EA. Altered structure of small cerebral arteries in patients with essential hypertension. J Hypertens. 2009;27(4):838–45.
56. Conway J. Hemodynamic aspects of essential hypertension in humans. Physiol Rev. 1984;64:617–60.
57. Hernandez N, Torres SH, Finol HJ, Vera O. Capillary changes in skeletal muscle of patients with essential hypertension. Anat Rec. 1999;256:425–32.
58. Debbabi H, Uzan L, Mourad JJ, Safar M, Levy BI. Increased skin capillary density in treated essential hypertensive patients. Am J Hypertens. 2006;19:477–83.
59. Paiardi S, Rodella LF, De Ciuceis C, Porteri E, Boari GE, Rezzani R, Rizzardi N, Platto C, Tiberio GA, Giulini SM, Rizzoni D, Agabiti-Rosei E. Immunohistochemical evaluation of microvascular rarefaction in hypertensive humans and in spontaneously hypertensive rats. Clin Hemorheol Microcirc. 2009;42(4):259–68.
60. Henrich HA, Romen W, Heimgartner W, Hartung E, Baumer F. Capillary rarefaction characteristic of the skeletal muscle of hypertensive patients. Klin Wochenschr. 1988;66:54–60.
61. Noon JP, Walker BR, Webb DJ, et al. Impaired micro-vascular dilatation and capillary rarefaction in young adults with a predisposition to high blood pressure. J Clin Invest. 1997;99:1873–9.
62. Gliemann L, Buess R, Nyberg M, Hoppeler H, Odriozola A, Thaning P, Hellsten Y, Baum O, Mortensen SP. Capillary growth, ultrastructure remodelling and exercise training in skeletal muscle of essential hypertensive patients. Acta Physiol (Oxf). 2015;214(2):210–20.
63. Greene AS, Amaral SL. Microvascular angiogenesis and the renin-angiotensin system. Curr Hypertens Rep. 2002;4:56–62.
64. Flammer AJ, Lüscher TF. Human endothelial dysfunction: EDRFs. Pflugers Arch. 2010;459(6):1005–13.
65. Taddei S, Virdis A, Ghiadoni L, Magagna A, Salvetti A. Vitamin C improves endothelium-dependent vasodilation by restoring nitric oxide activity in essential hypertension. Circulation. 1998;97:2222–9.
66. Virdis A, Bacca A, Colucci R, Duranti E, Fornai M, Materazzi G, Ippolito C, Bernardini N, Blandizzi C, Bernini G, Taddei S. Endothelial dysfunction in small arteries of essential hypertensive patients: role of cyclooxygenase-2 in oxidative stress generation. Hypertension. 2013;62(2):337–44.
67. Touyz RM, Briones AM. Reactive oxygen species and vascular biology: implications in human hypertension. Hypertens Res. 2011;34:5–14.
68. Hellsten Y, Jensen L, Thaning P, Nyberg M, Mortensen S. Impaired formation of vasodilators in peripheral tissue in essential hypertension is normalized by exercise training: role of adenosine and prostacyclin. J Hypertens. 2012;30(10):2007–14.
69. Suvorava T, Lauer N, Harm PD, Kojda G, Harm PD. Physical inactivity causes endothelial dysfunction in healthy young mice. J Am Coll Cardiol. 2004;44(6):1320–7.
70. Nyberg M, Jensen LG, Thaning P, Hellsten Y, Mortensen SP. Role of nitric oxide and prostanoids in the regulation of leg blood flow and blood pressure in humans with essential hypertension: effect of high intensity aerobic training. J Physiol. 2012;590(Pt 6):1481–94.
71. McEniery CM, Wilkinson IB, Jenkins DG, Webb DJ. Endogenous endothelin-1 limits exercise-induced vasodilation in hypertensive humans. Hypertension. 2002;40(2):202–6.
72. Barrett-O'Keefe Z, Ives SJ, Trinity JD, Morgan G, Rossman MJ, Donato AJ, Runnels S, Morgan DE, Gmelch BS, Bledsoe AD, Richardson RS, Wray DW. Endothelin-A-mediated vasoconstriction during exercise with advancing age. J Gerontol A Biol Sci Med Sci. 2015;70(5):554–65.
73. Cardillo C, Kilcoyne CM, Waclawiw M, Cannon RO III, Panza JA. Role of endothelin in the increased vascular tone of patients with essential hypertension. Hypertension. 1999;33(2):753–8.
74. Nyberg M, Mortensen SP, Hellsten Y. Physical activity opposes the age related increase in skeletal muscle and plasma endothelin-1 levels and normalizes plasma endothelin-1 levels in individuals with essential hypertension. Acta Physiol (Oxf). 2013;207(3):524–35.

75. Zhao W, Swanson SA, Ye J, Li X, Shelton JM, Zhang W, Thomas GD. Reactive oxygen species impair sympathetic vasoregulation in skeletal muscle in angiotensin II-dependent hypertension. Hypertension. 2006;48:637–43.
76. VongpatanasinW WZ, Arbique D, Arbique G, Adams-Huet B, Mitchell JH, Victor RG, Thomas GD. Functional sympatholysis is impaired in hypertensive humans. J Physiol. 2011;589:1209–20.
77. Mortensen SP, Nyberg M, Gliemann L, Thaning P, Saltin B, Hellsten Y. Exercise training modulates functional sympatholysis and α-adrenergic vasoconstrictor responsiveness in hypertensive and normotensive individuals. J Physiol. 2014;592(14):3063–73.
78. Maury E, Brichard S. Adipokine dysregulation, adipose tissue inflammation and metabolic syndrome. Mol Cell Endocrinol. 2010;314(1):1e16.
79. Baron AD, Brechtel G, Wallace P, Edelman SV. Rates and tissue sites of non-insulin- and insulin-mediated glucose uptake in humans. Am J Physiol. 1988;255:E769–74.
80. Stuart CA, McCurry MP, Marino A, South MA, Howell MEA, Layne AS, et al. Slow-twitch fiber proportion in skeletal muscle correlates with insulin responsiveness. J Clin Endocrinol Metab. 2013;98(5):2027e36.
81. Atkins KB, Johns D, Watts S, Clinton Webb R, Brosius FC 3rd. Decreased vascular glucose transporter expression and glucose uptake in DOCA-salt hypertension. J Hypertens. 2001;19(9):1581–7.
82. Natali N, Santoro D, Palombo C, Cerri M, Ghione S, Ferrannini. Impaired insulin action on skeletal muscle metabolism in essential hypertension. Hypertension. 1991;17:170–8.
83. De Ciuceis C, Flati V, Rossini C, Rufo A, Porteri E, Di Gregorio J, Petroboni B, La Boria E, Donini C, Pasini E, Rosei EA, Rizzoni D. Effect of antihypertensive treatments on insulin signalling in lympho-monocytes of essential hypertensive patients: a pilot study. Blood Press. 2014;23(6):330–8.
84. Duplain H, Burcelin R, Sartori C, Cook S, Egli M, Lepori M, et al. Insulin resistance, hyperlipidemia, and hypertension in mice lacking endothelial nitric oxide synthase. Circulation. 2001;104(3):342e5.
85. Han TS, Al-Gindan YY, Govan L, Hankey CR, Lean MEJ. Associations of body fat and skeletal muscle with hypertension. J Clin Hypertens. 2018;21:230–8.
86. Ahmetov I, et al. Gene polymorphisms and fiber-type composition of human skeletal muscle. Int J Sport Nutr Exerc Metab. 2012;22(4):292–303.
87. Ben Bachir-Lamrini L, Sempore B, Mayet MH, Favier RJ. Evidence of a slow-to-fast fiber type transition in skeletal muscle from spontaneously hypertensive rats. Am J Physiol. 1990;258:R352–7.
88. Nagatomo F, Gu N, Fujino H, Takeda I, Tsuda K, Ishihara A. Skeletal muscle characteristics of rats with obesity, diabetes, hypertension, and hyperlipidemia. J Atheroscler Thromb. 2009;16:576–85.
89. Lash JM, Bohlen G. Functional adaptations of rat skeletal muscles arterioles to aerobic exercise training. J Appl Physiol. 1992;72:2052–62.
90. Green DJ, Cable NT, Fox C, Rankin JM, Taylor RR. Modification of forearm resistance vessels by exercise training in young men. J Appl Physiol. 1994;77:1829–33.
91. Jensen L, Pilegaard H, Neufer PD, Hellsten Y. Effect of acute exercise and exercise training on VEGF splice variants in human skeletal muscle. Am J Physiol Regul Integr Comp Physiol. 2004;287(2):R397–402.
92. Høier B, Nordsborg N, Andersen S, et al. Pro- and anti-angiogenic factors in human skeletal muscle in response to acute exercise and training. J Physiol. 2012;590(Pt 3):595–606.
93. Gustafsson T, Knutsson A, Puntschart A, et al. Increased expression of vascular endothelial growth factor in human skeletal muscle in response to short-term one-legged exercise training. Pflügers Arch Eur J Physiol. 2002;444(6):752–9.
94. Gavin TP, Robinson CB, Yeager RC, England JA, Nifong LW, Hickner RC. Angiogenic growth factor response to acute systemic exercise in human skeletal muscle. J Appl Physiol. 2004;96:19–24.

95. Laughlin MH, Roseguini B. Mechanisms for exercise training-induced increases in skeletal muscle blood flow capacity: differences with interval sprint training versus aerobic endurance training. J Physiol Pharmacol. 2008;59(Suppl 7):71–88.
96. Gute D, Laughlin MH, Amann JF. Regional changes in capillary supply in skeletal muscle of interval sprint and low intensity, endurance trained rats. Microcirculation. 1994;1:183–93.
97. Mortensen SP, Egginton S, Madsen M, et al. Alpha adrenergic receptor blockade increases capillarization and fractional O2 extraction and lowers blood flow in contracting human skeletal muscle. Acta Physiol (Oxf). 2017;221(1):32–43.
98. Woodman CR, Muller JM, Laughlin MH, Price EM. Induction of nitric oxide synthase mRNA in coronary resistance arteries isolated from exercise-trained pigs. Am J Physiol. 1997;273:H2575–9.
99. Koller A, Huang A, Sun D, Kaley G. Exercise training augments flow-dependent dilation in rat skeletal muscle arterioles. Role of endothelial nitric oxide and prostaglandins. Circ Res. 1995;76:544–50.
100. Haga JH, Li Y-SJ, Chien S. Molecular basis of the effects of mechanical stretch on vascular smooth muscle cells. J Biomech. 2007;40:947–60.
101. Yan Z, Okutsu M, Akhtar YN, Lira VA. Regulation of exercise-induced fiber type transformation, mitochondrial biogenesis, and angiogenesis in skeletal muscle. J Appl Physiol (1985). 2011;110:264–74.
102. Higashi Y, Yoshizumi M. Exercise and endothelial function: role of endothelium-derived nitric oxide and oxidative stress in healthy subjects and hypertensive patients. Pharmacol Ther. 2004;102:87–96.
103. Kuru O, Sentürk UK, Koçer G, Ozdem S, Başkurt OK, Cetin A, Yeşilkaya A, Gündüz F. Effect of exercise training on resistance arteries in rats with chronic NOS inhibition. J Appl Physiol. 2009;107:896–902.
104. Higashi Y, Sasaki S, Kurisu S, Yoshimizu A, Sasaki N, Matsuura H, Kajiyama G, Oshima T. Regular aerobic exercise augments endothelium-dependent vascular relaxation in normotensive as well as hypertensive subjects: role of endothelium-derived nitric oxide. Circulation. 1999a;100(11):1194–202.
105. Higashi Y, Sasaki S, Sasaki N, Nakagawa K, Ueda T, Yoshimizu A, Kurisu S, Matsuura H, Kajiyama G, Oshima T. Daily aerobic exercise improves reactive hyperemia in patients with essential hypertension. Hypertension. 1999b;33(1 Pt 2):591–7.
106. Beck DT, Martin JS, Casey DP, Braith RW. Exercise training improves endothelial function in resistance arteries of young prehypertensives. J Hum Hypertens. 2014;28:303–9.
107. Hagberg JM, Park JJ, Brown MD. The role of exercise training in the treatment of hyperten-Sion: an update. Sports Med. 2000;30:193–206.
108. Melo RP, Martinho E, Michelini LC. Training-induced, pressure lowering effect in SHR wide effects on circulatory profile of exercised and nonexercised muscles. Hypertension. 2003;42:851–7.
109. Bátkai S, Thum T. MicroRNAs in hypertension: mechanisms and therapeutic targets. Curr Hypertens Rep. 2012;14:79–87.
110. Krek A, Grün D, Poy MN, Wolf R, Rosenberg L, Epstein EJ, MacMenamin P, da Piedade I, Gunsalus KC, Stoffel M, Rajewsky N. Combinatorial microRNA target predictions. Nat Genet. 2005;37:495–500.
111. Thomson JM, Newman M, Parker JS, Morin-Kensicki EM, Wright T, Hammond SM. Ex-tensive post-transcriptional regulation of microRNAs and its implications for cancer. Genes Dev. 2006;20:2202–7.
112. Zhao Y, Samal E, Srivastava D. Serum response factor regulates a muscle-specific microRNA that targets Hand2 during cardiogenesis. Nature. 2005;436:214–20.
113. Chen JF, Mandel EM, Thomson JM, Wu Q, Callis TE, Hammond SM, et al. The role of mi-croRNA-1 and microRNA-133 in skeletal muscle proliferation and differentiation. Nat Genet. 2006;38:228–33.
114. Giraldez AJ, Cinalli RM, Glasner ME, Enright AJ, Thomson JM, Baskerville S, et al. Mi-croRNAs regulate brain morphogenesis in zebrafish. Science. 2005;308:833–8.

115. Chen CZ, Li L, Lodish HF, Bartel DP. MicroRNAs modulate hematopoietic lineage differentiation. Science. 2004;303:83–6.
116. Hazebroek M, Stöger L, Wijnands E, Janssen BJ, Creemers EE, Pinto YM, Grimm D, Schürmann N, Vigorito E, Thum T, Stassen F, Yin X, Mayr M, de Windt LJ, Lutgens E, Wouters K, de Winther MP, Zacchigna S, Giacca M, van Bilsen M, Papageorgiou AP, Schroen B. Macrophage microRNA-155 promotes cardiac hypertrophy and failure. Circulation. 2013;128:1420–32.
117. Soci UP, Fernandes T, Rosa KT, Irigoyen MC, Phillips MI, Oliveira EM. The role of microRNA-208a in cardiac hypertrophy induced by aerobic physical training. FASEB J. 2013;27:975. Abstract.
118. Fernandes T, Soci UP, Oliveira EM. MiRNA-208a targeting Purβ gene regulates the β-MHC content in cardiac hypertrophy induced by exercise training. Circ Res. 2013;128:A21942.
119. Yannoutsos A, Levy BI, Safar ME, Slama G, Blacher J. Pathophysiology of hypertension: interactions between macro and microvascular alterations through endothelial dysfunction. J Hypertens. 2014;32:216–24.
120. Hartmann D, Thum T. MicroRNAs and vascular (dys)function. Vascul Pharmacol. 2011;55:92–105.
121. Wei Y, Schober A, Weber C. Pathogenic arterial remodeling: the good and bad of microRNAs. Am J Physiol Heart Circ Physiol. 2013;304:H1050–9.
122. Wu XD, Zeng K, Liu WL, Gao YG, Gong CS, Zhang CX, Chen YQ. Effect of aerobic exercise on miRNA-TLR4 signaling in atherosclerosis. Int J Sports Med. 2014;35:344–50.
123. Sun HX, Zeng DY, Li RT, Pang RP, Yang H, Hu YL, Zhang Q, Jiang Y, Huang LY, Tang YB, Yan GJ, Zhou JG. Essential role of microRNA-155 in regulating endothelium-dependent vasorelaxation by targeting endothelial nitric oxide synthase. Hypertension. 2012;60:1407–14.
124. Shi L, Fleming I. One miR level of control: microRNA-155 directly regulates endothelial nitric oxide synthase mRNA and protein levels. Hypertension. 2012;60:1381–2.
125. Ba'tkai S, Thum T. MicroRNAs in hypertension: mechanisms and therapeutics targets. Curr Hypertens Rep. Epub ahead of print November 4, 2011.
126. Sua'rez Y, Sessa WC. MicroRNAs as novel regulators of angiogenesis. Circ Res. 2009;104:442–54.
127. Wang S, Aurora AB, Johnson BA, Qi X, McAnally J, Hill JA, Richardson JA, Bassel-Duby R, Olson EN. The endothelial-specific microRNAmiR-126 governs vascular integrity and angiogenesis. Dev Cell. 2008;15:261–71.
128. Harris TA, Yamakuchi M, Ferlito M, Mendell JT, Lowenstein CJ. MicroRNA-126 regulates endothelial expression of vascular cell adhesion molecule 1. Proc Natl Acad Sci U S A. 2008;105:1516–21.
129. Urbich C, Kuehbacher A, Dimmeler S. Role of microRNAs in vascular diseases, inflammation, and angiogenesis. Cardiovasc Res. 2008;79:581–8.
130. Fish JE, Santoro MM, Morton SU, Yu S, Yeh RF, Wythe JD, Bruneau BG, Stainier DYR, Srivastava D. miR-126 regulates angiogenic signaling and vascular integrity. Dev Cell. 2008;15:272–84.
131. Fernandes T, Magalhães FC, Roque FR, Phillips MI, Oliveira EM. Exercise training prevents the microvascular rarefaction in hypertension balancing angiogenic and apoptotic factors: role of microRNAs-16, −21, and −126. Hypertension. 2012;59:513–20.
132. Dejean E, Renalier MH, Foisseau M, Agirre X, Joseph N, de Paiva GR, Al Saati T, Soulier J, Desjobert C, Lamant L, Prosper F, Felsher DW, Cavaille J, Prats H, Delsol G, Giuriato S, Meggetto F. Hypoxia microRNA-16 downregulation induces VEGF expression in anaplastic lymphoma kinase (ALK)-positive anaplastic large-cell lymphomas. Leukemia. 2011;25:1882–90.
133. Chamorro-Jorganes A, Araldi E, Penalva LO, Sandhu D, Fernández-Hernando C, Suárez Y. MicroRNA-16 and MicroRNA-424 regulate cell-autonomous angiogenic functions in endothelial cells via targeting vascular endothelial growth factor receptor-2 and fibroblast growth factor receptor-1. Arterioscler Thromb Vasc Biol. 2011;31:2595–606.

134. Weber M, Baker MB, Moore JP, Searles CD. MiR-21 is induced in endothelial cells by shear stress and modulates apoptosis and eNOS activity. Biochem Biophys Res Commun. 2010;393:643–8.
135. Nicole S, Standley C, Walker P, Hurlstone A, Fogarty KE, Lawson ND. microRNA-mediated integration of haemodynamics and VEGF signaling during angiogenesis. Nature. 2010;464:1196–200.
136. Qin B, Yang H, Xiao B. Role of microRNAs in endothelial inflammation and senescence. Mol Biol Rep. 2012;39:4509–18.
137. Ota H, Eto M, Ogawa S, Iijima K, Akishita M, Ouchi Y. SIRT1/eNOS axis as a potential target against vascular senescence, dysfunction and atherosclerosis. J Atheroscler Thromb. 2010;17:431–5.
138. Chen JF, Mandel EM, Thomson JM, Wu Q, Callis TE, Hammond SM, Conlon FL, Wang DZ. The role of microRNA-1 and microRNA-133 in skeletal muscle proliferation and differentiation. Nat Genet. 2006;38:228–33.
139. Motohashi N, Alexander MS, Shimizu-Motohashi Y, Myers JA, Kawahara G, Kunkel LM. Regulation of IRS1/Akt insulin signaling by microRNA-128a during myogenesis. J Cell Sci. 2013;126:2678–91.
140. Rao PK, Kumar RM, Farkhondeh M, Baskerville S, Lodish HF. Myogenic factors that regulate expression of muscle-specific microRNAs. Proc Natl Acad Sci U S A. 2006;103:8721–6.
141. Safdar A, Abadi A, Akhtar M, Hettinga BP, Tarnopolsky MA. miRNA in the regulation of skeletal muscle adaptation to acute endurance exercise in C57Bl/6J male mice. PLoS One. 2009;4:e5610.
142. van Rooij E, Quiat D, Johnson BA, Sutherland LB, Qi X, Richardson JA, Kelm RJ, Olson EN. A family of microRNAs encoded by myosin genes governs myosin expression and muscle performance. Dev Cell. 2009;17:662–73.
143. van Rooij E, Sutherland LB, Qi X, Richardson JA, Hill J, Olson EN. Control of stress-dependent cardiac growth and gene expression by a microRNA. Science. 2007;316:575–9.

6 Effect of Regular Physical Activity on Arterial Distensibility

F. Saladini

6.1 Introduction

According to all most recent guidelines [1, 2] physical activity represents one of the milestones of non-pharmacological treatment for blood pressure (BP) reduction. Epidemiological studies suggest that regular aerobic physical activity may be beneficial for both the prevention and treatment of hypertension [1, 2], diabetes [3] and ischemic heart disease [4], and to lower cardiovascular risk and mortality [5–7]. Thus, guidelines suggest performing at least 30 min of moderate to intense dynamic aerobic exercise (walking, jogging, cycling or swimming) on 5–7 days per week, or resistance exercises on 2–3 days per week [1, 2]. The protective role of regular exercise in attenuating cardiovascular disease and mortality risk may be due to several different factors including lower BP, reduced body mass index (BMI), improvement of lipid profile and insulin sensitivity [8–10]. The decrease in BP has been documented in several cross-sectional and longitudinal studies [5, 11–17] and remains one of the main mechanisms underlying the beneficial effect of physical activity on arterial distensibility.

6.2 Effect of Physical Activity on Blood Pressure and Hypertension

According to literature the positive effect of physical exercise on BP levels is well recognized, and recently not only aerobic exercise, but also resistance training and isometric training were shown to be associated with an improvement of BP levels [5]. Cornelissen et al. [5] examined 93 trials lasting ≥4 weeks, involving 105

F. Saladini (✉)
Cardiology Unit, Cittadella Town Hospital, Cittadella, Padova, Italy
e-mail: francesca.saladini@aulss6.veneto.it

P. Palatini et al. (eds.), *Exercise, Sports and Hypertension*, Updates in Hypertension and Cardiovascular Protection,
https://doi.org/10.1007/978-3-031-07958-0_6

endurance, 29 dynamic resistance, 14 combined and 5 isometric resistance groups, including an overall number of 5223 participants (3401 exercisers and 1822 controls). They observed that systolic BP decreased by −3.5 mmHg (confidence limits −4.6 to −2.3) after endurance training, −1.8 mmHg (−3.7 to −0.011) after dynamic exercise, −10.9 mmHg (−14.5 to −7.4) after isometric resistance while after combined training there was no significant reduction. For diastolic BP the reduction was −2.5 mmHg (−3.2 to −1.7) after endurance exercise, −3.2 mmHg (−4.5 to −2.0) after dynamic exercise, −6.2 mmHg (−10.3 to −2.0) after isometric and −2.2 mmHg (−3.9 to −0.48) after combined training. Moreover, they observed that the effect on BP levels after endurance training was greater in hypertensive subjects compared to pre-hypertensive or normotensive ones ($p < 0.0001$), while after dynamic exercise the effect was more evident among pre-hypertensives compared to the other subgroups [5]. According to literature the majority of data regards the effect of physical activity in general population while the effect of regular exercise in hypertensive patients is less known. Some evidence comes from the HARVEST study. One of the first evidences of the favourable effect of physical activity on hypertensive subjects came from Palatini et al. [11]. The authors investigated 796 young hypertensive subjects: 153 exercisers and 493 sedentary subjects. The former group presented lower 24 hBP (78.8 vs. 81.2 mmHg, $p < 0.001$ adjusted for BMI, alcohol consumption and smoking habit) and daytime diastolic BP (80.4 vs. 83.3 mmHg, $p < 0.0001$ adjusted for BMI, alcohol consumption and smoking habit) in comparison to the latter. Also heart rate was significantly lower in exercisers (24 h 68.2 ± 0.7 bpm; daytime 70.1 ± 0.7 bpm; night-time 59.7 ± 0.7 bpm) compared to non-exercisers (24 h 72.0 ± 0.4 bpm, $p < 0.0001$; daytime 74.5 ± 0.4 bpm, $p < 0.0001$; night-time 62.0 ± 0.4 bpm, $p = 0.004$ adjusted for age, body mass index, alcohol intake, and smoking habit) [11]. The beneficial effect of exercise was due not only to the weight loss among exercisers, but also to the decrease of sympathetic activity as documented by the lower level of urinary norepinephrine and reduced heart rate [11, 12]. The same authors demonstrated a positive effect of exercises on BP reduction also in a longitudinal study [13]. They examined the effect of physical activity among 572 male subjects (331 non-exercisers, 192 mild exercisers and 49 heavy exercisers) during 3 months of follow-up at the same level of physical activity and observed among the group of heavy exercisers a significant decrease in daytime systolic BP compared to sedentary ones (135.4 ± 0.6 mmHg among heavy exercisers, 134 ± 0.8 among mild exercisers, 132.2 ± 1.6 mmHg among sedentary subjects; $p < 0.05$ sedentary patients compared to heavy exercisers) indicating that thc anti-hypertensive effect of physical activity persisted after 3 months [13]. These data were confrmed by subsequent analyses also in adult general population [14, 15] and hypertensive subjects [14, 16]. As described in the review by Cardoso Jr. CG et al. [17], aerobic training both acute and chronic, resulted effective in reducing 24 h BP in normotensive and hypertensive subjects, while resistance training was not able to reduce level and was suggested to be integrated to aerobic training.

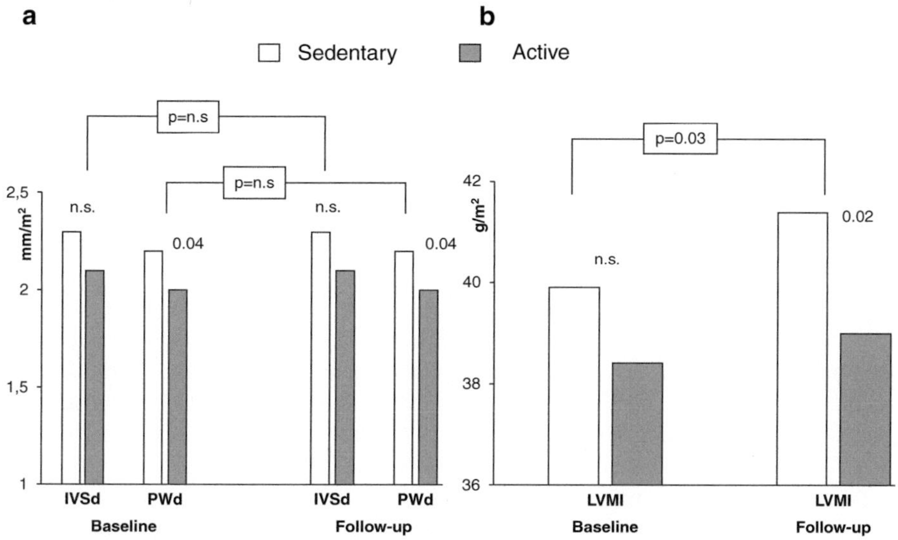

Fig. 6.1 Baseline and follow-up left interventricular septum thickness in diastole (IVSd), posterior wall thickness in diastole (PWd) (**a**), baseline and follow-up left ventricle mass indexed (LVMI) (**b**). (Adapted from Palatini P et al. [18])

Moreover, in the HARVEST study was demonstrated a beneficial effect of physical activity on target organ damage [18]. Palatini et al. investigated 454 subjects whose physical activity status was consistent during 8.3 years follow-up and observed a reduced left ventricle mass among exercises compared to sedentary ones; moreover, among sedentary participants there was an increase of left ventricle mass in comparison to baseline value, while among exercisers there was no significant changes compared to the baseline assessment (Fig. 6.1) [18]. Of note exercise resulted a protective factor for development of left ventricle hypertrophy (OR 0.26, 95%CI 0.07–0.09, $p = 0.033$) also after adjustment for age, sex, BMI, systolic and diastolic BP, hypertension duration, parental hypertension, follow-up length, smoking habits, coffee and alcohol intake, baseline left ventricle mass, BP and weight changes during follow-up [18]. Several mechanisms have been proposed as possible explanation for the positive effect of exercise for counteracting left ventricle hypertrophy. One of the first beneficial effects proposed was the reduction of BP caused by regular physical activity [19, 20], as well as changes on body weight [21, 22] even if in the paper by Palatini et al. [18] no significant changes in body weight was detected. According to literature other beneficial effect of exercise were haemodynamic changes on vascular resistance, blood volume and cardiac output [23], but also metabolic changes such as reduction of insulin resistance, as well as suppression of renin–angiotensin–aldosterone system [9, 24] and sympathetic activity as mentioned above [11, 12], are important determinants.

6.3 Effect of Physical Activity on Arterial Distensibility

As mentioned above exercise exerts a beneficial effect on target organ damage in particular among hypertensive subjects. One of the main target organs of hypertension that favours cardiovascular disease was impairment of arterial distensibility. Also on this target, physical activity exerts an important role counteracting atherosclerosis process. Again, evidence came from the HARVEST study. In 2011 Palatini et al. [25] explored the effect of regular physical activity on intima–media thickness on 87 stage I hypertensives during 6.5 years of follow-up. Exercisers presented lower values of mean intima–media thickness ($p = 0.01$), also comparing each single site: common carotid artery ($p = 0.01$), bulb (even if not significant $p = 0.13$) and internal carotid artery ($p = 0.05$); they also demonstrated lower maximum intima–media thickness ($p = 0.006$), again comparing each single site: common carotid artery (not statistically significant $p = 0.09$), bulb (not statistically significant $p = 0.21$) and internal carotid artery ($p = 0.01$) [25]. Moreover, in multivariate regression analysis the authors demonstrated that the beneficial effect of exercise on the reduction in cumulative time-related intima–media thickness was not attenuated by inclusion in the model of age, sex, height, smoking habit, baseline intima–media thickness value, total cholesterol, heart rate, systolic and diastolic BP and BMI: coefficient −0.28, S.E. 0.011, $p = 0.02$ [25]. The authors also explored the contribution of each explored potential mediator for the physical activity-related reduction in mean intima–media thickness progression (Fig. 6.2) and observed that total cholesterol and BP were the main contributors, followed by heart rare and BMI [25]. These data suggest that the anti-atherosclerotic action of physical activity on the

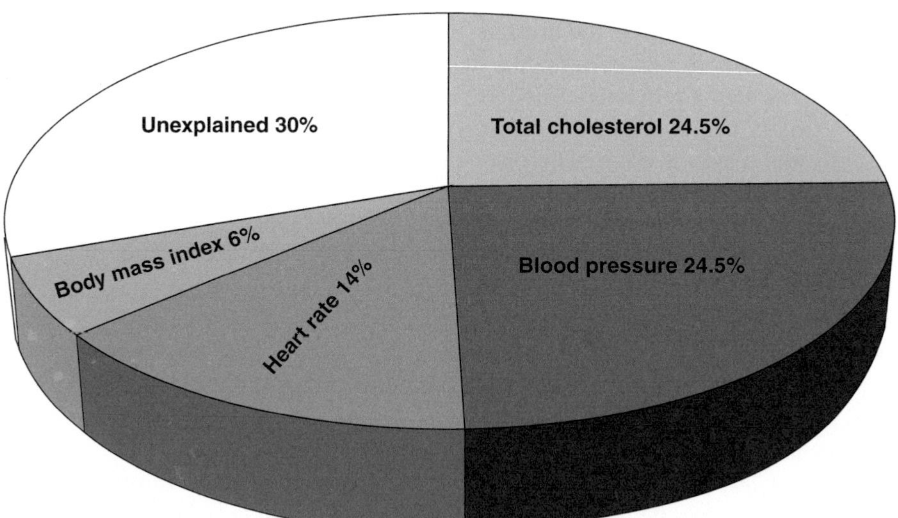

Fig. 6.2 Proportion of the physical activity–related reduction in mean intima–media thickness progression explained by each of the potential mediators. (Adapted from Palatini P et al. [25])

carotid artery of young subjects in the early stage of hypertension is mediated in substantial part by changes in known cardiovascular risk factors. Similar results were previous observed by Meyer et al. [26], investigating 96 young (mean age 14.2 ± 1.9) obese subjects. After 6 months of exercise program the authors observed improvements for intima–media thickness (0.44 ± 0.08 mm, $p = 0.012$, −6.3%) and flow mediated dilation (7.71 ± 2.53%, $p = 0.001$, +127%). This improvement correlated with reduction of risk factors such as body mass index (29.8 ± 5.93 kg/m^2 at the baseline, 27.2 ± 4.80 kg/m^2 after 6 month of intervention, $p < 0.001$), body fat mass (35.9 ± 6.99%, vs. 34.9 ± 9.71%, $p = 0.064$), waist–hip ratio (0.93 ± 0.12, vs. 0.87 ± 0.09, $p = 0.012$), ambulatory systolic BP (117.1 ± 7.1 mmHg, vs. 113.1 ± 7.7 mmHg, $p = 0.036$), insulin (13.8 ± 5.20 pmol/L, vs. 11.16 ± 4.61 pmol/L, $p = 0.008$), triglycerides (1.41 ± 1.14 mmol/L, vs. 1.04 ± 0.48 mmol/L, $p = 0.016$), low-density lipoprotein (2.71 ± 0.70 mmol/L, vs. 2.57 ± 0.66 mmol/L, $p = 0.025$), and low-degree inflammation (C-reactive protein (4.84 ± 6.31 mg/L, vs. 2.05 ± 2.44 mg/L, $p = 0.013$), fibrinogen (3.57 ± 0.75 g/L, vs. 3.24 ± 0.61 g/L, $p = 0.012$)) [26]. The mechanisms supposed by the authors to underlie the effect of exercise on the endothelium was the generalized impact of hemodynamic variables acting through vessel wall shear stress [27], upregulation of nitic-oxide-synthase gene expression [28, 29], and bioavailability of Nitric oxide. Other hormonal and inflammatory effects, such as the reduction of fibrinogen and C-reactive protein levels, and enhanced endothelial progenitor cells during exercise, could help to improve endothelial integrity [30]. On the opposite side other interventional studies failed to demonstrate positive changes of carotid intima–media thickness after training [31]. For example in the Finnish study (population based sample, aged 42–60 years of age) there was no statistically significant relation between self-reported leisure activity and intima–media thickness progression [32]. The reason for the differing results obtained in previous studies was hypothesized to be related to the different action of physical activity on carotid intima–media thickness according to age and relative risk factors of the study participants, suggesting a greater effect of exercise among younger patients and in the early phase of the disease [25].

Other interesting data on the protective effect of physical activity was demonstrated some years later again by the HARVEST study group [33]. The authors examined 366 subjects (sedentary $n = 264$ and physically active $n = 102$ subjects) by means of applanation tonometry to assess small and large artery compliance and augmentation index and were repeated in 151 subjects after 6 years of follow-up. The authors observed that both at the enrolment (Fig. 6.3) and at final evaluation (Table 6.1) arterial distensibility parameters were better among those patients who regularly performed physical activity in comparison to sedentary ones, even if the difference at the final evaluation was statistically significant only for small artery compliance after adjustment for age and sex [33]. However, when differences between baseline and final augmentation index were evaluated by means of one-way repeated measure ANCOVA analysis p for interaction (active vs. sedentary × basal versus follow-up) was 0.020; similarly also p for interaction for total peripheral resistances was 0.045 [33]. These results were in keeping with those obtained by Nettlefold et al. [34] in 102 normotensive children where moderate to

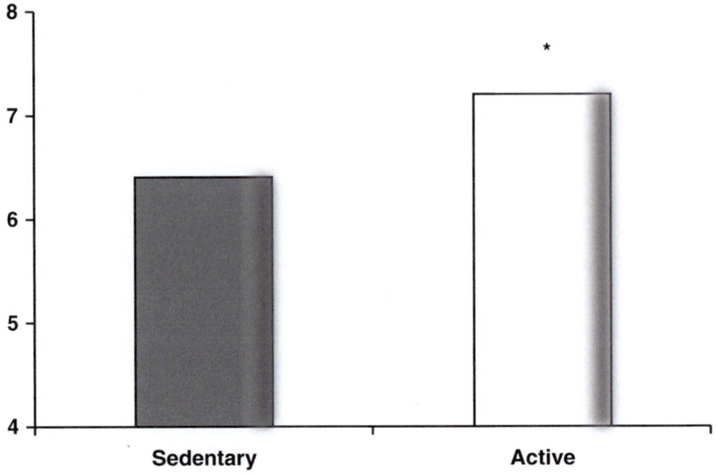

Model	Variables	P value*
Model 1	Age, sex, BMI, lifestyle factors, parental HT, SBP, DBP	0.0003
Model 2	Model 1+ CT, Glucose, TG	0.001
Model 3	Model 2+ HR	0.006

Fig. 6.3 Baseline small artery compliance in sedentary (n = 264) and active (n = 102) stage I hypertensive subjects from the HARVEST study. *BMI* body mass index, *Lifestyle factors* smoking habits, alcohol and coffee consumption, physical activity, *parental HT* parental hypertension, *SBP* systolic blood pressure, *DBP* diastolic blood pressure, *CT* total cholesterol, *Tg* serum triglycerides, *HR* heart rate. (Adapted by Saladini F et al. [33])

Table 6.1 Final assessment of haemodynamic and arterial distensibility parameters in sedentary and physically active stage I hypertensive from the HARVEST study

Variables	Sedentary subjects (n = 110)	Active subjects (n = 42)	P*
C1, mL/mmHg × 10	16.4 ± 4.5	17.0 ± 4.8	n.s.
C2, mL/mmHg × 100	6.2 ± 2.8	7.9 ± 2.5	0.009
AIx, %	25.8 ± 22.6	14.5 ± 0.24	n.s.
Carotid-radial PWV, m/s	8.8 ± 2.1	9.1 ± 2.2	n.s.
Peripheral resistance, dyne × s × cm^{-5}	1466.0 ± 236	1357.0 ± 228	n.s.
Cardiac output l/min	2.8 ± 0.2	2.9 ± 0.3	n.s.
Central SBP, mmHg	120.4 ± 15.0	118.2 ± 10.9	n.s.

Adapted by Saladini et al. [33]

Data are presented as mean ± standard deviation. *C1* large artery compliance, *C2* small artery compliance, *AIx* augmentation index, *PWV* pulse wave velocity, *SBP* systolic blood pressure. *P** value adjusted for age and sex, *n.s.* not statistically significant ($p > 0.05$)

vigorous physical activity was associated with lower small artery compliance but not lower large artery compliance; or data by McGavock et al. [35] that found a cross-sectional association between aerobic training and both large and small artery compliance, while no difference was found for total peripheral resistance according to physical activity status. Again, the mechanism underlying this favourable effect of exercise on arterial distensibility in young stage I hypertensives [33] was supposed to be the decreasing heart rate, which is recognized according to literature as a strong determinant of arterial distensibility [36–38], and the reduction in sympathetic activity mediated by physical training [39] that may reduce the peripheral vasoconstriction and prevent the long-term effects of sympathetic activity on the arterial wall. This was attested in the HARVEST study [33] by the drop in peripheral resistance and ambulatory diastolic BP after 6 years of follow-up in active participants which was consensual with the increase in small artery compliance. Prolonged sympathetic activation in hypertension may lead to small artery remodelling with a progressive increase in the wall–lumen ratio [40], while physical activity can have a favourable impact on the vascular tree in hypertension preventing the remodelling of the small arteries and promoting an increase in the cross-section of the microcirculation [41]. This may explain the reduction in vascular hyperresponsiveness seen in trained hypertensive individuals compared to sedentary hypertensives [42]. According to literature also humoral factors may contribute to the beneficial effect of exercise on arterial distensibility. Maeda et al. [43] observed that young subjects, after 8 weeks of exercise, had a significant reduction in endothelin 1 and an increase in nitric oxide concentrations, with an inverse correlation between the two biochemical factors. Indeed, a reduction of oxidative stress and an increased expression and activation of nitric oxide synthase [44] with enhanced endothelium-dependent dilation have been described in middle-aged endurance exercise-trained men compared to less active peers [45–47]. In addition, regular physical activity may improve vascular function by protecting the arterial tree from the adverse effects of traditional risk factors for cardiovascular disease. The role of decreased heart rate by regular aerobic training in determining improvement of arterial distensibility is debated in literature as contrasting results were described [48–57]. Previous studies showed that a progressive increase of heart rate through pacing was associated with a progressive increase of pulse wave velocity, indicating a cross-sectional association of heart rate and arterial stiffness [48]. In particular Tan et al. measured this effect, indicating a 0.17 m/s increase of PWV for each 10 beat/min increment in heart rate by pacing [48]. According to the authors the increased heart rate led to a decrease in stroke volume, resulting from a reduced diastolic filling time [49, 50] and ejection duration [50]. Moreover, the increase in heart rate led to an increased cardiac output which favoured an increase in mean arterial pressure in addition to an increase in both peripheral and central diastolic BP [48]. As pulse wave velocity is highly influenced by BP [58–61], much of the increase in pulse wave velocity was supposed by the authors to be attributable to the increase in BP [48]. Similar results were obtained by Tomiyama et al. [51] and by Benetos et al. [52] both in normotensive and in hypertensive subjects. Opposite results were described for the effect of heart rate on central systolic BP and augmentation index, in particular low resting heart rate was demonstrated to be associated with higher aortic systolic BP and augmentation index [53, 54]. This negative association has been attributed to a shift of the backward wave reflected from the periphery into late systole secondary to the prolongation of left ventricular ejection time and to increased stroke volume at lower rates [53, 55, 56]. These apparently contrasting results led some authors to suppose that the reduction of heart rate may be detrimental for endothelial function and cardiovascular disease [56]. The short-term and long-term effect of heart rate on arterial stiffness and central haemodynamic was explored by Palatini et al. within the frame of the HARVEST study [57]. The authors investigated the correlation of heart rate measured at the same time of arterial distensibility assessment with augmentation index (short-term correlation) and the correlation between night-time heart rate measured by 24-h BP recording performed 8 years before the arterial distensibility assessment with augmentation index (long-term correlation). They confirmed in the short term a negative correlation ($r = -0.407$, $p = 0.001$) between AIx and office heart rate, while a positive correlation in the long term ($r = 0.503$, $p = 0.0006$). Moreover, the authors observed that heart rate resulted an independent positive predictor of central systolic BP ($p = 0.014$), pressure amplification ($p = 0.004$) [57], suggesting that heart rate reduction in the long run has a favourable effect and not a detrimental one on all parameters of arterial distensibility and contributes to explain why aerobic physical activity, by decreasing heart rate, leads to a reduced risk of cardiovascular events and mortality in hypertension [62–64]. In summary elevated heart rate exposes the arteries to increased magnitude and frequency of mechanical load, which may eventually increase the stiffness of the vascular wall [65], as shown by the above-mentioned papers and it is thus possible that the increase in vascular stiffness favours the development of hypertension and cardiovascular disease in patients with tachycardia [66, 67].

6.4 Effect of Resistance and Combined Training Program on Arterial Distensibility

All the evidence reported above involved program of aerobic physical training, while results on the efficacy of resistance or combined programs seem to have contrasting results.

Several interventional [68, 69] studies and meta-analyses [70–73] investigated this issue coming to different data. Ashor et al. [70] in 2014 explored the effects of different exercise modalities (aerobic, resistance or combined) on pulse wave velocity and augmentation index according to the participants' or exercise characteristics in a meta-analysis involving 42 studies ($n = 1627$ participants). In keeping with previous results both arterial stiffness indexes were significantly reduced after aerobic training (−0.63 m/s, 95% CI: −0.90, −0.35, $p < 0.01$; −2.63%, 95% CI: −5.25 to −0.02, $p = 0.05$ respectively), while resistance training had no effect (−0.04 m/s, 95% CI: −0.42, to 0.34, $p = 0.82$ on pulse wave velocity; −1.69%, 95% CI: −4.11 to 0.72, $p = 0.17$ on augmentation index) as well as combined programs (−0.35 m/s, 95% CI: −0.82, 0.12, $p = 0.15$; only effect on pulse wave velocity was determined as studies on augmentation index were only a small number) [70]. These results were in apparent contrast to those previously published by Miyachi et al. [72] who observed a significant increase of arterial stiffness. However, these discrepancies may be explained by the heterogeneity of the studies considered as lower intensity rather than high intensity training [74], lower-limb rather than upper-limb training [75] and eccentric rather than concentric resistance training [76], and the combination of resistance with aerobic training [77] seem to lead to an improvement or at least no deterioration on endothelial function. Moreover, also the different populations involved may be responsible for different results as the increase of arterial stiffness is usually observed only in young participants or with higher intensity resistance exercise [70]. In particular, combined training induced positive modification in specific subsets of subjects [68]. Park et al. [68] explored effect of 12 weeks of moderate combined resistance ad aerobic exercise on 20 older and obese men and observed an improvement in pulse wave velocity (−0.27 (95% CI: −1.10, 0.59; $p < 0.001$) as well as body composition and cardiometabolic risk factors. The authors explained their positive results with a specific combination of the two types of training [68]. Resistance exercise training was demonstrated to worsen arterial stiffness in heavier subjects due to the excessive arterial wall stress [78]; however, in this interventional study aerobic exercise was performed after resistance exercise for minimizing the stiffening and more time of aerobic component was added too in the combined program [68]. This was consistent with the previous studies, showing that aerobic training after resistance training ameliorated arterial stiffness in young adults [77]. Other mechanisms advocated to underlie these favourable effects were again the increased nitric oxide bioavailability and/or decreased inflammatory responses [79], as well reduction of systolic BP levels [68].

6.5 Conclusions

Physical activity remains a milestone of nonpharmacological treatment for reducing cardiovascular disease burden. Exercise aids in reducing heart rate, blood pressure level and improving metabolic profile. This occurs through the impact of aerobic training on sympathetic activity and inflammation process, while evidence on resistance training are lacking despite it is practised combined to aerobic training. The great task for physicians remains the adherence of patients as documented by the low compliance of study participants in long-term studies [80, 81].

References

1. Williams B, Mancia G, Spiering W, Agabiti Rosei E, Azizi M, Burnier M, et al. 2018 ESC/ESH guidelines for the management of arterial hypertension. Eur Heart J. 2018;39(33):3021–104. https://doi.org/10.1093/eurheartj/ehy339.
2. Whelton PK, Carey RM, Aronow WS, Casey DE Jr, Collins KJ, Dennison Himmelfarb C, et al. 2017 ACC/AHA/AAPA/ABC/ACPM/AGS/APhA/ASH/ASPC/NMA/PCNA guideline for the prevention, detection, evaluation, and Management of High Blood Pressure in adults: a report of the American College of Cardiology/American Heart Association task force on

clinical practice guidelines. Hypertension. 2018;71(6):e13–e115. https://doi.org/10.1161/HYP.0000000000000065.
3. American Diabetes Association. Standards of medical care in Diabetes-2016. Diabetes Care. 2016;39(Suppl. 1):S1–S111.
4. Fihn SD, Blankenship JC, Alexander KP, Bittl JA, Byrne JG, Fletcher BJ, et al. 2014 ACC/AHA/AATS/PCNA/SCAI/STS focused update of the guideline for the diagnosis and management of patients with stable ischemic heart disease: a report of the American College of Cardiology/American Heart Association task force on practice guidelines, and the American Association for Thoracic Surgery, preventive cardiovascular nurses association, Society for Cardiovascular Angiography and Interventions, and Society of Thoracic Surgeons. J Am Coll Cardiol. 2014;64:1929–49. https://doi.org/10.1016/j.jacc.2014.07.017.
5. Cornelissen VA, Smart NA. Exercise training for blood pressure: a systematic review and meta-analysis. J Am Heart Assoc. 2013;2:e004473. https://doi.org/10.1161/JAHA.112.004473.
6. Leitzmann MF, Park Y, Blair A, Ballard-Barbash R, Mouw T, Hollenbeck AR, et al. Physical activity recommendations and decreased risk of mortality. Arch Intern Med. 2007;167:2453–60. https://doi.org/10.1001/archinte.167.22.2453.
7. Rossi A, Dikareva A, Bacon SL, Daskalopoulou SS. The impact of physical activity on mortality in patients with high blood pressure: a systematic review. J Hypertens. 2012;30:1277–88. https://doi.org/10.1097/HJH.0b013e3283544669.
8. Palatini P, Graniero G, Mormino P, Nicolosi L, Mos L, Visentin P, et al. Relation between physical training and ambulatory blood pressure in stage I hypertensive subjects. Results of the HARVEST trial. Circulation. 1994;90:2870–6. https://doi.org/10.1161/01.cir.90.6.2870.
9. Cornelissen VA, Fagard RH. Effects of endurance training on blood pressure, blood pressure-regulating mechanisms, and cardiovascular risk factors. Hypertension. 2005;46:667–75. https://doi.org/10.1161/01.HYP.0000184225.05629.51.
10. Fagard RH. Exercise therapy in hypertensive cardiovascular disease. Prog Cardiovasc Dis. 2011;53:404–11. https://doi.org/10.1016/j.pcad.2011.03.006.
11. Palatini P, Graniero GR, Mormino P, Nicolosi L, Mos L, Visentin P, et al. Relation between physical training and ambulatory blood pressure in stage I hypertensive subjects. Results of the HARVEST trial. Hypertension and ambulatory recording Venetia study. Circulation. 1994;90(6):2870–6. https://doi.org/10.1161/01.cir.90.6.2870.
12. Palatini P, Canali C, Graniero GR, Rossi G, de Toni R, Santonastaso M, et al. Relationship of plasma renin activity with caffeine intake and physical training in mild hypertensive men. HARVEST Study Group. Eur J Epidemiol. 1996;12(5):485–91. https://doi.org/10.1007/BF00144001.
13. Vriz O, Mos L, Frigo G, Sanigi C, Zanata G, Pegoraro F, et al. Effects of physical exercise on clinic and 24-hour ambulatory blood pressure in young subjects with mild hypertension. J Sports Med Phys Fitness. 2002;42(1):83–8. PMID: 11832879.
14. Wallace JP, Bogle PG, King BA, Krasnoff JB, Jastremski CA. The magnitude and duration of ambulatory blood pressure reduction following acute exercise. J Hum Hypertens. 1999;13:361–6. https://doi.org/10.1038/sj.jhh.1000797.
15. Park S, Jastremski CA, Wallace JP. Time of day for exercise on blood pressure reduction in dipping and nondipping hypertension. J Hum Hypertens. 2005;19:597–605. https://doi.org/10.1038/sj.jhh.1001901.
16. Ohkubo T, Hozawa A, Nagatomi R, Fujita K, Sauvaget C, Watanabe Y, et al. Effects of exercise training on home blood pressure values in older adults: a randomized controlled trial. J Hypertens. 2001;19:1045–52. https://doi.org/10.1097/00004872-200106000-00008.
17. Cardoso CG Jr, Gomides RS, Queiroz AC, Pinto LG, da Silveira LF, Tinucci T, et al. Acute and chronic effects of aerobic and resistance exercise on ambulatory blood pressure. Clinics (Sao Paulo). 2010;65(3):317–25. https://doi.org/10.1590/S1807-59322010000300013.
18. Palatini P, Visentin P, Dorigatti F, Guarnieri C, Santonastaso M, Cozzio S, et al. Regular physical activity prevents development of left ventricular hypertrophy in hypertension. Eur Heart J. 2009;30(2):225–32. https://doi.org/10.1093/eurheartj/ehn533.

19. Whelton SP, Chin A, Xin X, He J. Effect of aerobic exercise on blood pressure: a meta-analysis of randomized, controlled trials. Ann Intern Med. 2002;136(7):493–503. https://doi.org/10.7326/0003-4819-136-7-200204020-00006.
20. Kelley GA, Kelley KA, Tran ZV. Aerobic exercise and resting blood pressure: a meta-analytic review of randomized, controlled trials. Prev Cardiol. 2001;4(2):73–80. https://doi.org/10.1111/j.1520-037x.2001.00529.x.
21. MacMahon SW, Wilcken DE, Macdonald GJ. The effect of weight reduction on left ventricular mass. A randomized controlled trial in young, overweight hypertensive patients. N Engl J Med. 1986;314(6):334–9. https://doi.org/10.1056/NEJM198602063140602.
22. Himeno E, Nishino K, Nakashima Y, Kuroiwa A, Ikeda M. Weight reduction regresses left ventricular mass regardless of blood pressure level in obese subjects. Am Heart J. 1996;131(2):313–9. https://doi.org/10.1016/s0002-8703(96)90360-9.
23. Sasaki N, Matsuura H, Kajiyama G, Oshima T. Regular aerobic exercise augments endothelium-dependent vascular relaxation in normotensive as well as hypertensive subjects: role of endothelium-derived nitric oxide. Circulation. 1999;100(11):1194–202. https://doi.org/10.1161/01.cir.100.
24. Stewart KJ. Exercise training and the cardiovascular consequences of type 2 diabetes and hypertension: plausible mechanisms for improving cardiovascular health. JAMA. 2002;288(13):1622–31. https://doi.org/10.1001/jama.288.13.1622.
25. Palatini P, Puato M, Rattazzi M, Pauletto P. Effect of regular physical activity on carotid intima-media thickness. Results from a 6-year prospective study in the early stage of hypertension. Blood Press. 2011;20(1):37–44. https://doi.org/10.3109/08037051.2010.524080.
26. Meyer AA, Kundt G, Lenschow U, Schuff-Werner P, Kienast W. Improvement of early vascular changes and cardiovascular risk factors in obese children after a six-month exercise program. J Am Coll Cardiol. 2006;48(9):1865–70. https://doi.org/10.1016/j.jacc.2006.07.035.
27. Neibauer J, Cooke JP. Cardiovascular effects of exercise: role of endothelial shear stress. J Am Coll Cardiol. 1996;265:2679–87. https://doi.org/10.1016/j.jacc.2015.04.042.
28. Vita JA, Keaney JF. Endothelial function: a barometer for cardiovascular risk (editorial)? Circulation. 1993;88:2149–55. https://doi.org/10.1161/01.cir.88.5.2149.
29. Sessa WC, Pritchard K, Seyedi N, Wang J, Hintze TH. Chronic exercise in dogs increases coronary vascular nitric oxide production and endothelial cell nitric oxide synthase gene expression. Circ Res. 1994;74:349–53. https://doi.org/10.1161/01.res.74.2.349.
30. Laufs U, Werner N, Link A, et al. Physical training increases endothelial progenitor cells, inhibits neointima formation, and enhances angiogegenis. Circulation. 2004;109:220–6. https://doi.org/10.1161/01.CIR.0000109141.48980.37.
31. Nordstrom CK, Dwyer KM, Merz CN, Shircore A, Dwyer JH. Leisure time physical activity and early atherosclerosis: the Los Angeles atherosclerosis study. Am J Med. 2003;115:19–25. https://doi.org/10.1016/s0002-9343(03)00242-0.
32. Lakka TA, Laukkanen JA, Rauramaa R, Salonen R, Lakka HM. 12. Kaplan GA et al., cardiorespiratory fitness and the progression of carotid atherosclerosis in middle-aged men. Ann Intern Med. 2001;134:12–20. https://doi.org/10.7326/0003-4819-134-1-200101020-00008.
33. Saladini F, Benetti E, Mos L, Mazzer A, Casiglia E, Palatini P. Regular physical activity is associated with improved small artery distensibility in young to middle-age stage 1 hypertensives. Vasc Med. 2014;19(6):458–64. https://doi.org/10.1177/1358863X14556852.
34. Nettlefold L, McKay HA, Naylor PJ, Bredin SS, Warburton DE. The relationship between objectively measured physical activity, sedentary time, and vascular health in children. Am J Hypertens. 2012;25:914–9. https://doi.org/10.1038/ajh.2012.68.
35. McGavock JM, Anderson TJ, Lewanczuk RZ. Sedentary lifestyle and antecedents of cardiovascular disease in young adults. Am J Hypertens. 2006;19:701–7. https://doi.org/10.1016/j.amjhyper.2006.01.013.
36. Lantelme P, Mestre C, Lievre M, Gressard A, Milon H. Heart rate: an important confounder of pulse wave velocity assessment. Hypertension. 2002;39:1083–7. https://doi.org/10.1161/01.hyp.0000019132.41066.95.

37. Sa Cunha R, Pannier B, Benetos A, Siche JP, London GM, Mallion JM, Safar ME. Association between high heart rate and high arterial rigidity in normotensive and hypertensive subjects. J Hypertens. 1997;5:1423–30. https://doi.org/10.1097/00004872-199715120-00009.
38. Liang YL, Gatzka CD, Du XJ, Cameron JD, Kingwell BA, Dart AM. Effects of heart rate on arterial compliance in men. Clin Exp Pharmacol Physiol. 1999;6:342–6. https://doi.org/10.1046/j.1440-1681.1999.03039.x.
39. Wilkinson IB, McEniery CM. Arterial stiffness, endothelial function and novel pharmacological approaches. Clin Exp Pharmacol Physiol. 2004;31:795–9. https://doi.org/10.1111/j.1440-1681.2004.04074.x.
40. Dao HH, McMartens F, Zaor A, de Champlain J, Moreau P. Role of endothelin in the hypertrophic remodeling of small arteries induced by exogenous norepinephrine. Arch Mal Coeur Vaiss. 1999;92:1059–62.
41. Green DJ. Exercise training as vascular medicine: direct impacts on the vasculature in humans. Exerc Sport Sci Rev. 2009;37:196–202. https://doi.org/10.1097/JES.0b013e3181b7b6e3.
42. Palatini P, Bratti P, Palomba D, Saladini F, Zanatta N, Maraglino G. Regular physical activity attenuates the blood pressure response to public speaking and delays the development of hypertension. J Hypertens. 2010;28:1186–93.
43. Maeda S, Sugawara J, Yoshizawa M, Otsuki T, Shimojo N, Jesmin S, et al. Involvement of endothelin-1 in habitual exercise-induced increase in arterial compliance. Acta Physiol (Oxf). 2009;196:223–9. https://doi.org/10.1111/j.1748-1716.2008.01909.x.
44. Green DJ, Maiorana A, O'Driscoll G, Taylor R. Effect of exercise training on endothelium-derived nitric oxide function in humans. J Physiol. 2004;561:1–25. https://doi.org/10.1113/jphysiol.2004.068197.
45. DeSouza CA, Shapiro LF, Clevenger CM, Dinenno FA, Monahan KD, Tanaka H, et al. Regular aerobic exercise prevents and restores age-related declines in endothelium-dependent vasodilation in healthy men. Circulation. 2000;102:1351–7. https://doi.org/10.1161/01.cir.102.12.1351.
46. Taddei S, Galetta F, Virdis A, Ghiadoni L, Salvetti G, Franzoni F, et al. Physical activity prevents age-related impairment in nitric oxide availability in elderly athletes. Circulation. 2000;101:2896–901. https://doi.org/10.1161/01.cir.101.25.2896.
47. Eskurza I, Monahan KD, Robinson JA, Seals DR. Effect of acute and chronic ascorbic acid on flow-mediated dilatation with sedentary and physically active human ageing. J Physiol. 2004;556:315–24. https://doi.org/10.1113/jphysiol.2003.057042.
48. Tan I, Spronck B, Kiat H, et al. Heart rate dependency of large artery stiffness. Hypertension. 2016;68:236–42. https://doi.org/10.1161/HYPERTENSIONAHA.116.07462.
49. Noble MI, Wyler J, Milne EN, Trenchard D, Guz A. Effect of changes in heart rate on left ventricular performance in conscious dogs. Circ Res. 1969;24(2):285–95. https://doi.org/10.1161/01.res.24.2.285.
50. Weissler AM, Peeler RG, Roehll WH. Relationships between left ventricular ejection time, stroke volume, and heart rate in normal individuals and patients with cardiovascular disease. Am Heart J. 1961;62:367–78. https://doi.org/10.1016/0002-8703(61)90403-3.
51. Tomiyama H, Hashimoto H, Tanaka H, Matsumoto C, Odaira M, Yamada J, et al. Synergistic relationship between changes in the pulse wave velocity and changes in the heart rate in middle-aged Japanese adults: a prospective study. J Hypertens. 2010;28:687–94. https://doi.org/10.1097/HJH.0b013e3283369fe8.
52. Benetos A, Adamopoulos C, Bureau JM, Temmar M, Labat C, Bean K, et al. Determinants of accelerated progression of arterial stiffness in normotensive subjects and in treated hypertensive subjects over a 6-year period. Circulation. 2002;105:1202–7. https://doi.org/10.1161/hc1002.105135.
53. Wilkinson IB, Mohammad NH, Tyrrell S, Hall IR, Webb DJ, Paul VE, et al. Heart rate dependency of pulse pressure amplification and arterial stiffness. Am J Hypertens. 2002;15:24–30. https://doi.org/10.1016/s0895-7061(01)02252-x.
54. Courand PY, Lantelme P. Significance, prognostic value and management of heart rate in hypertension. Arch Cardiovasc Dis. 2014;107:48–57. https://doi.org/10.1016/j.acvd.2013.11.003.

55. McEniery CM, Yasmin HIR, Qasem A, Wilkinson IB, Cockcroft JR, Investigators ACCT. Normal vascular aging: differential effects on wave reflection and aortic pulse wave velocity: the Anglo-Cardiff collaborative trial (ACCT). J Am Coll Cardiol. 2005;46(9):1753–60. https://doi.org/10.1016/j.jacc.2005.07.037.
56. Messerli FH, Rimoldi SF, Bangalore S, Bavishi C, Laurent S. When an increase in central systolic pressure overrides the benefits of heart rate lowering. J Am Coll Cardiol. 2016;68:754–62. https://doi.org/10.1016/j.jacc.2016.03.610.
57. Palatini P, Saladini F, Mos L, Fania C, Mazzer A, Casiglia E. Low night-time heart rate is longitudinally associated with lower augmentation index and central systolic blood pressure in hypertension. Eur J Appl Physiol. 2018;118:543–50. https://doi.org/10.1007/s00421-017-3789-4.
58. Avolio AP, Chen SG, Wang RP, Zhang CL, Li MF, O'Rourke MF. Effects of aging on changing arterial compliance and left ventricular load in a northern Chinese urban community. Circulation. 1983;68:50–8. https://doi.org/10.1161/01.CIR.68.1.50.
59. Pruett JD, Bourland JD, Geddes LA. Measurement of pulse-wave velocity using a beat-sampling technique. Ann Biomed Eng. 1988;16:341–7. https://doi.org/10.1007/BF02364622.
60. Spronck B, Heusinkveld MH, Vanmolkot FH, Roodt JO, Hermeling E, Delhaas T, et al. Pressure-dependence of arterial stiffness: potential clinical implications. J Hypertens. 2015;33:330–8. https://doi.org/10.1097/HJH.0000000000000407.
61. Bramwell JC, Hill A. Velocity of transmission of the pulse-wave. Lancet. 1922;199:891–2.
62. Palatini P, Thijs L, Staessen JA, Fagard RH, Bulpitt CJ, Clement DL, et al. Predictive value of clinic and ambulatory heart rate for mortality in elderly subjects with systolic hypertension. Arch Intern Med. 2002;162:2313–21. https://doi.org/10.1001/archinte.162.20.2313.
63. Jouven X, Empana JP, Schwartz PJ, Desnos M, Courbon D, Ducimetiere P. Heart-rate profile during exercise as a predictor of sudden death. N Engl J Med. 2005;352:1951–8. https://doi.org/10.1056/NEJMoa043012.
64. Kolloch R, Legler UF, Champion A, Cooper-Dehoff RM, Handberg E, Zhou Q, et al. Impact of resting heart rate on outcomes in hypertensive patients with coronary artery disease: findings from the INternational VErapamil-SR/trandolapril STudy (INVEST). Eur Heart J. 2008;29:1327–34. https://doi.org/10.1093/eurheartj/ehn123.
65. Giannoglou GD, Chatzizisis YS, Zamboulis C, Parcharidis GE, Mikhailidis DP, Louridas GE, et al. Elevated heart rate and atherosclerosis: an overview of the pathogenetic mechanisms. Int J Cardiol. 2008;126:302–12. https://doi.org/10.1016/j.ijcard.2007.08.077.
66. Mancia G, Masi S, Palatini P, Tsioufis C, Grassi G. Elevated heart rate and cardiovascular risk in hypertension. J Hypertens. 2021;39(6):1060–9. https://doi.org/10.1097/HJH.0000000000002760.
67. Palatini P. Resting heart rate as a cardiovascular risk factor in hypertensive patients: an update. Am J Hypertens. 2021;34(4):307–17. https://doi.org/10.1093/ajh/hpaa187.
68. Park W, Jung WS, Hong K, Kim YY, Kim SW, Park HY. Effects of moderate combined resistance- and aerobic-exercise for 12 weeks on body composition, cardiometabolic risk factors, blood pressure, arterial stiffness, and physical functions, among obese older men: a pilot study. Int J Environ Res Public Health. 2020;17(19):7233. https://doi.org/10.3390/ijerph17197233.
69. Otsuki T, Namatame H, Yoshikawa T, Zempo-Miyaki A. Combined aerobic and low-intensity resistance exercise training increases basal nitric oxide production and decreases arterial stiffness in healthy older adults. J Clin Biochem Nutr. 2020;66(1):62–6. https://doi.org/10.3164/jcbn.19-81.
70. Ashor AW, Lara J, Siervo M, Celis-Morales C, Mathers JC. Effects of exercise modalities on arterial stiffness and wave reflection: a systematic review and meta-analysis of randomized controlled trials. PLoS One. 2014;9(10):e110034. https://doi.org/10.1371/journal.pone.0110034.
71. Lopes S, Afreixo V, Teixeira M, Garcia C, Leitão C, Gouveia M, Figueiredo D, Alves AJ, Polonia J, Oliveira J, Mesquita-Bastos J, Ribeiro F. Exercise training reduces arterial stiffness in adults with hypertension: a systematic review and meta-analysis. J Hypertens. 2021;39(2):214–22. https://doi.org/10.1097/HJH.0000000000002619.

72. Miyachi M. Effects of resistance training on arterial stiffness: a meta analysis. Br J Sports Med. 2013;47:393–6. https://doi.org/10.1136/bjsports-2012-090488.
73. Ceciliato J, Costa EC, Azevêdo L, Sousa JC, Fecchio RY, Brito LC. Effect of resistance training on arterial stiffness in healthy subjects: a systematic review and meta-analysis. Curr Hypertens Rep. 2020;22(8):51. https://doi.org/10.1007/s11906-020-01065-x.
74. Okamoto T, Masuhara M, Ikuta K. Effect of low-intensity resistance training on arterial function. Eur J Appl Physiol. 2011;111(5):743–8. https://doi.org/10.1007/s00421-010-1702-5.
75. Okamoto T, Masuhara M, Ikuta K. Upper but not lower limb resistance training increases arterial stiffness in humans. Eur J Appl Physiol. 2009;107(2):127–34. https://doi.org/10.1007/s00421-009-1110-x.
76. Okamoto T, Masuhara M, Ikuta K. Effects of muscle contraction timing during resistance training on vascular function. J Hum Hypertens. 2009;23(7):470–8. https://doi.org/10.1038/jhh.2008.152.
77. Okamoto T, Masuhara M, Ikuta K. Combined aerobic and resistance training and vascular function: effect of aerobic exercise before and after resistance training. J Appl Physiol. 2007;103(5):1655–61. https://doi.org/10.1152/japplphysiol.00327.2007.
78. DeVallance E, Fournier S, Lemaster K, Moore C, Asano S, Bonner D, et al. The effects of resistance exercise training on arterial stiffness in metabolic syndrome. Eur J Appl Physiol. 2016;116:899–910. https://doi.org/10.1007/s00421-016-3348-4.
79. Miyaki A, Maeda S. Arterial stiffness and lifestyle modification. J Phys Fit Sports Med. 2012;1:205–10.
80. Mora-Rodriguez R, Ramirez-Jimenez M, Fernandez-Elias VE, Guio de Prada MV, Morales-Palomo F, Pallares JG, Nelson RK, et al. Effects of aerobic interval training on arterial stiffness and microvascular function in patients with metabolic syndrome. J Clin Hypertens. 2018;20:11–8. https://doi.org/10.1111/jch.13130.
81. Koskinen J, Magnussen CG, Taittonen L, Räsänen L, Mikkilä V, Laitinen T, et al. Arterial structure and function after recovery from the metabolic syndrome: the cardiovascular risk in young Finns study. Circulation. 2010;121:392–400. https://doi.org/10.1161/CIRCULATIONAHA.109.894584.

7 Physiological Versus Pathological Left Ventricular Hypertrophy in the Hypertensive Athlete

Giacomo Merello, Luna Cavigli, and Flavio D'Ascenzi

7.1 Introduction

The athlete's heart represents a physiological adaptation to the increased physical workload induced by exercise. A common feature of this remodeling is left ventricular hypertrophy (LVH) (2). However, LVH is nonspecific and discriminating between physiological and pathological hypertrophy, such as in hypertrophic cardiomyopathy (HCM) or hypertension (HTN), can sometimes be challenging. Furthermore, although competitive athletes are commonly considered healthy, HTN can also be observed in this specific population, making evaluation of a competitive athlete with a concealed HTN even more challenging.

7.2 Athlete's Heart

The first description of the morphological changes induced by physical training on the heart is credited to Henschen in 1899, who first attributed the enlargement of the heart chambers of cross-country skiers to training [1]. In the subsequent years, there have been controversies about the real consequences on the health of this adaptation, but the more recent advances of echocardiography and cardiac magnetic resonance (CMR) have allowed for a more precise evaluation of the athlete's heart.

LVH is just one of the structural and functional changes that adapt to the increased physical workload induced by exercise. It is generally accompanied by an increase in ventricular chamber dimensions and volume associated with a normal systolic and diastolic function [2]. However, cardiac remodeling is not homogenous among

G. Merello · L. Cavigli · F. D'Ascenzi (✉)
Division of Cardiology, Department of Medical Biotechnologies,
University of Siena,
Siena, Italy
e-mail: g.merello@student.unisi.it; flavio.dascenzi@unisi.it

P. Palatini et al. (eds.), *Exercise, Sports and Hypertension*, Updates in Hypertension and Cardiovascular Protection,
https://doi.org/10.1007/978-3-031-07958-0_7

competitive athletes but depends on the type and level of training, body composition, sex, age, ethnicity, years of sports practice, and period of competitive season [3].

Three main patterns of LVH have been first described: concentric hypertrophy, eccentric hypertrophy, and concentric remodeling [4, 5]. In concentric LVH, left ventricular (LV) mass (LVM) predominantly increases by wall thickening in response to pressure overload. In contrast, when LVM predominantly increases because of chamber dilatation, hypertrophy is defined as eccentric. Concentric remodeling is defined as normal LVM in the presence of demonstrable LVH [4, 5]. According to Morganroth's theory, the type of remodeling corresponds to the hemodynamic overload imposed on the heart during exercise. Consequently, endurance sports would lead to eccentric LVH (as a consequence of volume overload and increased diastolic wall stress), while pressure overload and increased systolic stress induced by strength training to concentric LVH [5]. However, most sports disciplines are characterized by a varying degree of both isometric and isotonic components. Several factors (i.e., ethnicity, sex, age, and body size) are implicated in cardiac remodeling, making the correlation nonbinary [3]. An essential feature of physiological LVH is the reversibility with detraining: when athletes are detrained, a reverse remodeling of the LV is usually observed with a reduction in septal thickness of 15–33% starting from 3–4 months [4, 6].

Another common finding in athletes, particularly endurance athletes, is left atrial (LA) enlargement, which is related to LVM regardless of the type of LVH and seems to be associated with higher age, male gender, years of training, and increased LV volume [4, 7]. Competitive athletes have greater LA maximum volumes compared to controls and greater LA pre-P volume and LA minimum volume [8]. Despite this exercise-induced enlargement, LA function is normal, and this can be an essential parameter for distinguishing between physiologic and pathologic remodeling [9].

The physiologic remodeling induced by training is homogeneous among the cardiac chambers; as a consequence, training activity has an impact also on right chambers. Indeed, right ventricle (RV) and right atrium (RA) dilatation are common in athletes, as well as a mild tricuspid regurgitation [10]. In endurance-trained athletes, RV eccentric remodeling is common and usually associated with LV enlargement, with a balanced increase in RV and LV mass, leading to a harmonic remodeling typically observed in competitive athletes as a response to training-induced changes in hemodynamics [10, 11].

7.3 Hypertensive Heart Disease (HHD)

The structural changes induced by chronic arterial hypertension include hypertrophy of existing myocytes and the addition of sarcomeres, together with an increase in connective tissue, ultimately leading to an overall increase in LVM [12]. In addition to structural changes, functional compensations with neurohormonal recruitment of sympathetic or renin–angiotensin–aldosterone systems also ensue to normalize LV wall stress, preserve LV mechanical function, and ultimately protect cardiac output against an increasing afterload [13]. However, these compensatory mechanisms are harmful in the long term, leading to diastolic and/or systolic dysfunction, myocyte death, cardiac wall thickness decrease and LV dilatation [12].

LVH is a common phenotypic adaptation in response to increased afterload. The same LVH patterns can be found in hypertensive patients, and it is not clear whether a specific pattern develops in response to HTN, but factors such as pressure overload, volume overload, ethnicity, sex, obesity, sympathetic nervous system tone, and plasma renin level are supposed to play a role [14].

In hypertensive patients, LVH in advanced stages can be accompanied by LV dilation and a gradual decline in LV ejection fraction (EF), leading to dilated heart failure. However, patients with HTN may develop diastolic dysfunction and/or the clinical syndrome of heart failure even with preserved LV ejection fraction due to the remodeling of the extracellular matrix and the increase in LV filling pressures [15].

Hypertension also leads to arterial remodeling, a strong and independent predictor of cardiovascular disease [16]. The increased stress on the aortic wall leads to aortic root dilatation, increased arterial wall thickness, and arterial stiffness and coronary microangiopathy that may contribute to myocardial fibrosis in HTN patients [17, 18].

As mentioned above, myocardial fibrosis is a key feature of LVH in the context of hypertension. It is the result of excessive production and reduced degradation of collagen type I and type III fibers, which can be induced as a replacement of small foci of dead cardiomyocytes or as a reaction to a diversity of stimuli (mechanical, such as stretch, humoral, such as aldosterone, and chemical) [19]. CMR can detect myocardial fibrosis with late gadolinium enhancement (LGE) evaluation and with the more recent techniques of T1-mapping and extracellular volume fraction (ECV) quantification. LGE can be found in up to 45% of hypertensive patients, with a patchy distribution, although usually, the LGE pattern in HHD is diffuse and non-specific [20].

7.4 The Hypertensive Athlete

HTN is defined in the general population as systolic blood pressure (BP) values ≥140 mmHg and/or diastolic BP values ≥90 mmHg recurrently measured in the office [21]. Notably, the current American Guidelines lowered the threshold to define HTN to 130/80 mmHg [22]. HTN in children (from 1 to 17 years) is defined as systolic BP and/or diastolic BP persistently at least 95th percentile for sex, age and height measured on at least three separate occasions [23]. While the cutoffs have been identified in the general population, in competitive athletes, the upper limits of systolic and diastolic BP have not been clearly established. Caselli et al. reported in a population of 2040 Olympic athletes (aged 25 ± 6 years; male: 64%) a mean value of systolic BP of 110 ± 11 mmHg for female and 117 ± 10 mmHg for male athletes, while diastolic BP was 71 ± 7 and 75 ± 7 mmHg for females and males, respectively [24]. Although athletes are generally considered healthy subjects, high BP can be observed also in this population, with HTN being the most common abnormal finding during preparticipation evaluation [4]. The prevalence of HTN in the athletic population is unclear and varies among different studies due to different methods used to measure BP, different limits of normality and different study populations [4, 25]. Caselli et al. found in a large population of competitive athletes (2040 athletes, aged 18 to 40 years) a lower prevalence (i.e., 3%) as compared to a general population of similar age (11% in 493 subjects, aged 18 to 35 years) [24]. D'Ascenzi et al. observed a prevalence of 3.8% in a cohort of 1058 Olympic athletes (mean age 24 ± 6 years) [26]. However, other studies found even more significant differences, with the prevalence of HTN ranging from 0 to 80% [25].

Several factors can affect BP values in athletes, such as the use of BP increasing drugs (i.e., nonsteroidal anti-inflammatory drugs, stimulants), age (BP values being greater in older athletes), sex (with BP being greater in men), ethnicity, tobacco use, type of sport practiced, and family history of HTN [4, 26]. The influence of the type of sport is still debated: indeed, while some authors reported a higher incidence of HTN in strength than in endurance athletes [27], others found that the type of sport was not a significant determinant of BP [4, 24]. Another important factor seems to be the amount of training time, with a trend toward a higher BP in athletes training ≥10 h/week than in those training <10 h/week ($p = 0.058$) [25].

The clinical significance of hypertensive response during exercise testing in the athletic population is still debated. Some authors demonstrated that an excessive BP response during exercise was correlated to a greater incidence of HTN [28]. Unfortunately, there is currently no consensus about the values of systolic BP during exercise, mainly because of relevant differences in methods, classifications and testing procedures among the studies currently available [4]. In athletes undergoing stress testing, a hypertensive response to exercise may indicate underlying hypertension, even in those with normal resting BP levels [29]. Shultz et al. demonstrated that a systolic BP >150 mmHg achieved at stage 1 or 2 of the Bruce protocol was found to be the optimal threshold to reveal the presence of HTN confirmed by 24-h ambulatory BP independent of age, sex, and office BP level [28]. Moreover, Caselli et al. demonstrated that competitive athletes with high BP response during exercise (defined as >220 mmHg in males and >200 mmHg in females for peak systolic BP and/or > 85 mmHg in males and 80 mmHg in females for peak diastolic BP) had a hazard ratio of developing HTN in a follow-up period of 6.5 ± 2.8 years 3.6 times higher than those with normal BP response during exercise [30].

7.5 Clinical Tools for Distinguishing Between HHD and Athlete's Heart

The physiological remodeling induced by exercise on the heart may share some similarities with HHD. In addition, HTN can be found in athletes, making the differentiation between athlete's heart and HHD more complex. However, some relevant differences can be detected by noninvasive diagnostic techniques for an appropriate differential diagnosis between these two entities.

7.5.1 Twelve-Lead Resting Electrocardiogram (ECG)

Twelve-lead resting ECG is part of the preparticipation evaluation and is usually part of the routine evaluation of subjects with the suspicion of HTN [31]. Even though ECG has a low sensitivity for detecting LVH, it may provide helpful information for the differential diagnosis between athlete's heart and HHD [31]. The current recommendations for the interpretation of ECG in athletes suggest defining LVH by the presence of isolated QRS voltage criteria (SV1 + RV5 or RV6 > 3.5 mV) [31]. Although isolated LVH is a common finding in athletes, it could indicate a pathological finding when accompanied by T-wave inversion (TWI) ≥1 mm in depth in two or more contiguous leads in the anterior, lateral, inferolateral, or inferior leads [31]. Lateral or inferolateral TWI and ST depression is a recognized marker of the presence of pathological LVH, which can also be observed in HHD, with a prevalence of TWI of 11% in leads V5 and/or V6. Conversely, this finding is uncommon in competitive athletes [32], although in some cases, that is, TWI confined to leads V1–V4 in black athletes when preceded by J point and/or ST-segment elevation or TWI in leads V1–V3 in athletes aged <16 years or < 15 years are considered normal [33, 34]. Another ECG abnormality found in HTN patients is left anterior hemiblock, with HTN being its second most important cause [4, 35]. Conversely, left anterior hemiblock is not considered a typical finding in athletes [31].

A careful examination of ECG atrial parameters may also predict diastolic dysfunction, an earlier cardiac manifestation of HTN, providing new diagnostic markers, such as ventricular activation time, P-wave terminal force in V1, and P-wave dispersion [31, 36, 37].

7.5.2 Echocardiography

Echocardiography has a key role in the differential diagnosis between physiologic and pathologic hypertrophy in athletes, confirming the presence of LVM and assessing diastolic function, aortic size, and valvular heart function, essential data for the differential diagnosis. Furthermore, an essential difference between athlete's heart and HHD is the reverse remodeling in response to detraining: echocardiography, given its relatively low cost and being a "green" imaging technique, is extremely useful in monitoring the training-induced changes in LVM; notably, in HTN patients there is no significant reduction in septal thickness and LVM, unless with anti-hypertensive therapy [4].

In athletes, LVH is associated with normal systolic and diastolic function, while patients with HTN may develop systolic and/or diastolic dysfunction and/or heart failure, even with preserved LV EF [4]. Advanced echocardiographic techniques, such as speckle tracking echocardiography (STE), may be helpful for the characterization of LVH. Galderisi et al. studied with standard echocardiography and STE 19 sedentary controls, 22 top-level rowers, and 18 young newly diagnosed, never treated patients with HTN. They found that, despite an increase in LVM in both rowers and HTN patients, only the latter showed a reduction in global longitudinal strain (GLS, $-17.5 \pm 2.8\%$), while in the former and controls, LV GLS was normal ($-22.2 \pm 2.7\%$ and $-21.1 \pm 2.0\%$ respectively, $p < 0.0001$) [38]. Furthermore, LV GLS was strongly associated with LV diastolic function, independently from afterload changes and degree of LVH. Hypertensive patients with LVH have a lower longitudinal strain, peak systolic strain rate, and peak early diastolic strain rate than athletes [38].

The analysis of diastolic function can provide helpful information too. In early HTN, there is a mild "stiffening" and delayed relaxation of the myocardium, which affects peak early filling (E-wave) and late diastolic filling (A-wave), with a consequent reduced E/A ratio [15]. Conversely, competitive athletes do not exhibit diastolic dysfunction because LV relaxation and filling are normal or even supernormal ($E/A > 2$) [39]. Pulsed-wave Doppler and tissue Doppler imaging may be useful for distinguishing HHD from athlete's heart. Indeed, the athlete's heart is characterized by an increased e' velocity, while pathological LVH is usually characterized by reduced e' velocity. Notably, despite atrial dilatation, the ratio of transmitral early diastolic velocity to e' (E/e' ratio) is within the normal limits in the athlete while it is increased in HTN patients [38, 39].

The analysis of atrial function, particularly with STE, may be helpful, assuming that atrial dilation may also be present in the athlete and may overlap with pathological conditions. Indeed, despite the increase in LA size, LA stiffness is normal in athletes, supporting the hypothesis of a physiological remodeling induced by exercise [9]. Studies on the athletic population demonstrated that, while reservoir function did not differ between athletes and controls, LA active function tends to be lower in the former [39]. This finding was accompanied by a supernormal diastolic function related to LV filling shifting toward early diastole in the athlete's heart [39]. Conversely, HTN patients and even patients with masked hypertension show an impairment of LA phasic function and stiffness [40]. Remodeling of the aortic root may be expected in athletes because of hemodynamic overload associated with exercise training; however, the current literature does not support this hypothesis, and only a small proportion of athletes were found to have aortic dilatation [41]. Conversely, aortic dilatation is not an infrequent finding in patients with HTN [17] and may support the diagnosis of HTN in athletes.

7.5.3 Exercise Testing and CPET

Exercise testing is usually performed in clinical practice to assess exercise capacity and exercise-induced HTN [42]. This diagnostic tool may be used as a rapid and feasible screening test to identify suspected masked HTN that could be unmasked by the BP response to light exercise in untreated subjects. Cardiopulmonary exercise testing (CPET) can also be used for the identification of hypertensive response to exercise, adding further information about cardiopulmonary performance during exercise. The addition of ventilatory gas exchange measurements allows the assessment of aerobic capacity, and an inverse relationship between exercise capacity and progression from pre-HTN to HTN has been demonstrated [43]. Notably, elite athletes with high-normal and elevated BP have lower exercise capacity and lower peak oxygen consumption (VO_2) at anaerobic threshold than their normotensive counterparts [44].

7.5.4 Cardiac Magnetic Resonance

CMR is considered the gold-standard technique for quantifying LVM, wall thickness, and LV size, with the highest accuracy and reproducibility among all noninvasive techniques and can be extremely useful in differentiating between athlete's heart and pathological LVH [20]. Furthermore, CMR gives the unique opportunity to characterize myocardial tissue by the LGE technique. Tahir et al. studied LGE in triathletes and observed that LGE CMR imaging revealed focal nonischemic myocardial fibrosis in triathletes with higher peak exercise systolic BP than triathletes without high BP during exercise, suggesting that myocardial fibrosis appears to be related to exercise-induced HTN and myocardial hypertrophy [45]. Indeed, while biventricular insertion point LGE appears to be common in athletes and can be observed in up to 40% of athletes, except for veteran athletes, LGEs localized in other areas are uncommon, and their identification should raise the suspicion of a cardiac disorder [46]. Diffuse myocardial fibrosis may develop in HHD even before conventional MRI detectable LGE and ECV can identify myocardial fibrosis at an early stage in HTN patients [47].

Table 7.1 summarizes the main differences and similarities between athlete's heart and hypertensive heart disease.

Table 7.1 Differential diagnosis between athlete's heart and hypertensive heart disease

Differential diagnosis between hypertrophic cardiomyopathy and athlete's heart		
Athlete's heart	Findings	Hypertensive heart disease
ECG		
+–	Left ventricular hypertrophy	+–
–	Left axis deviation	+–
–	LBBB	+–
–	TWI in the inferolateral leads	+–
–	ST-T segment "strain"	+–
Echocardiography and cardiac magnetic resonance		
+–	LV hypertrophy	++
++	Regression of LV hypertrophy after detraining[a]	–
–	Aortic dilatation (more than mild)	+–
–	Reduction of LV function	+–
–	Diastolic dysfunction	++
–	Increased intracardiac filling pressures	++
–	Reduced LV e' velocity	++
+–	Atrial dilatation	+–
–	Reduced atrial function	+–
–	Reduced LV and LA deformation indexes	++
++	Balanced biventricular remodeling	–
++	Balanced biatrial remodeling	–
–	Patchy LGE	+–
Exercise testing		
–	Exercise-induced hypertension	++
Cardiopulmonary exercise testing		
–	Peak VO_2 lower than predicted	+–

++ usually observed, +– can be observed, –– usually not observed. *ECG* electrocardiogram, *LA* left atrial, *LBBB* left bundle branch block, *LGE* late gadolinium enhancement, *LV* left ventricular, *TWI* T-wave inversion, *TDI* tissue Doppler imaging

[a]A regression of left ventricular hypertrophy has been demonstrated in hypertensive patients after treatment and normalization of blood pressure

7.6 Conclusions

The diagnosis of HHD is not uncommon in competitive athletes and particularly in master athletes. Accordingly, the differential diagnosis between an athlete's heart and a hypertensive heart in an athlete is crucial to diagnose HTN early and adequately manage this condition. Several clinical tools are currently available to support the differential diagnosis, from 12-lead resting ECG to advanced cardiac imaging. The interpretation of the clinical data obtained by these tools is critical, and the knowledge of some peculiar clinical and morphological parameters of HHD and athlete's heart is helpful to distinguish between these two entities.

References

1. Maron BJ, Pelliccia A. The heart of trained athletes: cardiac remodeling and the risks of sports, including sudden death. Circulation. 2006;114:1633–44.
2. Galderisi M, Cardim N, D'Andrea A, et al. The multi-modality cardiac imaging approach to the Athlete's heart: an expert consensus of the European Association of Cardiovascular Imaging. Eur Heart J Cardiovasc Imaging. 2015;16:353.
3. Pelliccia A, Caselli S, Sharma S, et al. European Association of Preventive Cardiology (EAPC) and European Association of Cardiovascular Imaging (EACVI) joint position statement: recommendations for the indication and interpretation of cardiovascular imaging in the evaluation of the athlete's heart. Eur Heart J. 2018;39:1949–69.
4. D'Ascenzi F, Fiorentini C, Anselmi F, Mondillo S. Left ventricular hypertrophy in athletes: how to differentiate between hypertensive heart disease and athlete's heart. Eur J Prev Cardiol. 2020. https://doi.org/10.1177/2047487320911850. PMID: 33611377. Online ahead of print.
5. Morganroth J, Maron BJ, Henry WL, Epstein SE. Comparative left ventricular dimensions in trained athletes. Ann Intern Med. 1975;82:521–4.
6. Pelliccia A, Maron BJ, De Luca R, Di Paolo FM, Spataro A, Culasso F. Remodeling of left ventricular hypertrophy in elite athletes after long-term deconditioning. Circulation. 2002;105:944–9.
7. D'Andrea A, Riegler L, Cocchia R, et al. Left atrial volume index in highly trained athletes. Am Heart J. 2010;159:1155–61.
8. D'Ascenzi F, Pelliccia A, Natali BM, et al. Training-induced dynamic changes in left atrial reservoir, conduit, and active volumes in professional soccer players. Eur J Appl Physiol. 2015;115:1715–23.
9. D'Ascenzi F, Anselmi F, Focardi M, Mondillo S. Atrial enlargement in the Athlete's heart: assessment of atrial function may help distinguish adaptive from pathologic remodeling. J Am Soc Echocardiogr. 2018;31:148–57.
10. D'Ascenzi F, Pisicchio C, Caselli S, Di Paolo FM, Spataro A, Pelliccia A. RV remodeling in Olympic athletes. JACC Cardiovasc Imaging. 2017;10:385–93.
11. Scharhag J, Schneider G, Urhausen A, Rochette V, Kramann B, Kindermann W. Athlete's heart: right and left ventricular mass and function in male endurance athletes and untrained individuals determined by magnetic resonance imaging. J Am Coll Cardiol. 2002;40:1856–63.
12. Lovic D, Narayan P, Pittaras A, Faselis C, Doumas M, Kokkinos P. Left ventricular hypertrophy in athletes and hypertensive patients. J Clin Hypertens (Greenwich). 2017;19:413–7.
13. Lovic D, Manolis AJ, Lovic B, et al. The pathophysiological basis of carotid baroreceptor stimulation for the treatment of resistant hypertension. Curr Vasc Pharmacol. 2014;12:16–22.
14. Drazner MH. The progression of hypertensive heart disease. Circulation. 2011;123:327–34.
15. Schannwell CM, Schneppenheim M, Plehn G, Marx R, Strauer BE. Left ventricular diastolic function in physiologic and pathologic hypertrophy. Am J Hypertens. 2002;15:513–7.

16. Redheuil A, Wu CO, Kachenoura N, et al. Proximal aortic distensibility is an independent predictor of all-cause mortality and incident CV events: the MESA study. J Am Coll Cardiol. 2014;64:2619–29.
17. Milan A, Avenatti E, Tosello F, et al. Aortic root dilatation in essential hypertension: prevalence according to new reference values. J Hypertens. 2013;31:1189–95.
18. Nwabuo CC, Vasan RS. Pathophysiology of hypertensive heart disease: beyond left ventricular hypertrophy. Curr Hypertens Rep. 2020;22:11.
19. Gonzalez A, Ravassa S, Lopez B, et al. Myocardial remodeling in hypertension. Hypertension. 2018;72:549–58.
20. Mewton N, Liu CY, Croisille P, Bluemke D, Lima JA. Assessment of myocardial fibrosis with cardiovascular magnetic resonance. J Am Coll Cardiol. 2011;57:891–903.
21. Williams B, Mancia G, Spiering W, et al. 2018 ESC/ESH guidelines for the management of arterial hypertension. Eur Heart J. 2018;39:3021–104.
22. Whelton PK, Carey RM, Aronow WS, et al. 2017 ACC/AHA/AAPA/ABC/ACPM/AGS/APhA/ASH/ASPC/NMA/PCNA guideline for the prevention, detection, evaluation, and Management of High Blood Pressure in adults: executive summary: a report of the American College of Cardiology/American Heart Association task force on clinical practice guidelines. Hypertension. 2018;71:1269–324.
23. Lurbe E, Agabiti-Rosei E, Cruickshank JK, et al. 2016 European Society of Hypertension guidelines for the management of high blood pressure in children and adolescents. J Hypertens. 2016;34:1887–920.
24. Caselli S, Vaquer Sequi A, Lemme E, et al. Prevalence and management of systemic hypertension in athletes. Am J Cardiol. 2017;119:1616–22.
25. Berge HM, Isern CB, Berge E. Blood pressure and hypertension in athletes: a systematic review. Br J Sports Med. 2015;49:716–23.
26. D'Ascenzi F, Caselli S, Alvino F, et al. Cardiovascular risk profile in Olympic athletes: an unexpected and underestimated risk scenario. Br J Sports Med. 2019;53:37–42.
27. Naylor LH, George K, O'Driscoll G, Green DJ. The athlete's heart: a contemporary appraisal of the 'Morganroth hypothesis'. Sports Med. 2008;38:69–90.
28. Schultz MG, Picone DS, Nikolic SB, Williams AD, Sharman JE. Exaggerated blood pressure response to early stages of exercise stress testing and presence of hypertension. J Sci Med Sport. 2016;19:1039–42.
29. Sharman JE, LaGerche A. Exercise blood pressure: clinical relevance and correct measurement. J Hum Hypertens. 2015;29:351–8.
30. Caselli S, Serdoz A, Mango F, et al. High blood pressure response to exercise predicts future development of hypertension in young athletes. Eur Heart J. 2019;40:62–8.
31. Sharma S, Drezner JA, Baggish A, et al. International recommendations for electrocardiographic interpretation in athletes. Eur Heart J. 2018;39:1466–80.
32. Okin PM, Devereux RB, Nieminen MS, et al. Electrocardiographic strain pattern and prediction of cardiovascular morbidity and mortality in hypertensive patients. Hypertension. 2004;44:48–54.
33. D'Ascenzi F, Anselmi F, Berti B, et al. Prevalence and significance of T-wave inversion in children practicing sport: a prospective, 4-year follow-up study. Int J Cardiol. 2019;279:100–4.
34. Migliore F, Zorzi A, Michieli P, et al. Prevalence of cardiomyopathy in Italian asymptomatic children with electrocardiographic T-wave inversion at preparticipation screening. Circulation. 2012;125:529–38.
35. Elizari MV, Acunzo RS, Ferreiro M. Hemiblocks revisited. Circulation. 2007;115:1154–63.
36. Boles U, Almuntaser I, Brown A, Murphy RR, Mahmud A, Feely J. Ventricular activation time as a marker for diastolic dysfunction in early hypertension. Am J Hypertens. 2010;23:781–5.
37. Tanoue MT, Kjeldsen SE, Devereux RB, Okin PM. Relationship between abnormal P-wave terminal force in lead V1 and left ventricular diastolic dysfunction in hypertensive patients: the LIFE study. Blood Press. 2017;26:94–101.

38. Galderisi M, Lomoriello VS, Santoro A, et al. Differences of myocardial systolic deformation and correlates of diastolic function in competitive rowers and young hypertensives: a speckle-tracking echocardiography study. J Am Soc Echocardiogr. 2010;23:1190–8.
39. D'Ascenzi F, Cameli M, Zaca V, et al. Supernormal diastolic function and role of left atrial myocardial deformation analysis by 2D speckle tracking echocardiography in elite soccer players. Echocardiography. 2011;28:320–6.
40. Tadic M, Cuspidi C, Radojkovic J, Rihor B, Kocijanic V, Celic V. Masked hypertension and left atrial dysfunction: a hidden association. J Clin Hypertens (Greenwich). 2017;19:305–11.
41. Pelliccia A, Di Paolo FM, Quattrini FM. Aortic root dilatation in athletic population. Prog Cardiovasc Dis. 2012;54:432–7.
42. Niebauer J, Borjesson M, Carre F, et al. Recommendations for participation in competitive sports of athletes with arterial hypertension: a position statement from the sports cardiology section of the European Association of Preventive Cardiology (EAPC). Eur Heart J. 2018;39:3664–71.
43. Faselis C, Doumas M, Kokkinos JP, et al. Exercise capacity and progression from prehypertension to hypertension. Hypertension. 2012;60:333–8.
44. Mazic S, Suzic Lazic J, Dekleva M, et al. The impact of elevated blood pressure on exercise capacity in elite athletes. Int J Cardiol. 2015;180:171–7.
45. Tahir E, Starekova J, Muellerleile K, et al. Myocardial fibrosis in competitive triathletes detected by contrast-enhanced CMR correlates with exercise-induced hypertension and competition history. JACC Cardiovasc Imaging. 2018;11:1260–70.
46. Gati S, Sharma S, Pennell D. The role of cardiovascular magnetic resonance imaging in the assessment of highly trained athletes. JACC Cardiovasc Imaging. 2018;11:247–59.
47. Liu T, Song D, Dong J, et al. Current understanding of the pathophysiology of myocardial fibrosis and its quantitative assessment in heart failure. Front Physiol. 2017;8:238.

8 Atrial Fibrillation and Sports: Still a Challenging Problem

Luigi Sciarra, Mattia Petrungaro, Elena Cavarretta, Silvio Romano, Maria Penco, Pietro Delise, and Leonardo Calò

8.1 Introduction

Atrial fibrillation (AF) is the most common sustained arrhythmia encountered in clinical practice [1–3]. The prevalence is low among young people but it gets higher with increasing age: more than 95% of cases occur beyond the sixth decade of life. The presence of AF has been associated with higher risk of myocardial infarction, heart failure and all-cause mortality in many clinical settings [4, 5]. AF is usually associated with the classical cardiovascular disease risk factors such as diabetes,

L. Sciarra (✉) · L. Calò
Cardiology Department, Policlinico Casilino, Rome, Italy
e-mail: lui.sciarra@libero.it; leonardocalo.doc@gmail.com

M. Petrungaro
Cardiology Department, Faculty of Medicine and Psychology, Sant'Andrea Hospital, University of Rome Sapienza, Rome, Italy
e-mail: mattiapetrungaro@gmail.com

E. Cavarretta
Department of Medical-Surgical Sciences and Biotechnologies, Sapienza University, Rome, Italy

Mediterranea Cardiocentro, Naples, Italy
e-mail: Elena.Cavarretta@uniroma1.it

S. Romano · M. Penco
Cardiology, Department of Life, Health and Environmental Sciences, University of L'Aquila, L'Aquila, Italy
e-mail: silvio.romano@univaq.it; maria.penco@univaq.it

P. Delise
U.O. Cardiologia, Ospedale P. Pederzoli, Peschiera del Garda (VR), Italy
e-mail: pietro.delise@libero.it

P. Palatini et al. (eds.), *Exercise, Sports and Hypertension*, Updates in Hypertension and Cardiovascular Protection,
https://doi.org/10.1007/978-3-031-07958-0_8

aging, hypertension, obesity, ischemic heart disease, heart failure and extracardiac illnesses such as thyroid disease. However, this arrhythmia can affect even young people with structural normal hearts such as athletes [6, 7].

It is generally acknowledged that physical activity (PA) is associated with a reduction of the risk of cardiovascular disease and all-cause mortality [8]. Furthermore, moderate and regular PA, is considered a cornerstone in the prevention of AF through modifying many of its predisposing factors [9–13]. In fact, moderate, regular and aerobic physical activity can be considered a non-pharmacological therapeutic tool to cure AF [14, 15].

However, recently, some papers have raised doubts about the beneficial effects of PA on the prevention of AF and observed a higher incidence of AF in some elite athletes [16–19]. Therefore, the relationship between PA and AF could appear controversial [20–22], and, therefore, many questions can arise. What is the truth? Are these positions really contradictory?

8.2 Possible Mechanisms

AF is a multifactorial arrhythmia with a complex electrophysiology and various underlying arrhythmic mechanisms [23, 24] which can be different in single patients. In athletes, structural, functional and electrophysiological modifications induced by regular exercise can determine, at least theoretically, a favourable substrate for AF occurrence. There are several possible mechanisms that may favour the development of AF in athletes. However, nowadays, we can only make assumptions on this topic.

AF, just like any other arrhythmia, is generated by the interaction between triggers, arrhythmogenic substrate and modulating factors: the so-called Coumel's triangle [25]. Normally, the "trigger" is a premature ectopic beat often originating from inside the pulmonary veins ostia [26, 27] but, particularly in young people with structural normal hearts, it can be represented by a sustained supraventricular arrhythmia [24, 28, 29]. The "substrate" consists in morphological, structural and functional alterations that may favour the onset and the maintenance of the arrhythmia. The "modulating factors" are usually the sympathetic and vagal tone. It is obvious that those factors may be modified by practice of different types of sports.

8.2.1 Triggers Modification in Athletes

In general population, the most common triggers for paroxysmal AF have been identified in the presence of premature atrial contractions originating from pulmonary veins ectopy [26]. This is true also for athletes.

However, as already anticipated, in young subjects with structurally normal hearts (the vast majority of athletic population), AF trigger can be represented by the presence of other synchronised tachyarrhythmias. Supraventricular tachyarrhythmias, such as atrioventricular nodal re-entrant tachycardia, atrial tachycardia or atrioventricular re-entrant tachycardia through an accessory pathway, may generate atrial flutter or AF: the so-called "tachycardia-induced tachycardia" or "tachycardia-induced

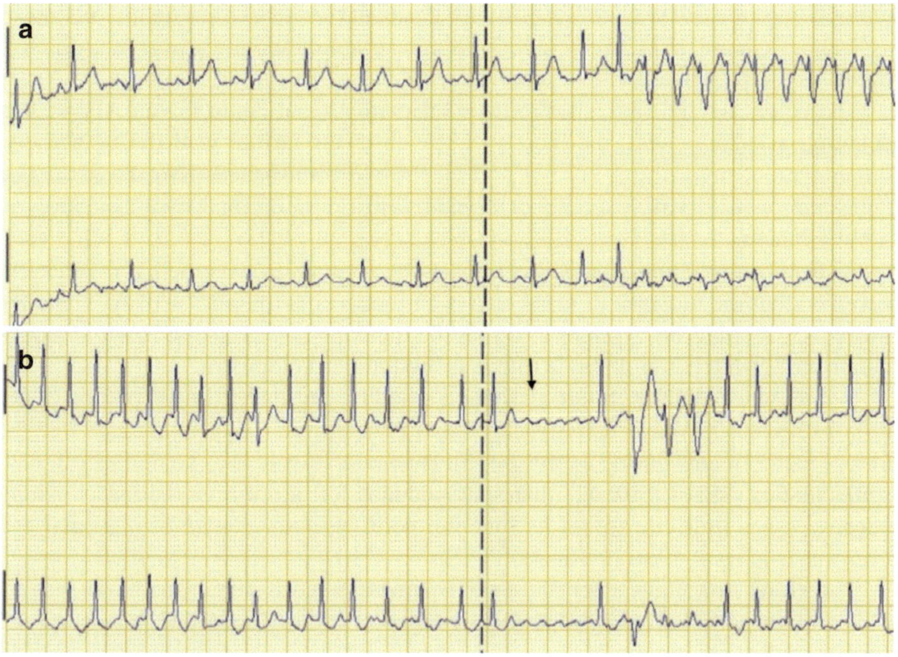

Fig. 8.1 ECG tracings refer to a young male athlete (cross country skier; 23 years) with recurrent episodes of sustained palpitations at rest. Patient was highly symptomatic for arrhythmic sustained palpitations. Recordings have been obtained by an external loop recorder. In (**a**) arrhythmia onset is displayed. The arrhythmia starts as a regular sequence of QRS, with aberrancy of conduction. In (**b**) it can be observed that the regular arrhythmia degenerates into an irregular sequence of QRS. The arrow clearly indicates the presence of atrial fibrillating waves. In this case the ECG tracings help to define the exact mechanism of the arrhythmia. A supraventricular regular tachycardia induces an atrial fibrillation. The patient underwent an electrophysiological study that showed the presence of a concealed accessory pathway responsible for atrio-ventricular re-entrant tachycardia and atrial fibrillation. He was successfully treated by trans-catheter ablation of the accessory pathway

AF" [30, 31] (Fig. 8.1). In this case it is very important to identify the underlying tachycardia even in view of planning an efficient therapy like ablation.

Nevertheless, currently available data are inconclusive and insufficient to affirm if atrial premature beats or other tachyarrhythmias can increase with PA and whether they may play a role in the pathogenesis of AF in athletes.

In fact, neither Baldesberger et al. [32] nor Elliot et al. [33] found an increased incidence of atrial ectopy in their study in former professional cyclists.

8.2.2 Substrate Modification in Athletes

Endurance exercise can induce several structural, functional, and electrophysiological adaptations in the heart such as left ventricular hypertrophy [34], atrial enlargement [35], and right ventricular enlargement [36]. This morphological and functional remodelling of cardiac chambers usually disappears with detraining and is known as "athlete's heart" [37]. Many functional and structural modifications of "Athlete's Heart" could play a key role in promoting AF.

Therefore, among these sport-related adaptations that could favour AF, we can count atrial enlargement, the increased stretch of the atrium wall during activity, inflammation, myocardial fibrosis and electrolyte disturbances (Na, K, Mg). The latter can occur during exercise combined with a non-optimal hydro-electrolytic replenishment.

As far as morphological modifications of the atrium are concerned, it is generally accepted that the increase of atrial size is an independent predictor of AF [38, 39]. Moreover, it could be hypothesised that the increase in exercise-induced hemodynamic atrial stretch could play a role in arrhythmia development.

In endurance athletes, bi-atrial dilation could be caused by the adaptation of the atria to regular physical activity, in order to accommodate the increased cardiac output requirements during exercise [35]. However, its role is to be defined. In fact, some studies suggest [40, 41] that sport-induced left atrial remodelling is benign because it has little impact on its function with the maintenance of a normal and even super-normal diastolic function [42].

Therefore, nowadays scientific evidence must be considered unable to prove a direct relationship between AF and sport-induced atrial remodelling or stretch, and further studies are required.

Fibrosis and inflammation can also be involved in the etiopathogenesis of AF in athletes. Both inflammation and fibrosis are well-established risk factors for the development of AF in different clinical conditions [16, 43, 44]. Strenuous endurance exercise can cause cardiac hypertrophy, inflammation and fibrosis. On the other hand, regular physical activity has been demonstrated also to induce a systemic chronic anti-inflammatory status [45, 46]. Therefore, the relationship between sport, inflammation and AF is controversial, and it needs to be better investigated and defined.

Studies in animal models suggested that atrial fibrosis could contribute to exercise-induced AF pathogenesis. Some experimental papers underlined the relationship between intense training, increased AF inducibility and modest atrial interstitial fibrosis [47, 48]. In active or former athletes, higher levels of profibrotic plasmatic biomarkers such as galectin-3 [49], ST2 [50], some microRNAs [51], and collagen turnover peptides [52] have been documented, but their real role in the development of AF remains uncertain.

Even if fascinating, at the present time the scientific background seems not to be adequate to sustain that increased atrial fibrosis may be directly responsible for a higher AF burden in athletes.

8.2.3 Modulating Factors Modifications in Athletes

In athletes, both vagal and sympathetic tone can be modified. In fact, another cardiovascular adaptation to regular exercise is an increased vagal tone [53]: as a consequence many athletes manifest sinus bradycardia at rest and some atrio-ventricular conduction disturbances [54]. Physical effort increases sympathetic tone with a consequent downregulation at rest, which makes the vagal tone dominant [55, 56]. This condition is reversible after detraining. Enhanced vagal tone can favour the onset and maintenance of AF also in normal hearts [16, 26, 57].

However, there are other forms of AF such as an adrenergic form. Increased sympathetic drive may trigger ectopic atrial activity and increase susceptibility to AF induction [26]. Undoubtedly, a higher sympathetic tone is present in athletes during competition or during intense effort, but it is very rare for AF to arise during a race. From a speculative point of view, changes in autonomic tone could lead to arrhythmias in athletes. This topic is very interesting and the role of sympatho-vagal balance in athletes suffering for AF needs further investigation.

8.3 Association Between AF and Sport: A Summary of the Literature

In the last decades, many papers have been published supporting a possible increased incidence of AF in people practicing sports. One of the first experiences was published by Karjalainen et al. [16] who reported a higher prevalence of AF in a cohort of 300 former top-level runners (5.3%) than in controls (0.9%). This result was confirmed a few years later by two studies conducted by Mont et al. [19, 58]. They concluded that vigorous endurance exercise could be a risk factor for AF in men. Again, also Furlanello et al. [18] supported the relationship between high-level of sport and AF. More recently, the Physicians' Health Study [59] enrolled 16,921 men undergoing vigorous exercise with a follow-up of 12 years. The authors found that AF incidence increased with the frequency of exercise and, in particular, men joggers who trained 7 days/week had a 20% higher risk of AF [59]. Furthermore, a meta-analytic study carried out by Abdulla and Nielsen [60] showed that long-term endurance exercise is associated with increased AF risk. Finally, another study [61] showed that AF incidence was higher in swimmers over 60 years than in a general internal medicine population, in spite of the latter cohort having a higher prevalence of cardiovascular risk factors such as diabetes mellitus and hypertension.

Therefore, an overall evaluation of these studies, despite their heterogeneity, seems to indicate that endurance sports could favour the development of AF. As a consequence, the scientific community wondered whether heavy PA could paradoxically be harmful to health. In order to answer this question, Marijon E. et al. [62] investigated mortality in top-level athletes. They observed a significantly lower mortality (40% less) among 786 cyclists participants in the Tour de France (between 1947 and 2012), compared with the general male population. In addition, a study [63] of 15,000 Olympic champions from nine different country concluded that endurance sports athletes had increased survival. The above findings appear of difficult interpretation: is it possible that high-intensity sports can increase AF incidence and, at the same time, reduce total mortality?

It should be noted that, if on the one hand some scientific studies support a causal relationship between sport and AF, there is scientific evidence raising doubts about this relationship.

In fact, a large meta-analysis encompassing 95,526 subjects [64] compared the incidence of atrial fibrillation in people who trained with those who had a sedentary lifestyle: there was no evidence of association between regular PA and higher incidence of AF. Moreover, this meta-analysis provided additional evidence to the already known beneficial effects of regular exercise on cardiovascular risk.

In a recent prospective cohort study, Albrecht M. et al. [65], in the Rotterdam Study, analysed total PA (different types of sports were considered) in 7018 people aged 55 years and older, with a median follow-up of 12.3 years. Then, according to PA estimated in MET-h/week, the study population was divided into tertiles; the low group was used as reference. The authors observed that neither total PA nor any of the included PA types were associated with increased AF risk. Furthermore, the absence of a relationship was also documented by comparing the AF events between the low and high tertile.

Therefore, the current state of scientific knowledge does not allow definitive conclusions on the relationship between AF and sports. However, there is no doubt that mild-to-moderate physical activity is beneficial and is not associated with AF risk. This statement is confirmed by numerous studies such as for example the Cardiovascular Health Study [66] that investigated the incidence of AF in a population of 5446 adults performing regular physical activity followed for over 12 years. The results showed that, unlike high-intensity exercise, light to moderate physical activity was associated with a lower incidence of AF, particularly leisure-time activity and walking.

Even less is known about the incidence of atrial fibrillation in women also due the fact that women have been excluded from many studies. In spite of this limitation, according to some studies there is no evidence of an increase in the incidence of atrial fibrillation in female endurance athletes.

In the Swedish Mammograph Cohort study [67], which evaluated the physical activity in 36,513 women for a median follow-up of 12 years, the incidence of AF resulted lower in those who trained over 4 h weekly versus those exercising less than 1 h per week. The beneficial role of sport in women was confirmed also in the Women's Health Initiative Observational Study [68]. In this study strenuous PA (>15 MET) has also been shown to have a protective role against AF in women.

This different relationship between sport and AF in males and females seems to be confirmed by a recent prospective study on about 400,000 individuals (mean age 56 ± 8 years; females 52.4%) from UK biobank cohort [69]. Among males, a high dose of vigorous PA was associated with a 12% increase in AF unlike low or moderate PA. In contrast, for female participants, vigorous PA was associated with an 8–16% lower AF incidence. Therefore, in women, it appears that any intensity of sport is associated with a lower risk of AF.

Finally, in a very recent and extensive meta-analysis (23 unique cohorts with two million people), Kunutsor et al. [70] confirmed that the AF/PA relationship is sex-related: an increased risk of AF was reported in men while a reduced risk was reported in women.

8.4 Comment

From a general evaluation of the available data in the literature, we can assume that the relationship between sport and AF appears controversial. On the one hand, some papers reported a clear association between AF incidence and sport, on the other hand, other studies arose some doubts about this relationship. Despite these apparent contradictory data, a comprehensive and objective evaluation of this issue cannot ignore the increasing evidence of higher rates of AF in men practicing endurance activities. But, from a pure speculative point of view, could we imagine that some confounding factors may have influenced the homogeneity of the available data? Can we hypothesise that the higher incidence of AF reported in some studies, could have been caused by a selection bias? Generally, sportsmen undergo more frequent medical examinations than the general population even if asymptomatic. This is particularly true in Italy where athletes have to undergo routine medical workout because of legislative obligations. Such a factor could have influenced, at least in part, the estimate of AF incidence. Prospective and controlled trials about this subject are lacking, and are very welcome in order to better clarify this question.

Moreover, could it be easier to diagnose this arrhythmia in sportsmen? Symptoms related to AF could be more easily perceived during physical activity than at rest. In other words, an athlete could appreciate earlier a reduction in physical performance, and this could induce him or her to undergo clinical evaluation.

Furthermore, the prevalence of AF in athletes could be influenced by the significant diffusion of sports activity in master populations. It is well known that the prevalence of the arrhythmia increases with age (3). Thus, it is possible that the high prevalence of AF in some athletic populations may have been, at least in part, influenced by an increased prevalence of master athletes. It could be interesting to investigate in prospective studies the real prevalence of AF in master athletes, and to analyse the prevalence of cardiovascular risk factors in sport practitioners with or without AF.

Another controversial issue is the use of illicit substances. Doping phenomenon is far from being solved and its diffusion is anything but decreasing even in recreational athletes. Many illicit substances, like for instance sympathetic agonists, could influence the onset of AF. However, the dark nature of doping hinders any scientific conclusion and thus this problem remains speculative.

Nonetheless, from a pure theoretical point of view, some kind of sports may favour the development of pathophysiological factors known to facilitate the onset and sustainment of AF (see paragraph 2) and, as already stated in this chapter, increasing scientific evidence seems to suggest that certain types of sports, in particular endurance sports, may facilitate the onset of AF. Thus, the relationship PA-AF is complex, and it seems to be influenced by the intensity and the duration of PA. Therefore, the connection between AF and sport may be a "U-shaped relationship": in this case, both a sedentary lifestyle and a strenuous and long-time endurance physical activity may favour the onset of AF. In fact, a lower risk of AF was reported practicing sports at moderate intensity or duration, but not when exercising vigorously [71]. But can we identify a maximum safety limit for endurance activities? Based on current scientific evidence it cannot be defined with certainty. Elosua et al. [72] claimed that more than 1500 h/lifetime of sport was associated with an increased risk of AF. According to Calvo et al. [73] the safety threshold for endurance sports should be set at 2000 h/lifetime. However, even if a definite "safety" limit is hardly identifiable, we can generally assume that "much is too much", particularly in predisposed subjects.

Nevertheless, despite significant cardiac remodelling, most endurance athletes do not develop AF. Why? Probably other factors are important in the development of AF: while in non-athletes, the classic cardiovascular risk factors seem to significantly contribute to the development of AF, in athletes it is possible to hypothesise that a genetic predisposition can play a crucial role. In fact, some studies have identified several single nucleotide polymorphisms associated with an increased risk of atrial fibrillation, even if in non-athletes [74, 75]. Therefore, it could be possible that some genetic polymorphisms amplify the risk of AF when combined with the presence of a sport-induced substrate (athlete's heart). Further studies are warrantied to better clarify this aspect.

Another controversial issue is the relationship between FA and sports in women. With the limitation that women have been excluded from many studies, it does not seem to be any evidence of an increased AF incidence in female endurance athletes. Female sex seems to be a protective factor against AF even in athletes. But even on this issue confirmation coming from solid scientific data is required.

8.5 Conclusive Considerations

In conclusion, there seems to be enough evidence to state that regular mild-to-moderate physical exercise has a strong preventive effect against AF and, conversely, a sedentary lifestyle is a recognised risk factors for the occurrence of this arrhythmia. It is well known that exercise is one of the most powerful lifestyle intervention strategies for the primary and secondary prevention of cardiovascular disease. The prescription of PA should be encouraged also in patients suffering from AF. As physicians, our role is to promote a physically active lifestyle, to increase the quality of lives and to facilitate the prevention of many diseases, including cardiovascular ones and, in particular, AF. We believe that generating doubts about the beneficial effect of sports could be somewhat dangerous, and not scientifically justified.

According to the literature, there is not enough scientific evidence to sustain that sport can be the cause itself of AF. However, it is reasonable to affirm that some kind of regular physical activity, and in particular high-intensity endurance sports, may have a facilitating effect on AF induction in predisposed men. On the other hand, preliminary data seem to confirm a preventive effect of female sex against the onset of AF even in the athletic population.

Large prospective clinical studies are strongly desired to improve our knowledge on the pathophysiological relationship between physical activity and AF in order to allow a prompt identification of athletes at risk of developing the arrhythmia. Our main goal is to be able in the near future to identify the type of sport that could be pro-arrhythmic in a given patient, performing an individualised sport prescription.

References

1. Heeringa J, van der Kuip DA, Hofman A, et al. Prevalence, incidence and lifetime risk of atrial fibrillation: the Rotterdam study. Eur Heart J. 2006;27:949–53.
2. Go AS, Hylek EM, Phillips KA, et al. Prevalence of diagnosed atrial fibrillation in adults: national implications for rhythm management and stroke prevention: the AnTicoagulation and risk factors in atrial fibrillation (ATRIA) study. JAMA. 2001;285:2370–5.
3. Hindricks G, Potpara T, Dagres N, Arbelo E, Bax JJ, Blomström-Lundqvist C, Boriani G, Castella M, Dan GA, Dilaveris PE, Fauchier L, Filippatos G, Kalman JM, La Meir M, Lane DA, Lebeau JP, Lettino M, Lip GYH, Pinto FJ, Thomas GN, Valgimigli M, Van Gelder IC, Van Putte BP, Watkins CL, ESC Scientific Document Group. 2020 ESC guidelines for the diagnosis and management of atrial fibrillation developed in collaboration with the European Association for Cardio-Thoracic Surgery (EACTS): the task force for the diagnosis and management of atrial fibrillation of the European Society of Cardiology (ESC) developed with the special contribution of the European heart rhythm association (EHRA) of the ESC. Eur Heart J. 2021;42(5):373–498.
4. Ruddox V, Sandven I, Munkhaugen J, et al. Atrial fibrillation and the risk for myocardial infarction, all-cause mortality and heart failure: a systematic review and meta-analysis. Eur J Prev Cardiol. 2017;24:1555–66.
5. Bayturan O, Puri R, Tuzcu EM, et al. Atrial fibrillation, progression of coronary atherosclerosis and myocardial infarction. Eur J Prev Cardiol. 2017;24:373–81.
6. Kopecky SL, Gersh BJ, McGoon MD, et al. The natural history of lone atrial fibrillation: a population-based study over three decades. N Engl J Med. 1987;317:669–74.
7. Brand FN, Abbott RD, Kannel WB, Wolf PA. Characteristics and prognosis of lone atrial fibrillation: 30-year follow-up in the Framingham study. JAMA. 1985;254:3449–53.
8. Williams PT. Dose-response relationship of physical activity to premature and total all-cause and cardiovascular disease mortality in walkers. PLoS One. 2013;8:e78777.
9. Pathak RK, Elliott A, Middeldorp ME, Meredith M, Mehta AB, Mahajan R, Hendriks JML, Twomey D, Kalman JM, Abhayaratna WP, Lau DH, Sanders P. Impact of CARDIOrespiratory FITness on arrhythmia recurrence in obese individuals with atrial fibrillation: the CARDIO-FIT study. J Am Coll Cardiol. 2015;66:985996.
10. Du X, Dong J, Ma C. Is atrial fibrillation a preventable disease? J Am Coll Cardiol. 2017;69:19681982.
11. Mozaffarian D, Furberg CD, Psaty BM, Siscovick D. Physical activity and incidence of atrial fibrillation in older adults: the cardiovascular health study. Circulation. 2008;118:800807.
12. Rienstra M, Hobbelt AH, Alings M, Tijssen JGP, Smit MD, Brugemann J, Geelhoed B, Tieleman RG, Hillege HL, Tukkie R, Van Veldhuisen DJ, Crijns H, Van Gelder IC, IR. Targeted therapy of underlying conditions improves sinus rhythm maintenance in patients with persistent atrial fibrillation: results of the RACE 3 trial. Eur Heart J. 2018;39:29872996.
13. Elliott AD, Maatman B, Emery MS, Sanders P. The role of exercise in atrial fibrillation prevention and promotion: finding optimal ranges for health. Heart Rhythm. 2017;14:17131720.
14. Reed JL, Mark AE, Reid RD, Pipe AL. The effects of chronic exercise training in individuals with permanent atrial fibrillation: a systematic review. Can J Cardiol. 2013;29(12):1721–8.
15. Osbak PS, Mourier M, Kjaer A, Henriksen JH, Kofoed KF, Jensen GB. A randomized study of the effects of exercise training on patients with atrial fibrillation. Am Heart J. 2011;162(6):1080–7.
16. Karjalainen J, Kujala UM, Kaprio J, Sarna S, Viitasalo M. Lone atrial fibrillation in vigorously exercising middle aged men: case-control study. BMJ. 1998;316:1784–5.

17. Coelho A, Palileo E, Ashley W, et al. Tachyarrhythmias in young athletes. J Am Coll Cardiol. 1986;7:237–43.
18. Furlanello F, Bertoldi A, Dallago M, et al. Atrial fibrillation in elite athletes. J Cardiovasc Electrophysiol. 1998;9(Suppl):S63–8.
19. Mont L, Sambola A, Brugada J, et al. Long-lasting sport practice and lone atrial fibrillation. Eur Heart J. 2002;23:477–82.
20. Ofman P, Khawaja O, Rahilly-Tierney CR, et al. Regular physical activity and risk of atrial fibrillation: a systematic review and meta-analysis. Circ Arrhythm Electrophysiol. 2013;6:252–6.
21. Kwok CS, Anderson SG, Myint PK, et al. Physical activity and incidence of atrial fibrillation: a systematic review and meta-analysis. Int J Cardiol. 2014;177:467–76.
22. Zhu WG, Wan R, Din Y, et al. Sex differences in the association between regular physical activity and incident atrial fibrillation: a meta-analysis of 13 prospective studies. Clin Cardiol. 2016;39:360–7.
23. Van Gelder IC, Hobbelt AH, Marcos EG, Schotten U, Cappato R, Lewalter T, Schwieler J, Rienstra M, Boriani G. Tailored treatment strategies: a new approach for modern management of atrial fibrillation. J Intern Med. 2016;279(5):457–66.
24. Sciarra L, Rebecchi M, De Ruvo E, De Luca L, Zuccaro LM, Fagagnini A, Corò L, Allocca G, Lioy E, Delise P, Calò L. How many atrial fibrillation ablation candidates have an underlying supraventricular tachycardia previously unknown? Efficacy of isolated triggering arrhythmia ablation. Europace. 2010;12(12):1707–12.
25. Coumel P, Leenhardt A. Mental cardiac arrhythmias and the autonomic nervous system. J Cardiovasc Electrophysiol. 1993;4:338–55.
26. Haïssaguerre M, Jaïs P, Shah DC, Takahashi A, Hocini M, Quiniou G, Garrigue S, Le Mouroux A, Le Métayer P, Clémenty J. Spontaneous initiation of atrial fibrillation by ectopic beats originating in the pulmonary veins. N Engl J Med. 1998;339(10):659–66.
27. Adragão P, Cavaco D, Aguiar C, Palos J, Morgado F, Ribeiras R, Abecasis M, Neves J, Bonhorst D, Seabra-Gomes R. Ablation of pulmonary vein foci for the treatment of atrial fibrillation; percutaneous electroanatomical guided approach. Europace. 2002;4(4):391–9.
28. Brugada J, Mont L, Matas M, Navarro-Lopez F. Atrial fibrillation induced by atrio-ventricular nodal reentrant tachycardia. Am J Cardiol. 1997;79:681–2.
29. Delise P, Gianfranchi L, Paparella N, Brignole M, Menozzi C, Themistoclakis S, et al. Clinical usefulness of slow pathway ablation in patients with both paroxysmal atrioventricular nodal reentrant tachycardia and atrial fibrillation. Am J Cardiol. 1997;79:1421–3.
30. Prystowsky EN. Tachycardia-induced tachycardia: a mechanism of initiation of atrial fibrillation. In: Di Marco J, Prystowsky EN, editors. Atrial arrhythmias. State of the art. Armonk, NY: Futura Publishing; 1995. p. 81–95.
31. Delise P, Gianfranchi L, Paparella N, et al. Clinical usefulness of slow pathway ablation in patients with both paroxysmal atrioventricular nodal reentrant tachycardia and atrial fibrillation. Am J Cardiol. 1997;79:1421–3.
32. Baldesberger S, Bauersfeld U, Candinas R, Seifert B, Zuber M, Ritter M, et al. Sinus node disease and arrhythmias in the long-term follow-up of former professional cyclists. Eur Heart J. 2008;29:71–8.
33. Elliott AD, Mahajan R, Linz D, et al. Atrial remodeling and ectopic burden in recreational athletes: implications for risk of atrial fibrillation. Clin Cardiol. 2018;41:843–8.
34. Arbab-Zadeh A, Perhonen M, Howden E, et al. Cardiac remodeling in response to 1 year of intensive endurance training. Circulation. 2014;130:2152–61.
35. Wilhelm M, Roten L, Tanner H, Wilhelm I, Schmid J-P, Saner H. Atrial remodeling, autonomic tone, and lifetime training hours in nonelite athletes. Am J Cardiol. 2011;108:580–5.
36. Thompson P. Exercise and the heart: the good, the bad and the ugly. Dialog Cardiovasc Med. 2002;7:140–58.
37. Brosnan MJ, Rakhit D. Differentiating athlete's heart from cardiomyopathies—the left side. Heart Lung Circ. 2018;27(9):1052–62.
38. Vaziri SM, Larson MG, Benjamin EJ, Levy D. Echocardiographic predictors of nonrheumatic atrial fibrillation. The Framingham Heart Study. Circulation. 1994;89:724–30.

39. Neuberger H-R, Schotten U, Blaauw Y, et al. Chronic atrial dilatation, electrical remodeling, and atrial fibrillation in the goat. J Am Coll Cardiol. 2006;47:644–53.
40. D'Ascenzi F, Cameli M, Zacà V, Lisi M, Santoro A, Causarano A, Mondillo S. Supernormal diastolic function and role of left atrial myocardial deformation analysis by 2D speckle tracking echocardiography in elite soccer players. Echocardiography. 2011 Mar;28(3):320–6.
41. Brugger N, Krause R, Carlen F, Rimensberger C, Hille R, Steck H, Wilhelm M, Seiler C. Effect of lifetime endurance training on left atrial mechanical function and on the risk of atrial fibrillation. Int J Cardiol. 2014;170(3):419–25.
42. Gabrielli L, Enríquez A, Córdova S, Yáñez F, Godoy I, Corbalán R. Assessment of left atrial function in hypertrophic cardiomyopathy and athlete's heart: a left atrial myocardial deformation study. Echocardiography. 2012;29:943–9.
43. Dzeshka MS, Lip GY, Snezhitskiy V, Shantsila E. Cardiac fibrosis in patients with atrial fibrillation: mechanisms and clinical implications. J Am Coll Cardiol. 2015;66:943–59.
44. Aviles RJ, Martin DO, Apperson-Hansen C, Houghtaling PL, Rautaharju P, Kronmal RA, et al. Inflammation as a risk factor for atrial fibrillation. Circulation. 2003;108:3006–10.
45. Scheffer DDL, Latini A. Exercise-induced immune system response: anti-inflammatory status on peripheral and central organs. Biochim Biophys Acta Mol Basis Dis. 2020;1866(10):165823.
46. Wang J, Liu S, Li G, Xiao J. Exercise regulates the immune system. Adv Exp Med Biol. 2020;1228:395–408.
47. Guasch E, Benito B, Qi X, et al. Atrial fibrillation promotion by endurance exercise: demonstration and mechanistic exploration in an animal model. J Am Coll Cardiol. 2013;62:68–77.
48. Aschar-Sobbi R, Izaddoustdar F, Korogyi AS, et al. Increased atrial arrhythmia susceptibility induced by intense endurance exercise in mice requires TNFα. Nat Commun. 2015;6:6018.
49. Hättasch R, Spethmann S, de Boer RA, et al. Galectin-3 increase in endurance athletes. Eur J Prev Cardiol. 2014;21:1192–9.
50. Roca E, Nescolarde L, Lupón J, et al. The dynamics of cardiovascular biomarkers in non-elite marathon runners. J Cardiovasc Transl Res. 2017;10:206–8.
51. Baggish AL, Hale A, Weiner RB, et al. Dynamic regulation of circulating microRNA during acute exhaustive exercise and sustained aerobic exercise training. J Physiol. 2011;589:3983–94.
52. Lindsay MM, Dunn FG. Biochemical evidence of myocardial fibrosis in veteran endurance athletes. Br J Sports Med. 2007;41:447–52.
53. Okazaki K, Iwasaki KI, Prasad A, et al. Dose-response relationship of endurance training for autonomic circulatory control in healthy seniors. J Appl Physiol. 1985;2005(99):1041–9.
54. Cooper JP, Fraser AG, Penny WJ. Reversibility and benign recurrence of complete heart block in athletes. Int J Cardiol. 1992;35:118–20.
55. Zeppilli P, Santini C. L'elettrocardiogramma nell'atleta. In: Zeppilli P, editor. Cardiologia dello Sport. Roma: CESI; 1990. p. 121–40.
56. Zeppilli P, Manno V. Vagotonia fisiologica e non fisiologica nell'atleta. G Ital Cardiol. 1987;17:865–73.
57. Carpenter A, Frontera A, Bond R, Duncan E, Thomas G. Vagal atrial fibrillation: what is it and should we treat it? Int J Cardiol. 2015;201:415–21.
58. Molina L, Mont L, Marrugat J, Berruezo A, Brugada J, Bruguera J, Rebato C, Elosua R. Long-term endurance sport practice increases the incidence of lone atrial fibrillation in men: a follow-up study. Europace. 2008;10(5):618–23.
59. Aizer A, Gaziano JM, Cook NR, et al. Relation of vigorous exercise to risk of atrial fibrillation. Am J Cardiol. 2009;103:1572–7.
60. Abdulla J, Nielsen JR. Is the risk of atrial fibrillation higher in athletes than in the general population? A systematic review and meta-analysis. Europace. 2009;11(9):1156–9.
61. Schreiner AD, Keith BA, Abernathy KE, Zhang J, Brzezinski WA. Long-term, competitive swimming and the association with atrial fibrillation. Sports Med Open. 2016;2:42.
62. Marijon E, Tafflet M, Antero-Jacquemin J, El Helou N, Berthelot G, Celermajer DS, Bougouin W, Combes N, Hermine O, Empana JP, Rey G, Toussaint JF, Jouven X. Mortality of French participants in the tour de France (1947-2012). Eur Heart J. 2013;34(40):3145–50.

63. Clarke PM, Walter SJ, Hayen A, Mallon WJ, Heijmans J, Studdert DM. Survival of the fittest: retrospective cohort study of the longevity of Olympic medallists in the modern era. BMJ. 2012;13(345):e8308.
64. Ofman P, Khawaja O, Rahilly-Tierney CR, Peralta A, Hoffmeister P, Reynolds MR, Gaziano JM, Djousse L. Regular physical activity and risk of atrial fibrillation: a systematic review and meta-analysis. Circ Arrhythm Electrophysiol. 2013;6(2):252–6.
65. Albrecht M, Koolhaas CM, Schoufour JD, van Rooij FJA, Kavousi M, Ikram MA, et al. Physical activity types and atrial fibrillation risk in the middle-aged and elderly: the Rotterdam study. Eur J Prev Cardiol. 2018;25(12):1316–23.
66. Mozaffarian D, Furberg CD, Psaty BM, Siscovick D. Physical activity and incidence of atrial fibrillation in older adults: the cardiovascular health study. Circulation. 2008;118:800–7.
67. Drca N, Wolk A, Jensen-Urstad M, Larsson SC. Physical activity is associated with a reduced risk of atrial fibrillation in middle-aged and elderly women. Heart. 2015;101(20):1627–30.
68. Azarbal F, Stefanick ML, Salmoirago-Blotcher E, et al. Obesity, physical activity, and their interaction in incident atrial fibrillation in postmenopausal women. J Am Heart Assoc. 2014;3:e001127.
69. Elliott AD, Linz D, Mishima R, Kadhim K, Gallagher C, Middeldorp ME, Verdicchio CV, Hendriks JML, Lau DH, La Gerche A, Sanders P. Association between physical activity and risk of incident arrhythmias in 402 406 individuals: evidence from the UK biobank cohort. Eur Heart J. 2020;41(15):1479–86.
70. Kunutsor SK, Seidu S, Mäkikallio TH, Dey RS, Laukkanen JA. Physical activity and risk of atrial fibrillation in the general population: a meta-analysis of 23 cohort studies involving about 2 million participants. Eur J Epidemiol. 2021;36(3):259–74.
71. Centurión OA, Candia JC, Scavenius KE, García LB, Torales JM, Miño LM. The association between atrial fibrillation and endurance physical activity: how much is too much? J Atr Fibrill. 2019;12(3):2167.
72. Elosua R, Arquer A, Mont L, Sambola A, Molina L, Garcia-Moran E, et al. Sport practice and the risk of lone atrial fibrillation: a case-control study. Int J Cardiol. 2006;108:332–7.
73. Calvo N, Ramos P, Montserrat S, et al. Emerging risk factors and the dose-response relationship between physical activity and lone atrial fibrillation: a prospective case-control study. Europace. 2016;18:57–63.
74. Tucker NR, Clauss S, Ellinor PT. Common variation in atrial fibrillation: navigating the path from genetic association to the mechanism. Cardiovasc Res. 2016;109(4):493–501.
75. Christophersen I, Ellinor P. Genetics of atrial fibrillation: from families to genomes. J Hum Genet. 2016;61:61–70.

Metabolic Syndrome: Effect of Physical Activity on Arterial Elasticity

9

F. Saladini

9.1 Introduction

Metabolic syndrome (MetS) is defined by WHO as a pathologic condition characterized by abdominal obesity, insulin resistance, a concurrence of disturbed glucose and insulin metabolism, hypertension and hyperlipidemia [1]; it has a high prevalence all over the world [2–4] and has become one of the major health hazards of modern world [4] because of the well-known association with cardiovascular disease (CVD) [1]. General population studies have shown that about one-quarter to one-third of adults have MetS and its prevalence continues to increase [5, 6], and this pathological condition is not peculiar to adulthood as it is becoming frequent also among children and adolescents [7]. In particular, the increased sedentary lifestyle is a major driving force for the high prevalence of MetS [8]. MetS is associated with a chronic inflammatory and prothrombotic state [1] and with increased oxidative stress [9], which promote vascular arterial wall remodeling and arterial stiffness (AS) [10, 11]. A large number of studies have documented that AS increases with the number of MetS components [4, 12, 13] as each risk factor acts independently through different mechanisms with adverse effects on the structure and function of the vascular system. Physical activity and exercise represent key components of energy expenditure and energy balance, but the benefit of exercise in preventing MetS goes beyond the immediate benefit of caloric expenditure [14]. Several authors observed a favorable effect of regular physical activity on arterial elasticity [15, 16], which is confined to aerobic training. In a recent meta-analysis, aerobic but not resistance exercise was associated with a significant reduction of AS [16]. The protective role of physical activity may be independent from the isolated effect on

F. Saladini (✉)
Cardiology Unit, Cittadella Town Hospital, Cittadella, Padova, Italy
e-mail: francesca.saladini@aulss6.veneto.it

P. Palatini et al. (eds.), *Exercise, Sports and Hypertension*, Updates in Hypertension and Cardiovascular Protection,
https://doi.org/10.1007/978-3-031-07958-0_9

weight loss [15], because it includes other beneficial effects such as blood pressure (BP) reduction [17] and improvement of lipid profile [17, 18].

9.2 Mechanisms Underlying Metabolic Syndrome and Arterial Distensibility Impairment

Among modifiable risk factors, several authors demonstrated that MetS and its components are strictly related to the risk of AS [9, 12, 19]. In a recent paper by Gong and coworkers [20], the authors examined the relationship between components of MetS and AS, measured by means of pulse wave velocity (PWV). They examined 680 subjects (mean age 58.4 years) divided according to the number of MetS components, and they observed that the level of PWV progressively increased with increasing number of MetS components. Stepwise multiple regression analysis revealed that age, gender, the number of MetS components, heart rate as well as serum uric acid level were significant determinants of PWV ($p < 0.05$). In the subgroups stratified by age, systolic BP correlated with PWV in hypertensives younger than 55 years, while in nonhypertensives the correlation was found after 60 years of age. The authors concluded that AS became significant with the increasing number of MetS components, which was independent of age, gender and BP; moreover, the presence of hypertension played the most important role in the progress of AS even compared with age [20]. The above results are in keeping with those of the TRIPLE A-Stiffness study [21], a multicenter longitudinal study performed in a large European population. In this study, the authors investigated the values of AS according to the presence or absence of MetS and observed a higher PWV in patients with MetS (9.65 ± 2.57 m/s) compared to those without it (8.42 ± 2.09 m/s), a difference that remained statistically significant also after adjustment for age and sex ($p < 0.001$) [21]. Moreover, the authors explored the effect of different MetS components on AS and observed that the presence of any of these five components (waist circumference, triglycerides, HDL cholesterol, BP, and serum glucose) was associated with higher PWV values (all $p < 0.0001$ age and sex adjusted). In multivariate analysis adjusted for age and sex, older age (R^2 (%) 11.2 $p < 0.0001$), BP (R^2 (%) 1 $p < 0.0001$), glycemia (R^2 (%) 1.4 $p < 0.0001$), and HDL cholesterol (R^2 (%) 0.7 $p < 0.0003$) components were demonstrated to be independent determinants of high PWV [21]. The relationship between MetS components and AS was also documented in a study by Lopes-Vincente et al. [12]. The authors examined 64 patients with 3 to 5 components of MetS ($n = 8$ with 5 components, $n = 27$ with 4 components and $n = 29$ with 3 factors) and 17 control subjects. The increase in the number of risk factors caused a progressive impairment in PWV: mean value was 7.2 ± 0.3 m/s in control group, 7.5 ± 0.2 m/s in the group with three risk factors (p = n.s vs controls), 7.9 ± 0.2 m/s in the group with four risk factors ($p = 0.047$ vs controls) and 8.5 ± 0.4 m/s in the group with five risk factors ($p = 0.011$ vs controls and $p = 0.012$ vs group with three risk factors) [12].

The above data highlight the important role of increased BP as component of MetS in determining increased AS. The role of hypertension in determining impairment of endothelial function was recently demonstrated among young stage I hypertensive subjects from the HARVEST study [22]. Among 40 middle-age hypertensives (mean age 49.7 years) whose BP had been kept at target by pharmacological treatment and/or lifestyle modifications for a mean of 7.5 years, the authors observed that, despite good BP control (mean office BP 133.7 ± 9.0/81.2 ± 7.0 mmHg), these hypertensive subjects presented impaired endothelial function documented by lower carotid distensibility coefficient, carotid compliance coefficient and flow mediated dilation in comparison to a group of age and sex matched normotensive subjects (Table 9.1) [22]. Moreover, in logistic regression analysis hypertensive status was a significant predictor of local carotid vascular stiffness with an odds ratio of 14.98 (95%CI, 2.60–18.55) $p < 0.0005$ for crude data and an odds ratio of 13.04 (2.27–74.96), $p = 0.004$ after adjustment for age, flow-mediated dilation, serum osteoprotegerin, and body mass index. Of note, hypertensive status remained a significant predictor also after the adjustment for systolic and diastolic BP or mean BP ($p < 0.017$ for both analyses) [22]. Several mechanisms were supposed to explain the impairment of endothelial function despite apparently good BP control, both with drugs or nonpharmacological measures: some genetic peculiarities of the hypertensive participants, may justify these differences [22]. In addition, hypertension may accelerate the atherosclerotic process not only through hemodynamic factors but also through the release of humoral factors such as angiotensin II and endothelin-1. This favors oxidative stress in the arterial wall, due to overexpression of adhesion molecules and inflammatory mediators, thereby accelerating endothelial dysfunction [23]. These mechanisms may promote atherosclerotic vascular damage among hypertensives [24], despite good BP control [25], a hypothesis supported by the increased levels of inflammatory biomarkers, such as serum osteoprotegerin, an independent risk factor for the progression of carotid atherosclerosis and the onset of CVD in population-based studies [26] as well as in patients with hypertension [27] or MetS [28]. The inflammatory process with activated monocytes could induce the overexpression of serum osteoprotegerin by vascular cells [29], promoting smooth cell migration/proliferation, thereby favoring carotid intima media thickness progression [24].

Another important mechanism underlying both MetS and progression of AS is the high level of sympathetic activity that may act as a trigger for both these clinical

Table 9.1 Arterial compliance and distensibility among hypertensive and normotensive subjects. Adapted from Saladini et al. [22]

Variables	Normotensive subjects ($n = 40$)	Hypertensive subjects ($n = 40$)	p
CDC, 10^{-3}/kPa	36.97 ± 8.5	24.50 ± 9.0	< 0.0005
CCC, mm^2/kPa	1.28 ± 0.36	0.92 ± 0.34	< 0.0005
FMD, %	9.2 ± 2.9	5.7 ± 2.4	< 0.0005

Data are presented as mean value ± SD. p: t-test for normally distributed data or Mann-Whitney test for not normally distributed data. *CDC* carotid distensibility coefficient, *CCC* carotid compliance coefficient, *FMD* flow mediated dilation conditions. In the paper by Gong et al. [20] heart rate, an indirect marker of sympathetic activity, was found to be an independent risk factor for PWV in all subjects, similar to what was previously found by other authors [30, 31] in diabetic patients [32]. Higher heart rate, an index of sympathetic overactivity, was recognized as having a relationship with several risk factors, including BMI, dyslipidemia, and increased glucose [30]. Among young stage I hypertensive subjects from the HARVEST study it was clearly demonstrated the role of elevated heart rate, measured either in the office or with 24 h ambulatory monitoring, as a significant predictor of body weight and body weight gain during 7 years of follow-up [33]. The same group elegantly demonstrated that sympathetic predominance (measured by spectral analysis of heart rate variability during standing and during Stroop's color mental test) may favor the development of sustained hypertension and hypercholesterolemia early in life, and lead to increased susceptibility to vascular complications [34]. The authors examined 163 stage 1 hypertensives during 6 years of follow-up and observed that those with sympathetic predominance presented a higher percentage of subjects who developed hypertension requiring antihypertensive treatment (23.7 vs 9.6%; $p = 0.02$), higher level of total cholesterol ($p = 0.035$ for group × time interaction at repeated-measure ANCOVA), and impaired large artery compliance ($p < 0.001$) compared to those with normal autonomic nervous system activity [34]. These data were in keeping with those previously observed in the young general population of the Tecumseh study. Again, participants with sympathetic predominance presented high BP, waist–hip ratio, and total cholesterol compared to the rest of the subjects [35]. According to these findings sympathetic predominance adversely affects not only BP elevation, but also the lipid profile, another important risk factor for atherosclerosis [34, 36]. The association between sympathetic overactivity and cholesterol level has been attributed to stimulation of the enzyme 3-hydroxy-3-methyl-glutaryl coenzyme A reductase [37] and to increased lipolysis through stimulation of adipocyte beta-adrenoceptors [38], and the induction of the atherosclerosis to the damage to elastin fibers, resulting in replacement with collagen declining elasticity and compliance [35].

Another important component of MetS that favors AS is visceral obesity associated with sedentary lifestyle. Again, increased sympathetic activity with the associated fast heart rate enhances activity of the renin–angiotensin–aldosterone system and production of inflammatory cytokines, reduces the nitric oxide availability, and increases reactive oxygen species, promoting impairment of endothelial function and AS [39]. In addition, MetS and obesity are associated with high levels of leptin and decreased adiponectin that increase vascular smooth muscle cell proliferation and migration, thereby favoring the production of collagen [40].

9.3 Effect of Physical Activity on Arterial Distensibility

According to all recent guidelines [41, 42], physical activity represents one of the milestones of nonpharmacological treatment for prevention of hypertension and reduction of high BP. Epidemiological studies suggest that regular aerobic physical activity may be beneficial also for both the prevention and treatment of diabetes [43] and ischemic heart disease [44], and for lowering cardiovascular risk and mortality in general [45–47]. In this respect, guidelines suggest performing at least 30 min of moderate to intense dynamic aerobic exercise (walking, jogging, cycling, or swimming) on 5–7 days/week, and/or resistance exercises on 2–3 days/week [41, 42]. The protective role of regular exercise in attenuating CVD and mortality risk may be due to several different factors including lower BP, reduced BMI, improvement of lipid profile and insulin sensitivity [48–50]. The decrease in BP has been documented in several meta-analytic studies. Cornelissen et al. [45] investigated the effect of at least 4 weeks of exercise on BP in healthy subjects, examining different types of physical activity: endurance, dynamic resistance, combined training, and isometric resistance. All types of exercise, except combined training, were able to reduce both systolic and diastolic BP: endurance −3.5 (confidence limits −4.6 to −2.3)/−2.5 (−3.2 to −1.7) mmHg, dynamic resistance −1.8 (−3.7 to −0.011)/−3.2 (−4.5 to −2.0) mmHg and isometric resistance −10.9 (−14.5 to −7.4)/−6.2 (−10.3 to −2.0) mmHg, while combined training showed a significant reduction only in diastolic BP: −2.2 (−3.9 to −0.48) mmHg. Of note, the BP reduction with aerobic exercise was particularly elevated among hypertensive individuals: −8.3 (−10.7 to −6.0)/−5.2 (−6.8 to −3.4) mmHg [45]. Another important mechanism that contributes to the reduction of CV risk is the effect of exercise on metabolic variables. The influence of chronic aerobic endurance training on body fatness, waist circumference, lipid profile, glucose, and HOMA index was reported in another meta-analysis by Cornelissen and coauthors [49]. The authors observed that all components of the MetS were improved by exercise, but the strongest effects were found for HDL-cholesterol (net change 0.032 mmol/L, $p < 0.05$), serum glucose (−0.15 mmol/L, <0.001), fasting insulin (−1.4 IU/L, $p < 0.005$), and the HOMA index (−0.31, $p < 0.01$). These effects can explain why aerobic physical activity can retard the age-related decline in arterial elasticity measured with PWV [50], as shown in a recent meta-analysis [16]. Although there were some neutral studies, the majority of published data was in favor of a beneficial effect of aerobic exercise on PWV (−0.63 m/s, 95% CI: −0.90, −0.35) [16]. In addition, exercise proved effective in improving small artery compliance in adults [51]. In 151 subjects arterial distensibility parameters were assessed at the baseline and after 6 years of follow-up and the authors observed an improvement of all compliance parameters among nonsedentary subjects compared to sedentary ones

Table 9.2 Changes in arterial compliance and stiffness parameters in sedentary and active young stage I hypertensives during 6 years of follow-up. Adapted from Saladini et al. [51]

Variables	Sedentary subjects ($n = 111$)	Active subjects ($n = 40$)	P*
C1, mL/mmHg × 10	+2.1 ± 4.7	+1.5 ± 4.7	n.s.
C2, mL/mmHg × 100	−0.28 ± 0.23	+ 0.69 ± 0.39	0.047
AIx, %	5.8 ± 0.2	−3.9 ± 0.2	0.0125
PWV, m/s	+0.5 ± 1.3	−0.5 ± 0.1	n.s.
Peripheral resistance, dyne × s × cm^{-5}	−19.8 ± 239.1	−107.4 ± 237.9	0.0251

Data are presented as mean ± SEM. *C1* large artery compliance, *C2* small artery compliance, *AIx* augmentation index, *PWV* carotid to radial pulse wave velocity. *P** value adjusted age, sex, presence/absence of antihypertensive therapy, and time within the first and second assessment

(Table 9.2) [51]. These results were in keeping with those obtained by Nettlefold et al. in a cross-sectional study of 102 normotensive children in whom moderate to vigorous physical activity was associated with higher small artery compliance [52] or data by McGavock et al. that found a cross-sectional association between aerobic training and both large and small artery compliance [53]. Moreover, a higher incidence of hypertension needing treatment was observed among the sedentary patients (59.1%) compared to the nonsedentary ones (42.2%) ($\chi 2 = 8.5$, $p = 0.003$) [51]. Similar results were found by the same authors some years later in patients with high serum uric acid [54]. Patients examined were 1156 participants from the HARVEST with a mean age of 33.0 ± 8.6 years, during 11.4 years of follow-up, divided according to their physical activity status: $n = 713$ sedentary and $n = 443$ active. For the sedentary patients in the top serum uric acid tertile (serum uric acid >5.60 mg/dL), the risk of hypertension was 1.44 (95% CI, 1.11–1.88) compared with those of the bottom tertile (serum uric acid <4.32 mg/dL). In contrast, no association between serum uric acid tertile and risk of hypertension was found among the active participants. No difference in the prediction of hypertension was found between the active participants grouped according to whether they had serum uric acid below or above the median value ($p = 0.40$) or below or above the lower limit of the top serum uric acid tertile ($p = 0.86$) [54]. One of the main mechanisms underlying the favorable effect of exercise on AS is the reduction of heart rate. Studies in human beings have shown that there is a progressive increase in PWV with increasing heart rate with pacing independent from pressure changes [55], documenting that heart rate is cross-sectionally associated with AS. This effect has been quantified as an increase of 0.17 m/s for each 10 beats/min increment in heart rate [55]. A positive association between heart rate and AS has been documented also in longitudinal studies by Tomiyama et al. [56] and by Benetos et al. [57], either among normotensive or hypertensive subjects. However, opposite effect was observed for heart rate on other determinants of arterial distensibility such as central systolic BP and augmentation index (AIx) [58, 59]. This negative relationship has been attributed to a shift of the backward wave reflected from the periphery into late systole secondary to the prolongation of left ventricle ejection time and to the increase in stroke volume at low heart rates [58, 60]. This finding led some authors to claim that heart rate reduction in hypertension is detrimental because it may favor the risk of CV events [60]. Recently, the short-term and long-term effects of heart rate on arterial distensibility parameters were explored by Palatini et al. [61]. The authors confirmed the negative relationship of heart rate with AIx recorded at the same time (Fig. 9.1a), being AIx 19.9 ± 2.5% in the bottom nighttime heart rate quintile (heart rate < 57.4 bpm), 14.8 ± 1.4% in the intermediate quintiles (heart rate ≥ 57.4 and ≤ 72.3 bpm), and 5.0 ± 2.7% in the top quintile (heart rate > 72.3 bpm). In contrast, ambulatory heart rate turned out to be an independent positive predictor of AIx (Fig. 9.1b) and central BP measured 8 years later [61]. These findings suggest that heart rate reduction in the long run have a favorable effect and not a detrimental one on all parameters of arterial distensibility and contribute to explain why people with lower hear rate have a reduced risk of CV events and mortality in hypertension. In other words, training induced

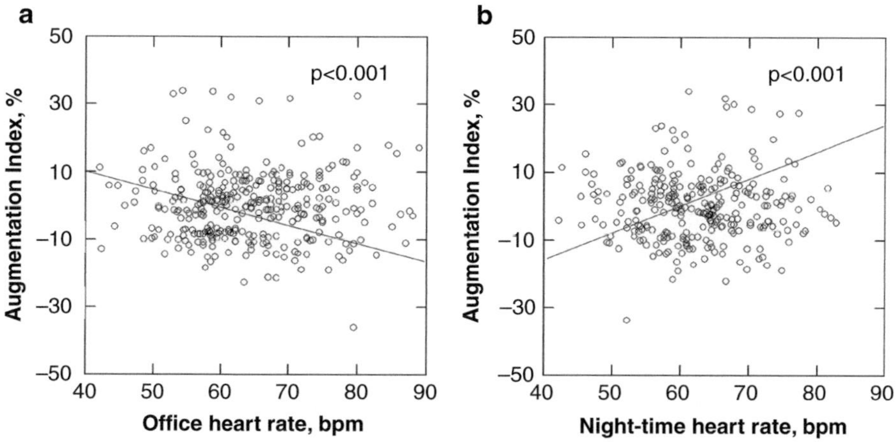

Fig. 9.1 Relationship of AIx with office heart rate measured at the same time (**a**) and with ambulatory heart rate measured 8 years before the arterial elasticity assessment (**b**), after eliminating the effect of age, sex, BMI, height, mean blood pressure, *PWV* small artery compliance, left ventricular ejection duration, lifestyle factors. Adapted from Palatini et al. [62]

bradycardia results to have an unfavorable effect on central hemodynamics measured within the same session, due to the prolongation of ejection fraction so that the reflected wave may return in systole. However, in the long term, it improves small artery compliance and reduces peripheral resistance [61]. Other mechanisms by which physical activity exerts a positive effect on AS is the effect of on sympathetic tone. As observed in the HARVEST study [54], active subjects presented lower plasma renin activity compared to sedentary participants (3.2 ± 0.7 versus 4.8 ± 0.4 ng/mL/h, $p = 0.050$), suggesting a reduction in sympathetic tone among active compared to sedentary ones. These findings were in keeping with previous findings that described lower norepinephrine values in physically trained individuals, pointing to a role of blunted sympathetic activity in determining the training related decrease in plasma renin activity [62–64]. The reduction of sympathetic tone associated with physical activity can improve endothelial function and arterial elasticity and decrease peripheral vasoconstriction, preventing small artery remodeling with an increase in the lumen–wall ratio [65] and cross-sectional area of the microcirculation [66]. Also, humoral factors may contribute to the beneficial effect of dynamic sport activities on small artery distensibility. Maeda et al. [67] after 8 weeks of exercise observed a reduction in endothelin-1 and an increase in nitric oxide concentrations with an inverse correlation between these two factors. A reduction of oxidative stress and an increased expression and activation of nitric oxide synthase [68] with enhanced endothelium-dependent dilation have been described in middle-aged endurance exercise trained men compared to less active peers [69, 70]. In addition, regular physical activity may improve vascular function by protecting the arterial tree from the adverse effects of traditional risk factors for CVD [71].

9.4 Effect of Physical Activity on Arterial Stiffness in Patients with the Metabolic Syndrome

The above evidence highlights the important role of physical activity on AS and this is particularly true among people with MetS. Indeed, several cross-sectional and longitudinal studies have demonstrated that exercise has beneficial effects on arterial distensibility in this clinical condition [72–75, 78]. Within a group of participants with the MetS, Pasha et al. [72] observed that carotid β-stiffness index was lower in the individuals who performed regular physical activity than in those who were sedentary. In the former, the β-stiffness index was similar to that in a group of healthy individuals, indicating that physical activity may be effective in mitigating the adverse effects of high BP, visceral adiposity and metabolic abnormalities on the vessel wall. In a similar study, Bohn and coworkers [73] explored the effect of different levels of physical activity (sedentary, light, moderate-to-vigorous), among 197 middle-age patients (116 without and 81 with MetS). Patients with MetS had higher PWV compared to patients without MetS (10.2 ± 1.9 m/s vs 8.3 ± 1.5 m/s, $p < 0.001$). However, participants with MetS who were more sedentary, showed significantly greater PWV than those who were more active and people without MetS regardless of the level of physical activity [73]. These cross-sectional data have been confirmed also by longitudinal studies. Tanabe et al. [74] investigated 188 middle-age men and women with overweight or obesity that underwent lifestyle modifications for several months including low calory diet and/or exercise. They observed that after 6 months weight loss was higher among those who underwent a high-intensity program compared to those who underwent a moderate- or low-intensity program, while PWV was reduced in all groups with no differences according to the intensity level of the program (114.3 ± 16.3, 82.6 ± 15.2, and 98.8 ± 90.4 cm/s, respectively), indicating the importance of weight loss, one of the components of MetS to improve AS [74]. Similarly, Pekas et al. [75] investigated 57 elderly postmenopausal women who performed regularly combined resistance and aerobic exercise training for 1 year versus a sedentary cohort ($n = 44$) of similar age. They observed significant differences for PWV, systolic BP, low-density lipoprotein, and body fat percentage, which were significantly lower ($p < 0.05$) in active women compared to sedentary ones (Table 9.3) [75]. Several mechanisms have been suggested by the authors as being responsible for the significantly lower PWV and BP in the active compared to the sedentary group, including reduced inflammation and improved nitric oxide bioavailability [75]. Elevated levels of proinflammatory markers, such as C-reactive protein, have been demonstrated to be associated with increased prevalence of AS, high BP, and CVD development [76]. Aerobic training was shown to reduce C-reactive protein in postmenopausal women, thereby supporting the use of exercise to reduce systemic inflammation and likelihood of disease development [77]. Considering that inflammation is associated with AS and hypertension, reduction in inflammation by means of physical activity may serve as a mechanism for vascular protection. Similar results were obtained also in a study

Table 9.3 Differences in blood pressure, arterial stiffness parameter, and lipid profile among sedentary ($n = 44$) and active ($n = 57$) women. Adapted by Pekas et al. [75]

Variables	Sedentary subjects ($n = 44$)	Active subjects ($n = 57$)	*P**
PWV, m/s	12.8 ± 1.8	12.1 ± 2.0	0.041
SBP, mmHg	137.0 ± 33.0	120.0 ± 15.0	0.03
DBP, mmHg	68.0 ± 15.0	67.7 ± 10.0	n.s.
TC, mg/dL	284.6 ± 112.5	287.3 ± 116.9	n.s
HDL-c, mg/dL	48.3 ± 9.8	47.9 ± 11.7	n.s.
LDL-c, mg/dL	110.9 ± 27.7	94.9 ± 23.5	0.023
Tg, mg/dL	173.0 ± 61.9	176.9 ± 80.4	n.s.
Body fat percentage, %	33.0 ± 7.0	27.0 ± 7.0	0.028

Data are presented as mean ± SD. *PWV* pulse wave velocity, *SBP* systolic blood pressure, *DBP* diastolic blood pressure, *TC* total cholesterol, *HDL-c* high density lipoprotein cholesterol, *LDL-c* low density lipoprotein cholesterol, *Tg* serum triglycerides, *n.s.* not statistically significant $p > 0.05$. *p value for t-test

with long-term follow-up by Koskinen et al. [78] in a longitudinal analysis of the Young Finns Study. After 6 years of follow-up, participants with Mets who performed regular physical activity and recovered from the MetS had higher carotid artery distensibility compared with MetS people who remained sedentary and still had the MetS at study end [78].

In summary, according to all the evidences mentioned above, several mechanisms can explain the favorable effect of exercise on arterial distensibility in people with MetS: exercise decreases heart rate, levels of inflammatory cytokines, improving arterial elasticity, and remodulates the effects of MetS on several other humoral factors, such as nitric oxide, leptin, adiponectin, and reactive oxygen species, which have an important impact on the arterial structure and endothelial function [39]. Thus, special attention should be paid by clinicians to people with MetS in whom the adverse effect of metabolic disturbances on the arteries can be offset by a program of physical activity.

9.5 Conclusions

Regular physical activity has shown beneficial effects both in general populations and in several clinical conditions and should thus be recommended to every subject for the prevention of CVD. However, implementing a long-lasting program of physical training is a challenging task because of the low compliance to exercise shown by participants in long-term studies [17, 78]. Special attention should be paid by health-care personnel to patients with MetS who are at high risk of CV events. A number of studies have shown that exercise can reduce body weight and BP and improve the metabolic profile in these patients with a direct beneficial effect on arterial elasticity. In addition, physical activity can counteract the pathogenetic mechanisms underlying AS and thus it represents one of the best tools for restoring arterial structure and function in patients with MetS.

References

1. Alberti KGMM, Eckel RH, Grundy SM, Zimmet PZ, Cleeman JI, Donato KA, et al. Harmonizing the metabolic syndrome: a joint interim statement of the international diabetes federation task force on epidemiology and prevention; National Heart, Lung, and Blood Institute; American Heart Association; world heart federation; international atherosclerosis society; and International Association for the Study of obesity. Circulation. 2009;120:1640–5. https://doi.org/10.1161/CIRCULATIONAHA.109.192644.
2. Beltran-Sanchez H, Harhay MO, Harhay MM, McElligott S. Prevalence and trends of metabolic syndrome in the adult U.S. population, 1999–2010. J Am Coll Cardiol. 2013;62(8):697–703. https://doi.org/10.1016/j.jacc.2013.05.064.
3. Aguilar M, Bhuket T, Torres S, Liu B, Wong RJ. Prevalence of the metabolic syndrome in the United States, 2003–2012. JAMA. 2015;313(19):1973–4. https://doi.org/10.1001/jama.2015.4260.
4. Saklayen MG. The global epidemic of the metabolic syndrome. Curr Hypertens Rep. 2018;20(2):12. https://doi.org/10.1007/s11906-018-0812-z.
5. Alberti KG, Zimmet P, Shaw J, IDF Epidemiology Task Force Consensus Group. The metabolic syndrome—a new worldwide definition. Lancet. 2005;366:1059–62. https://doi.org/10.1016/S0140-6736(05)67402-8.
6. Ford ES, Giles WH. A comparison of the prevalence of the metabolic syndrome using two proposed definitions. Diabetes Care. 2003;26:575–81. https://doi.org/10.2337/diacare.26.3.575.
7. DeBoer MD. Assessing and managing the metabolic syndrome in children and adolescents. Nutrients. 2019;11(8):1788. https://doi.org/10.3390/nu11081788.
8. Stokes A, Preston SH. Deaths attributable to diabetes in the United States: comparison of data sources and estimation approaches. PLoS One. 2017;12(1):e0170219. https://doi.org/10.1371/journal.pone.0170219.
9. Slivovskaja I, Ryliskyte L, Serpytis P, Navickas R, Badarienė J, Celutkiene J, et al. Aerobic training effect on arterial stiffness in metabolic syndrome. Am J Med. 2018;131:148–55. https://doi.org/10.1016/j.amjmed.2017.07.038.
10. Scuteri A, Najjar SS, Muller DC, Andres R, Hougaku H, Metter EJ, et al. Metabolic syndrome amplifies the age-associated increases in vascular thickness and stiffness. J Am Coll Cardiol. 2004;43:1388–95. https://doi.org/10.1016/j.jacc.2003.10.061.
11. Scuteri A, Cunha PG, Rosei EA, Badariere J, Bekaert S, Cockcroft JR, et al. Arterial stiffness and influences of the metabolic syndrome: a cross-countries study. Atherosclerosis. 2014;233:654–60. https://doi.org/10.1016/j.atherosclerosis.2014.01.041.
12. Lopes-Vicente WRP, Rodrigues S, Cepeda FX, Jordão CP, Costa-Hong V, Dutra-Marques ACB, et al. Arterial stiffness and its association with clustering of metabolic syndrome risk factors. Diabetol Metab Syndr. 2017;9:87. https://doi.org/10.1186/s13098-017-0286-1.
13. Kim M, Kim M, Yoo HJ, Lee SY, Lee SH, Lee JH. Age-specific determinants of pulse wave velocity among metabolic syndrome components, inflammatory markers, and oxidative stress. J Atheroscler Thromb. 2018;25:178–85. https://doi.org/10.5551/jat.39388.
14. Bird SR, Hawley JA. Update on the effects of physical activity on insulin sensitivity in humans. BMJ Open Sport Exerc Med. 2017;2(1):e000143. https://doi.org/10.1136/bmjsem-2016-000143.
15. Joo HJ, Cho SA, Cho JY, Lee S, Park JH, Yu CW, et al. Different relationship between physical activity, arterial stiffness, and metabolic status in obese subjects. J Phys Act Health. 2017;14:716–25. https://doi.org/10.1123/jpah.2016-0595.
16. Ashor AW, Lara J, Siervo M, Celis-Morales C, Mathers JC. Effects of exercise modalities on arterial stiffness and wave reflection: a systematic review and meta-analysis of randomized controlled trials. PLoS One. 2014;9:e110034. https://doi.org/10.1371/journal.pone.0110034.
17. Mora-Rodriguez R, Ramirez-Jimenez M, Fernandez-Elias VE, Guio de Prada MV, Morales-Palomo F, Pallares JG, Nelson RK, et al. Effects of aerobic interval training on arterial

stiffness and microvascular function in patients with metabolic syndrome. J Clin Hypertens. 2018;20:11–8. https://doi.org/10.1111/jch.13130.

18. Donley DA, Fournier SB, Reger BL, DeVallance E, Bonner DE, Olfert IM, et al. Aerobic exercise training reduces arterial stiffness in metabolic syndrome. J Appl Physiol. 2014;116:1396–404. https://doi.org/10.1152/japplphysiol.00151.2014.
19. Nilsson PM. Arterial stiffness, the metabolic syndrome, and the brain. Am J Hypertens. 2017;31:24–6. https://doi.org/10.1093/ajh/hpx152.
20. Gong J, Xie Q, Han Y, Chen B, Li L, Zhou G, et al. Relationship between components of metabolic syndrome and arterial stiffness in Chinese hypertensives. Clin Exp Hypertens. 2020;42(2):146–52. https://doi.org/10.1080/10641963.2019.1590385.
21. Topouchian J, Labat C, Gautier S, Bäck M, Achimastos A, Blacher J, et al. Effects of metabolic syndrome on arterial function in different age groups: the advanced approach to arterial stiffness study. J Hypertens. 2018;36(4):824–33. https://doi.org/10.1097/HJH.0000000000001631.
22. Saladini F, Rattazzi M, Faggin E, Palatini P, Puato M. Carotid elasticity is impaired in stage 1 hypertensive patients with well-controlled blood pressure levels. J Hum Hypertens. 2021. https://doi.org/10.1038/s41371-021-00584-7
23. Masoura C, Pitsavos C, Aznaouridis K, Skoumas I, Vlachopoulos C, Stefanadis C, et al. Arterial endothelial function and wall thickness in familial hypercholesterolemia and familial combined hyperlipidemia and the effect of statins. A systematic review and meta-analysis. Atherosclerosis. 2011;214:129–38. https://doi.org/10.1016/j.atherosclerosis.2010.10.008.
24. Hansson GK. Inflammation, atherosclerosis, and coronary artery disease. N Engl J Med. 2005;352:1685–95. https://doi.org/10.1056/NEJMra043430.
25. Puato M, Boschetti G, Rattazzi M, Zanon M, Pesavento R, Faggin E, et al. Intima-media thickness remodelling in hypertensive subjects with long-term well-controlled blood pressure levels. Blood Press. 2017;26(1):48–53. https://doi.org/10.1080/08037051.2016.1184964.
26. Vik A, Mathiesen EB, Brox J, Wilsgaard T, Njølstad I, Jørgensen L, et al. Relation between serum osteoprotegerin and carotid intima media thickness in a general population—the Tromso study. J Thromb Haemost. 2010;8:2133–9. https://doi.org/10.1111/j.1538-7836.2010.03990.x.
27. Puato M, Rattazzi M, Zanon M, Benetti E, Faggin E, Palatini P, et al. Predictors of vascular remodeling in hypertensive subjects with well-controlled blood pressure levels. J Hum Hypertens. 2015;29:561–5. https://doi.org/10.1038/jhh.2014.121.
28. Musialik K, Szulińska M, Hen K, Skrypnik D, Bogdański P. The relation between osteoprotegerin, inflammatory processes, and atherosclerosis in patients with metabolic syndrome. Eur Rev Med Pharmacol Sci. 2017;21:4379–85.
29. Scuteri A, Stuehlinger MC, Cooke JP, Wright JG, Lakatta EG, Anderson DE, et al. Nitric oxide inhibition as a mechanism for blood pressure increase during salt loading in normotensive postmenopausal women. J Hypertens. 2003;21(7):1339–46. https://doi.org/10.1097/00004872-200307000-00023.
30. Chandra P, Sands RL, Gillespie BW, Levin NW, Kotanko P, Kiser M, et al. Relationship between heart rate variability and pulse wave velocity and their association with patient outcomes in chronic kidney disease. Clin Nephrol. 2014;81(01):9–19. https://doi.org/10.5414/cn108020.
31. Logan JG, Kim SS. Resting heart rate and aortic stiffness in normotensive adults. Korean Circ J. 2016;46(6):834–40. https://doi.org/10.4070/kcj.2016.46.6.834.
32. Kang MK, Yu JM, Chun KJ, Choi J, Choi S, Lee N, et al. Association of female sex and heart rate with increased arterial stiffness in patients with type 2 diabetes mellitus. Anatol J Cardiol. 2017;18(5):347–52. https://doi.org/10.14744/AnatolJCardiol.2017.7773.
33. Palatini P, Mos L, Santonastaso M, Zanatta N, Mormino P, Saladini F, et al. Resting heart rate as a predictor of body weight gain in the early stage of hypertension. Obesity (Silver Spring). 2011;19(3):618–23. https://doi.org/10.1038/oby.2010.191.
34. Palatini P, Longo D, Zaetta V, Perkovic D, Garbelotto R, Pessina AC. Evolution of blood pressure and cholesterol in stage 1 hypertension: role of autonomic nervous system activity. J Hypertens. 2006 Jul;24(7):1375–81. https://doi.org/10.1097/01.hjh.0000234118.25401.1c.

35. Palatini P, Majahalme S, Amerena J, Nesbitt S, Vriz O, Michieletto M, et al. Determinants of left ventricular structure and mass in young subjects with sympathetic over-activity. The Tecumseh Offspring Study. J Hypertens. 2000;18(6):769–75. https://doi.org/10.1097/00004872-200018060-00016.
36. Lantelme P, Milon H, Gharib C, Gayet C, Fortrat JO. White coat effect and reactivity to stress: cardiovascular and autonomic nervous system responses. Hypertension. 1998;31:1021–9. https://doi.org/10.1161/01.hyp.31.4.1021.
37. Mahley RW, Weisgraber KH, Farese RV. Disorders of lipid metabolism. In: Wilson JD, editor. Williams textbook of endocrinology. Philadelphia: Saunders; 1996. p. 109–1153.
38. Arner P, Wahrenberg H, Lönnqvist F, Angelin B. Adipocyte beta-adrenoceptor sensitivity influences plasma lipid levels. Aterioscler Thromb Vasc Biol. 1993;13:967–72. https://doi.org/10.1161/01.atv.13.7.967.
39. Saladini F, Palatini P. Arterial distensibility, physical activity and the metabolic syndrome. Curr Hypertens Rep. 2018;20(5):39. https://doi.org/10.1007/s11906-018-0837-3.
40. Van den Munckhof ICL, Holewijn S, de Graaf J, et al. Sex differences in fat distribution influence the association between BMI and arterial stiffness. J Hypertens. 2017;35:1219–25. https://doi.org/10.1097/HJH.0000000000001297.
41. Williams B, Mancia G, Spiering W, Agabiti Rosei E, Azizi M, Burnier M, et al. 2018 ESC/ESH guidelines for the management of arterial hypertension. Eur Heart J. 2018;39(33):3021–104. https://doi.org/10.1093/eurheartj/ehy339.
42. Whelton PK, Carey RM, Aronow WS, Casey DE Jr, Collins KJ, Dennison Himmelfarb C, et al. 2017 ACC/AHA/AAPA/ABC/ACPM/AGS/APhA/ASH/ASPC/NMA/PCNA guideline for the prevention, detection, evaluation, and Management of High Blood Pressure in adults: a report of the American College of Cardiology/American Heart Association task force on clinical practice guidelines. Hypertension. 2018;71(6):e13–e115. https://doi.org/10.1161/HYP.0000000000000065.
43. American Diabetes Association. Standards of medical Care in Diabetes-2016. Diabetes Care. 2016;39(Suppl. 1):S1–S111.
44. Fihn SD, Blankenship JC, Alexander KP, Bittl JA, Byrne JG, Fletcher BJ, et al. 2014 ACC/AHA/AATS/PCNA/SCAI/STS focused update of the guideline for the diagnosis and management of patients with stable ischemic heart disease: a report of the American College of Cardiology/American Heart Association Task Force on Practice Guidelines, and the American Association for Thoracic Surgery, Preventive Cardiovascular Nurses Association, Society for Cardiovascular Angiography and Interventions, and Society of Thoracic Surgeons. J Am Coll Cardiol. 2014;64:1929–49. https://doi.org/10.1016/j.jacc.2014.07.017.
45. Cornelissen VA, Smart NA. Exercise training for blood pressure: a systematic review and meta-analysis. J Am Heart Assoc. 2013;2:e004473. https://doi.org/10.1161/JAHA.112.004473.
46. Leitzmann MF, Park Y, Blair A, Ballard-Barbash R, Mouw T, Hollenbeck AR, et al. Physical activity recommendations and decreased risk of mortality. Arch Intern Med. 2007;167:2453–60. https://doi.org/10.1001/archinte.167.22.2453.
47. Rossi A, Dikareva A, Bacon SL, Daskalopoulou SS. The impact of physical activity on mortality in patients with high blood pressure: a systematic review. J Hypertens. 2012;30:1277–88. https://doi.org/10.1097/HJH.0b013e3283544669.
48. Palatini P, Graniero G, Mormino P, Nicolosi L, Mos L, Visentin P, et al. Relation between physical training and ambulatory blood pressure in stage I hypertensive subjects. Results of the HARVEST trial. Circulation. 1994;90:2870–6. https://doi.org/10.1161/01.cir.90.6.2870.
49. Cornelissen VA, Fagard RH. Effects of endurance training on blood pressure, blood pressure-regulating mechanisms, and cardiovascular risk factors. Hypertension. 2005;46:667–75. https://doi.org/10.1161/01.HYP.0000184225.05629.51.
50. Fagard RH. Exercise therapy in hypertensive cardiovascular disease. Prog Cardiovasc Dis. 2011;53:404–11. https://doi.org/10.1016/j.pcad.2011.03.006.
51. Saladini F, Benetti E, Mos L, Mazzer A, Casiglia E, Palatini P. Regular physical activity is associated with improved small artery distensibility in young to middle-age stage 1 hypertensives. Vasc Med. 2014;19:458–64. https://doi.org/10.1177/1358863X14556852.

52. Nettlefold L, McKay HA, Naylor PJ, Bredin SS, Warburton DE. The relationship between objectively measured physical activity, sedentary time, and vascular health in children. Am J Hypertens. 2012;25:914–9. https://doi.org/10.1038/ajh.2012.68.
53. McGavock JM, Anderson TJ, Lewanczuk RZ. Sedentary lifestyle and antecedents of cardiovascular disease in young adults. Am J Hypertens. 2006;19:701–7. https://doi.org/10.1016/j.amjhyper.2006.01.013.
54. Saladini F, Mos L, Fania C, Garavelli G, Casiglia E, Palatini P. Regular physical activity prevents development of hypertension in young people with hyperuricemia. J Hypertens. 2017;35(5):994–1001. https://doi.org/10.1097/HJH.0000000000001271.
55. Tan I, Spronck B, Kiat H, Barin E, Resnik KD, Delhaas T, et al. Heart rate dependency of large artery stiffness. Hypertension. 2016;68:236–42. https://doi.org/10.1161/HYPERTENSIONAHA.116.07462.
56. Tomiyama H, Hashimoto H, Tanaka H, Matsumoto C, Odaira M, Yamada J, et al. Synergistic relationship between changes in the pulse wave velocity and changes in the heart rate in middle-aged Japanese adults: a prospective study. J Hypertens. 2010;28:687–94. https://doi.org/10.1097/HJH.0b013e3283369fe8.
57. Benetos A, Adamopoulos C, Bureau JM, Temmar M, Labat C, Bean K, et al. Determinants of accelerated progression of arterial stiffness in normotensive subjects and in treated hypertensive subjects over a 6-year period. Circulation. 2002;105:1202–7. https://doi.org/10.1161/hc1002.105135.
58. Wilkinson IB, Mohammad NH, Tyrrell S, Hall IR, Webb DJ, Paul VE, et al. Heart rate dependency of pulse pressure amplification and arterial stiffness. Am J Hypertens. 2002;15:24–30. https://doi.org/10.1016/s0895-7061(01)02252-x.
59. Courand PY, Lantelme P. Significance, prognostic value and management of heart rate in hypertension. Arch Cardiovasc Dis. 2014;107:48–57. https://doi.org/10.1016/j.acvd.2013.11.003.
60. Messerli FH, Rimoldi SF, Bangalore S, Bavishi C, Laurent S. When an increase in central systolic pressure overrides the benefits of heart rate lowering. J Am Coll Cardiol. 2016;68:754–62. https://doi.org/10.1016/j.jacc.2016.03.610.
61. Palatini P, Saladini F, Mos L, Fania C, Mazzer A, Casiglia E. Low night-time heart rate is longitudinally associated with lower augmentation index and central systolic blood pressure in hypertension. Eur J Appl Physiol. 2018;118:543–50. https://doi.org/10.1007/s00421-017-3789-4.
62. Palatini P, Canali C, Graniero GR, Rossi G, de Toni R, Santonastaso M, et al. Relationship of plasma renin activity with caffeine intake and physical training in mild hypertensive men. Eur J Epidemiol. 1996;12(5):485–91. https://doi.org/10.1007/BF00144001.
63. Fagard R, Grauwels R, Groeseneken D, Lijnen P, Staessen J, Vanhees L, et al. Plasma levels of renin, angiotensin II and 6-ketoprostaglandin F1 α in endurance athletes. J Appl Physiol. 1985;59:947–52. https://doi.org/10.1152/jappl.1985.59.3.947.
64. Jennings G, Nelson L, Nestel P, Esler M, Korner P, Burton D, et al. The effects of changes in physical activity on major cardiovascular risk factors, hemodynamics, sympathetic function and glucose utilization in man: a controlled study of four levels of activity. Circulation. 1986;73:30–40. https://doi.org/10.1161/01.cir.73.1.30.
65. Dao HH, McMartens F, Zaor A, de Champlain J, Moreau P. Role of endothelin in the hypertrophic remodeling of small arteries induced by exogenous norepinephrine. Arch Mal Coeur Vaiss. 1999;92:1059–62.
66. Green DJ. Exercise training as vascular medicine: direct impacts on the vasculature in humans. Exerc Sport Sci Rev. 2009;37:196–202. https://doi.org/10.1097/JES.0b013e3181b7b6e3.
67. Maeda S, Sugawara J, Yoshizawa M, Otsuki T, Shimojo N, Jesmin S, et al. Involvement of endothelin-1 in habitual exercise-induced increase in arterial compliance. Acta Physiol (Oxf). 2009;196:223–9. https://doi.org/10.1111/j.1748-1716.2008.01909.x.
68. Green DJ, Maiorana A, O'Driscoll G, Taylor R. Effect of exercise training on endothelium-derived nitric oxide function in humans. J Physiol. 2004;561:1–25. https://doi.org/10.1113/jphysiol.2004.068197.

69. Taddei S, Galetta F, Virdis A, Ghiadoni L, Salvetti G, Franzoni F, et al. Physical activity prevents age-related impairment in nitric oxide availability in elderly athletes. Circulation. 2000;101:2896–901. https://doi.org/10.1161/01.cir.101.25.2896.
70. Eskurza I, Monahan KD, Robinson JA, Seals DR. Effect of acute and chronic ascorbic acid on flow-mediated dilatation with sedentary and physically active human ageing. J Physiol. 2004;556:315–24. https://doi.org/10.1113/jphysiol.2003.057042.
71. Tolezani EC, Costa-Hong V, Correia G, Mansur AJ, Drager LF, Bortolotto LA. Determinants of functional and structural properties of large arteries in healthy individuals. Arq Bras Cardiol. 2014;103:426–32. https://doi.org/10.5935/abc.20140124.
72. Pasha EP, Birdsill AC, Oleson S, Haley AP, Tanaka H. Physical activity mitigates adverse effect of metabolic syndrome on vessels and brain. Brain Imaging Behav. 2018;12(6):1658–68. https://doi.org/10.1007/s11682-018-9830-3.
73. Bohn L, Ramoa A, Silva G, Silva N, Abreu SM, Ribeiro F, et al. Sedentary behavior and arterial stiffness in adults with and without metabolic syndrome. Int J Sports Med. 2017;38:396–401. https://doi.org/10.1055/s-0043-101676.
74. Tanabe Y, Nakata Y, Zempo-Miyaki A, Hieda MY, Choi Y, Fujii N, et al. Different degree of intervention in 6-month weight-loss support and arterial stiffness: secondary analysis of a randomized controlled trial. Obes Res Clin Pract. 2021;15(1):93–5. https://doi.org/10.1016/j.orcp.2020.11.006.
75. Pekas EJ, Shin J, Son WM, Headid RJ 3rd, Park SY. Habitual combined exercise protects against age-associated decline in vascular function and lipid profiles in elderly postmenopausal women. Int J Environ Res Public Health. 2020;17(11):3893. https://doi.org/10.3390/ijerph17113893.
76. Hage FG. C-reactive protein and hypertension. J Hum Hypertens. 2014;28:410–5. https://doi.org/10.1038/jhh.2013.111.
77. Campbell PT, Campbell KL, Wener MH, Wood BL, Potter JD, McTiernan A, et al. A yearlong exercise intervention decreases CRP among obese postmenopausal women. Med Sci Sports Exerc. 2009;41:1533–9. https://doi.org/10.1249/MSS.0b013e31819c7feb.
78. Koskinen J, Magnussen CG, Taittonen L, Räsänen L, Mikkilä V, Laitinen T, et al. Arterial structure and function after recovery from the metabolic syndrome: the cardiovascular risk in young Finns study. Circulation. 2010;121:392–400. https://doi.org/10.1161/CIRCULATIONAHA.109.894584.

10 Effect of Exercise Training on Clinical Outcomes in Patients with Diabetes

Angelo Avogaro

10.1 Introduction

Type 2 diabetes mellitus (DM2) is a common metabolic disorder worldwide and it is principally determined by the combination of defective insulin secretion by the pancreatic β-cells and insulin resistance, that is, the inability of insulin-sensitive tissues to respond to insulin. Nonetheless, the pathophysiology of DM2 is far more complex and several organs and systems may contribute to the disease. Conversely, in type 1 diabetes (DM1) there is a complete insulin deficiency due to autoimmune-driven destruction of the β-cells: insulin resistance may or may not be present.

The hallmark of diabetes is hyperglycemia that leads to long-term microvascular complications such as retinopathy, chronic kidney disease, and neuropathy. However, notably in DM2, a more widespread metabolic derangement including chronic subclinical inflammation, hypertension, and obesity is frequently present: their combination along with hyperglycemia leads to macrovascular complications. Patients with DM2 have from two- to threefold increased risk of coronary heart disease, ischemic stroke, and other vascular disease-related deaths. Once prediabetes and DM are identified, a lifestyle modification should be applied: in this context physical activity is of paramount importance [1].

10.2 The Priceless Value of Exercise in Diabetes Prevention

High-caloric diets lead to an imbalance between caloric intake and consumption, thus contributing to a progressive weight gain. Although weight gain is the most important and phenotypically detectable effect, the intake of large amounts of fats

A. Avogaro (✉)
Department of Medicine, The University of Padova, Padua, Italy
e-mail: angelo.avogaro@unipd.it

P. Palatini et al. (eds.), *Exercise, Sports and Hypertension*, Updates in Hypertension and Cardiovascular Protection,
https://doi.org/10.1007/978-3-031-07958-0_10

and carbohydrates induces a surge of both reactive oxygen species (ROS) and of inflammatory molecules, which beget insulin resistance and beta-cell dysfunction. Once weight gain eventually results in obesity, there is a substantial risk of DM2: obesity is the strongest risk factor for DM2 and is associated with insulin resistance [2]. Therefore, exercise is of paramount importance for diabetes prevention: the incidence of DM2 is inversely correlated to physical activity [3]. Warburton and colleagues showed an inverse relationship between exercise and DM2 incidence; the most active participants to exercise had a 42% risk reduction than the least active [4]. It has been shown a dose–response relationship between exercise intensity and incidence of DM2: Manson and colleagues showed that women who had at least a weekly vigorous exercise had a 16% reduced risk of developing DM2 when controlled for age and body mass index [5]. In Hu and associates in the Nurses' Health Study demonstrated a 34% reduction in diabetes incidence for each hour per day of brisk walking [6].

In the Henry Ford Exercise Testing Project, people who achieved ≥12 metabolic equivalents (METs) had a 54% lower risk of incident DM2 compared to people achieving <6 METs (controlled for multiple variables). In men with cardiorespiratory fitness levels greater than 31.0 mL of oxygen per kilogram per minute who exercised at moderate intensity (>5.5 METs) for more than 40 min/week, there was a decreased incidence of DM2 [7].

The Diabetes Prevention Program (DPP) Intensive Lifestyle showed that there was a 16% reduction in diabetes risk per kilogram of weight loss among people allocated to the intensive lifestyle intervention arm [8]. A relationship between exercise dose, weight status, and diabetes incidence, was observed in a systematic review that showed positive biological interaction on an additive scale [9]. This observation was further shown in a meta-analysis of 9 prospective cohort studies by Cloostermans et al., where there was a 7.4-fold increased risk of T2D in those who were obese and with a low physical activity level when compared to normal weight, highly active individuals [10].

In DPP, those who met the physical activity goal (150 min of moderate-intensity activity/week) had a 46% reduction in diabetes incidence, despite not always meeting weight loss goals. This effect was similarly seen in other international studies when intensive lifestyle intervention was used for the prevention of diabetes. In the Da Qing IGT and Diabetes Study, a reduction was observed in the incidence of diabetes by 33% in the diet-only group, 47% in the exercise-only group, and 38% in the diet-plus-exercise group, underlining the paramount importance of exercise in DM2 prevention [11].

Physical activity can dramatically improve also cardiovascular risk factors associated with prediabetes and diabetes. In the DPP, patients who received intensive lifestyle intervention had decreased blood pressure, LDL cholesterol, and triglyceride levels compared to the metformin-treated and placebo groups after 5 years. Improved fitness had a favorable effect on HbA1c, and HDL, triglycerides, and diastolic blood pressure, beyond the effect of weight change. Indeed, a sedentary lifestyle is a powerful risk factor for DM2: walking 2–3 h a week or at least 40 min a week reduces the risk of conversion to DM2 by more than 30% [12]. For this very reason, weight loss is a cornerstone therapy both to prevent and to normalize glucose concentration. Moreover, there is no antidiabetic treatment that can be successful over time if a regular lifestyle is not thoroughly implemented in patients with DM2. This is true not only for DM2 but also for DM1. Although it has been the established exercise is a hallmark of treatment as defined by the 2021 Standards of Medical Care in Diabetes, up to 40% of patients with DM2 are physically inactive (<10 min/week of moderate or vigorous activity within work, transportation, or leisure time) [13].

10.3 The Inestimable Value of Exercise in Diabetes Management

Exercise has multiple, positive effects in patients with DM, both type 1 and type 2 (Fig. 10.1). Exercise improves insulin action with a consequent increase in glucose uptake by peripheral insulin-sensitive tissues. Muscle contraction itself and the contraction-mediated skeletal muscle blood flow leads to glucose uptake via insulin-dependent and independent mechanisms: contraction stimulates glucose transporter (GLUT4) and their translocation on cell membrane stimulates facilitated transport of glucose into the muscle [14]. There are other several relevant and positive effects of exercise in patients with DM. Endurance training stimulates the oxidation of dietary fatty acids and increases intramuscular triacylglycerol turnover. An important role of exercise-mediated perturbations is mediated by interleukin-6 (IL-6) released in response to exercise: this cytokine stimulates the mobilization of

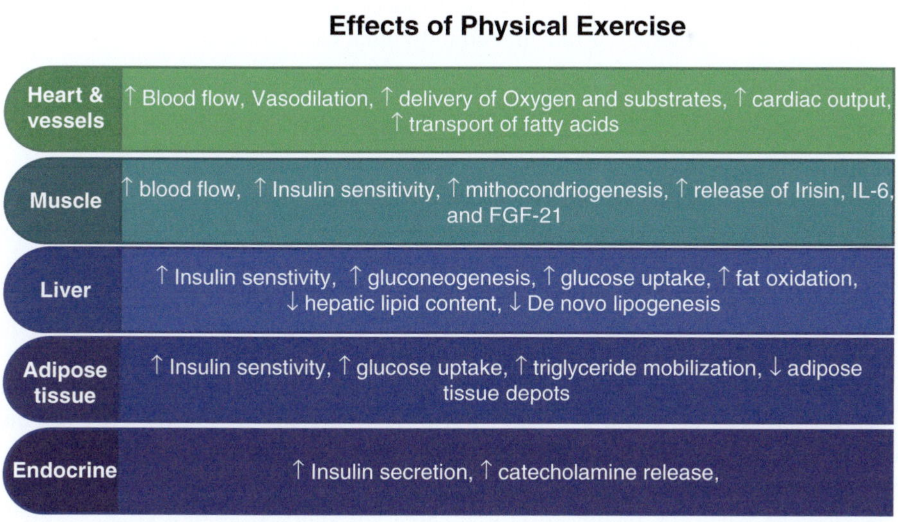

Fig. 10.1 The numerous systemic effects of exercise. (*IL-6* interleukin-6, *FGF-21* fibroblast growth factor-21)

intramuscular triacylglycerol, fatty acid oxidation, translocation of GLUT4 from the cytosol to the membrane, and ameliorates skeletal muscle insulin sensitivity [15].

Exercise increases the mobilization of hepatic glycogen into plasma, followed by increased rates of gluconeogenesis: as a consequence, there is an increased uptake of the gluconeogenic precursors such as lactate, pyruvate, glycerol. The liver also produces ketones, which can be oxidized in the presence of relative insulin deficiency such as during a low-carbohydrate diet. During exercise, in the adipose tissue, and increased mobilization of FFA is observed because of increased release of catecholamines, via sympathetic nervous system activation [16]. Interestingly, exercise activates significant muscle-adipose tissue crosstalk: the former releases IL-6, fibroblast growth factor (FGF)-21, and irisin that can modify adipose tissue metabolism, oxidative capacity, and glucose uptake [17]. Insulin secretion is also altered by exercise: one bout of exercise can lower insulin secretion, showing that insulin secretion is tightly regulated by exercise-driven pathways and contraction can facilitate glucose entry into muscle independently of insulin [18].

Notably, resistance exercise tends to acutely increase blood glucose, whereas aerobic exercise causes a larger initial decrease in blood glucose [19]. Thus, it is not clear which type of exercise is best for patients with DM: physical activity guidelines suggest the combination of resistance and aerobic activity. In one randomized control trial of sedentary individuals with T2D, a combination of aerobic and resistance training for 9 months significantly lowered HgbA1c levels compared to a nonexercise control group [20]. Similarly, high-intensity interval training (HIIT) session (10 min of intense exercise) reduces postprandial hyperglycemia in patients with DM2 [21]. At the same time, any type of exercise is beneficial. Individuals with T2D who engage in exercise have a decrease in HgbA1c by 0.67%, regardless of the type of exercise (structured aerobic, resistance, or combined exercise training): therefore, the best therapy is one that an individual can maintain.

10.4 Exercise on Diabetes Outcomes

The Look AHEAD (Action for Health in Diabetes) examined whether an intensive lifestyle intervention for weight loss would decrease cardiovascular morbidity and mortality among patients with DM2 overweight or obese [22]. Eligible patients were randomly assigned to participate in an intensive lifestyle intervention aimed at achieving and maintaining weight loss of at least 7% by focusing on reduced caloric intake and increased physical activity or to receive diabetes support and education. Specific intervention strategies included a calorie goal of 1200–1800 kcal/day (with <30% of calories from fat and >15% from protein), the use of meal-replacement products, and at least 175 min of moderate-intensity physical activity/week. Unfortunately, the trial was stopped early based on a futility analysis when the median follow-up was 9.6 years, despite a greater weight loss in the intervention group, a greater reduction in glycated hemoglobin, and a greater initial improvement in fitness and all cardiovascular risk factors, except for low-density–lipoprotein cholesterol levels. The primary outcome occurred in 403 patients in the intervention group and 418 in the control group (HR in the intervention group, 0.95; 95% confidence interval, 0.83–1.09; $p = 0.51$).

Notably, investigators of the study examined whether the incidence of cardiovascular disease in Look AHEAD varied by changes in weight or fitness. Individuals who lost at least 10% of their body weight in the first year of the study had a 21% lower risk of the primary outcome (adjusted HR 0.79, 95% CI 0.64–0.98; $p = 0.034$) [23]. Blomster and colleagues analyzed the effect of physical activity, categorized as none, mild, moderate, or vigorous, and the number of sessions within a week in 11,140 patients from the ADVANCE (Action in Diabetes and Vascular Disease: Preterax and Diamicron modified release Controlled Evaluation) trial [24]. They found that, compared to patients who undertook no or mild physical activity, those reporting moderate to vigorous activity had a 28% decreased risk for cardiovascular events, 15% for microvascular events, and 17% for all-cause mortality.

Observational studies have shown an inverse linear dose–response relationship between physical activity amount and mortality [25]. Exercise capacity can also predict mortality in people with DM [26]. Conversely, a reduced exercise capacity in people with DM2 is associated with the development of future cardiovascular events. Complications are positively affected by exercise: men with DM1 and with a history of higher levels of physical activity had a lower prevalence of nephropathy and neuropathy [27]. In the Finish Diabetic Nephropathy (FinnDiane) Study, low intensity of self-reported leisure-time physical activity in DM1 was associated with a greater degree of renal dysfunction, proteinuria, CVD, and retinopathy [28]. Bohn et al. also found an inverse relationship between physical activity level and both retinopathy and microalbuminuria in people with DM1 [29].

10.5 Exercise and Diabetes: What the Guidelines Say

Aerobic training such as running, jogging, brisk walking, swimming, and cycling increase mitochondrial density, insulin sensitivity, the reactivity of blood vessels, and cardiopulmonary fitness. Exercise does improve some parameters that are frequently altered in patients with DM2 such as muscular strength. Resistance training improves muscle mass, body composition, strength, physical function, mental health, bone mineral density, insulin sensitivity, blood pressure, lipid profiles, and cardiovascular health [30]. Resistance exercise can also minimize the risk of exercise-induced hypoglycemia in patients with DM1: in this context, if performed together, performing resistance exercise first results in less hypoglycemia than vice versa. Resistance exercise (free weights or weight machines) increases strength in adults with DM2 by about 50% and improves HbA1c by 0.57% [31]. Exercise should not always be seen as strenuous, problematic, and cumbersome obligation but it can also be part of small changes in daily life: as an example, prolonged sitting interrupted by brief (#5 min) bouts of standing every 20–30 min, improves glycemic control in sedentary overweight/obese [32]. Interrupting prolonged sitting with 15 min of postmeal walking and with 3 min of light walking improves glycemic control. Homemade calisthenic exercise can increase strength, flexibility, and overall fitness [33]. Unfortunately, the glycemic response to exercise is not uniform and cannot be uniformly predicted: this depends also on the amount and the timing of carbohydrate ingested before the exercise, by the type of exercise, and by the type of antidiabetic treatment. For these reasons, blood glucose concentrations should always be checked before exercise is undertaken, especially in patients with DM1. The target range for blood glucose before exercise should ideally be between 90 and 250 mg/dL (Fig. 10.2). Of paramount importance reductions in basal and/or bolus insulin doses should always be considered before exercising. The use of continuous glucose monitoring (CGM) may help patients to determine the glycemic response for a given type and intensity of exercise for a given baseline glucose level [32].

Therefore, the American Diabetes Association Guidelines endorse aerobic activity bouts that should ideally last at least 10 min, with the goal of 30 min/day or more, most days of the week for adults with DM2. If possible, activities should increase in intensity, frequency, and/or duration to at least 150 min/week of moderate-intensity exercise. Low-volume HIIT (short bursts of very intense activity interspersed with longer periods of recovery at low to moderate intensity) is an alternative approach to continuous aerobic activity. For resistance exercise training, adults with diabetes should engage in a minimum of 2 nonconsecutive days/week, but preferably 3 (Fig. 10.3). It has been shown that nonexercise activity thermogenesis (NEAT), the energy required for activities other than sleeping, eating, or sports-like exercise, is of great importance in determining weight loss. NEAT reduces total

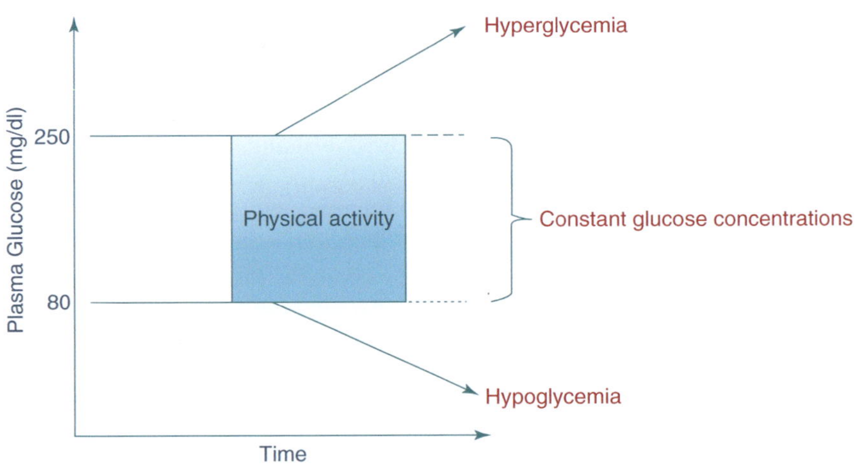

Fig. 10.2 The glycemic responses to exercise according to the baseline glucose concentrations

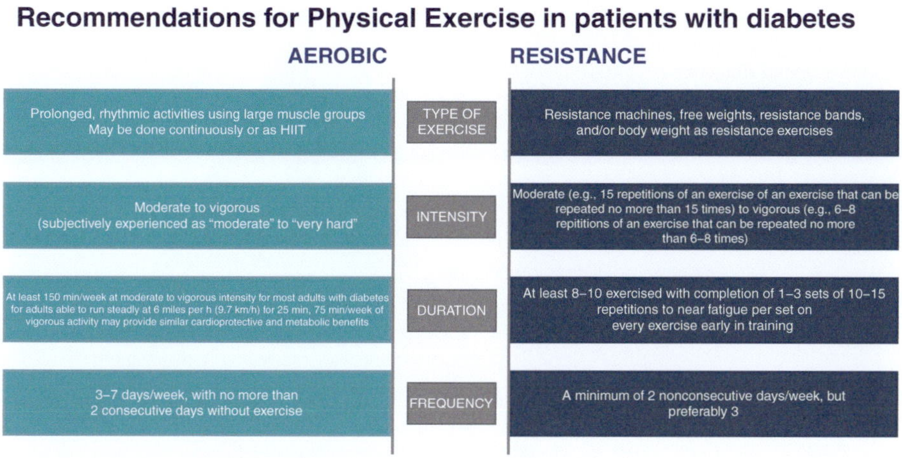

Fig. 10.3 American Diabetes Association recommendations for physical exercise in patients with diabetes

daily sitting time. Increasing nonexercise activity, even in brief (3–15 min) bouts, is effective in acutely reducing postprandial hyperglycemia and improving glycemic control in those with diabetes.

10.6 Conclusions

The prescription of and adherence to physical exercise is of paramount importance in persons with either prediabetes or diabetes (Fig. 10.4), and in a hypothetical hierarchy is by far more important than the antidiabetic treatment. Physical activity is not only a part of the management of glycemic control and overall health but also allows for significant durability of antidiabetic therapies, which shortly fail without a significant lifestyle modification. Recommendations should be personalized to each patient and should be feasible: all persons should be encouraged to decrease the total amount of daily sedentary time along with proper consumption of an adequate amount of healthy food. Food quality should win over quantity; even little physical activity is better than nothing.

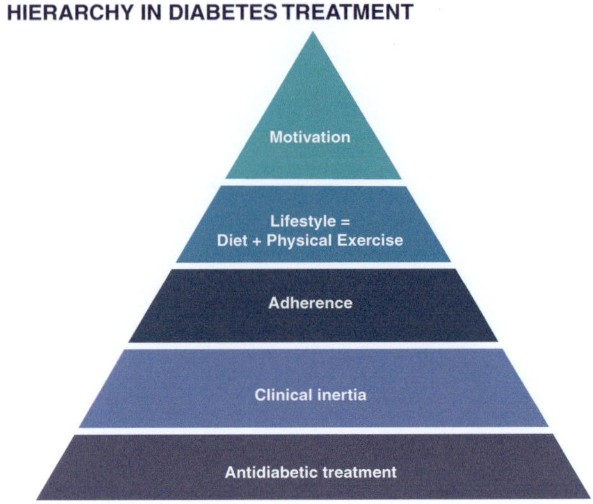

Fig. 10.4 The hierarchic importance of the different components of diabetes management

Acknowledgments None.

Funding None.

Author Contributions A.A. performed study design, data collection, analysis, manuscript writing, and revision.

Conflict of Interest A.A. received research grants, lecture or advisory board fees from: Merck Sharp & Dome, AstraZeneca, Novartis, Boehringer-Ingelheim, Sanofi, Mediolanum, Janssen, Novo Nordisk, Lilly, Servier, and Takeda.

Statement All human studies in the present review have been reviewed by the appropriate ethics committee and have therefore been performed in accordance with the ethical standards laid down in an appropriate version of the 1964 Declaration of Helsinki.

References

1. American Diabetes Association. 5. Lifestyle management: standards of medical care in diabetes-2019. Diabetes Care. 2019;42(Suppl 1):S46–60.
2. Inaishi J, Saisho Y. Beta-cell mass in obesity and type 2 diabetes, and its relation to pancreas fat: a mini-review. Nutrients. 2020;12(12):3846. https://doi.org/10.3390/nu12123846.
3. Teich T, Zaharieva DP, Riddell MC. Advances in exercise, physical activity, and diabetes mellitus. Diabetes Technol Ther. 2019;21(S1):S112–22. https://doi.org/10.1089/dia.2019.2509.
4. Warburton DE, Nicol CW, Bredin SS. Health benefits of physical activity: the evidence. CMAJ. 2006;174(6):801–9. https://doi.org/10.1503/cmaj.051351.
5. Manson JE, Nathan DM, Krolewski AS, Stampfer MJ, Willett WC, Hennekens CH. A prospective study of exercise and incidence of diabetes among US male physicians. JAMA. 1992;268(1):63–7.
6. Hu FB, Sigal RJ, Rich-Edwards JW, Colditz GA, Solomon CG, Willett WC, et al. Walking compared with vigorous physical activity and risk of type 2 diabetes in women: a prospective study. JAMA. 1999;282(15):1433–9. https://doi.org/10.1001/jama.282.15.1433.

7. Shaya GE, Juraschek SP, Feldman DI, Brawner CA, Ehrman JK, Keteyian SJ, et al. Relation of exercise capacity to risk of development of diabetes in patients on statin therapy (the Henry Ford Exercise Testing Project). Am J Cardiol. 2017;120(5):769–73. https://doi.org/10.1016/j.amjcard.2017.05.048.
8. Crandall JP, Knowler WC, Kahn SE, Marrero D, Florez JC, Bray GA, et al.; Diabetes Prevention Program Research Group. The prevention of type 2 diabetes. Nat Clin Pract Endocrinol Metab. 2008;4(7):382–93. https://doi.org/10.1038/ncpendmet0843
9. Aune D, Norat T, Leitzmann M, Tonstad S, Vatten LJ. Physical activity and the risk of type 2 diabetes: a systematic review and dose-response meta-analysis. Eur J Epidemiol. 2015;30(7):529–42. https://doi.org/10.1007/s10654-015-0056-z.
10. Cloostermans L, Wendel-Vos W, Doornbos G, Howard B, Craig CL, Kivimäki M, et al. Independent and combined effects of physical activity and body mass index on the development of Type 2 diabetes—a meta-analysis of 9 prospective cohort studies. Int J Behav Nutr Phys Act. 2015;12:147. https://doi.org/10.1186/s12966-015-0304-3.
11. Gong Q, Zhang P, Wang J, Ma J, An Y, Chen Y, et al.; Da Qing Diabetes Prevention Study Group. Morbidity and mortality after lifestyle intervention for people with impaired glucose tolerance: 30-year results of the Da Qing Diabetes Prevention Outcome Study. Lancet Diabetes Endocrinol. 2019;7(6):452–61. https://doi.org/10.1016/S2213-8587(19)30093-2
12. Hu FB. Sedentary lifestyle and risk of obesity and type 2 diabetes. Lipids. 2003;38(2):103–8. https://doi.org/10.1007/s11745-003-1038-4.
13. Cronin O, Keohane DM, Molloy MG, Shanahan F. The effect of exercise interventions on inflammatory biomarkers in healthy, physically inactive subjects: a systematic review. QJM. 2017;110(10):629–37. https://doi.org/10.1093/qjmed/hcx091.
14. Egan B, Zierath JR. Exercise metabolism and the molecular regulation of skeletal muscle adaptation. Cell Metab. 2013;17(2):162–84. https://doi.org/10.1016/j.cmet.2012.12.012.
15. Fischer CP. Interleukin-6 in acute exercise and training: what is the biological relevance? Exerc Immunol Rev. 2006;12:6–33.
16. Blum JW, Eichinger H. Epinephrine and norepinephrine related to cardiorespiratory and metabolic changes in calves during physical exercise. Horm Metab Res. 1988;20(12):738–42. https://doi.org/10.1055/s-2007-1010935.
17. Benedini S, Dozio E, Invernizzi PL, Vianello E, Banfi G, Terruzzi I, et al. Irisin: a potential link between physical exercise and metabolism—an observational study in differently trained subjects, from elite athletes to sedentary people. J Diabetes Res. 2017;2017:1039161. https://doi.org/10.1155/2017/1039161.
18. Holmstrup M, Fairchild T, Keslacy S, Weinstock R, Kanaley J. Multiple short bouts of exercise over 12-h period reduce glucose excursions more than an energy-matched single bout of exercise. Metabolism. 2014;63(4):510–9. https://doi.org/10.1016/j.metabol.2013.12.006.
19. Fry AC. The role of resistance exercise intensity on muscle fibre adaptations. Sports Med. 2004;34(10):663–79. https://doi.org/10.2165/00007256-200434100-00004.
20. Colberg SR, Sigal RJ, Yardley JE, Riddell MC, Dunstan DW, Dempsey PC, et al. Physical activity/exercise and diabetes: a position statement of the American Diabetes Association. Diabetes Care. 2016;39(11):2065–79. https://doi.org/10.2337/dc16-1728.
21. Jelleyman C, Yates T, O'Donovan G, Gray LJ, King JA, Khunti K, Davies MJ. The effects of high-intensity interval training on glucose regulation and insulin resistance: a meta-analysis. Obes Rev. 2015;16(11):942–61. https://doi.org/10.1111/obr.12317.
22. Look AHEAD Research Group, Wing RR, Bolin P, Brancati FL, Bray GA, Clark JM, Coday M, et al. Cardiovascular effects of intensive lifestyle intervention in type 2 diabetes. N Engl J Med. 2013;369(2):145–54. https://doi.org/10.1056/NEJMoa1212914. Erratum in: N Engl J Med. 2014;370(19):1866.
23. Look AHEAD Research Group, Gregg EW, Jakicic JM, Blackburn G, Bloomquist P, Bray GA, Clark JM, et al. Association of the magnitude of weight loss and changes in physical fitness with long-term cardiovascular disease outcomes in overweight or obese people with type 2 diabetes: a post-hoc analysis of the Look AHEAD randomised clinical trial. Lancet Diabetes Endocrinol. 2016;4(11):913–21. https://doi.org/10.1016/S2213-8587(16)30162-0

24. Blomster JI, Chow CK, Zoungas S, Woodward M, Patel A, Poulter NR, et al. The influence of physical activity on vascular complications and mortality in patients with type 2 diabetes mellitus. Diabetes Obes Metab. 2013;15(11):1008–12. https://doi.org/10.1111/dom.12122.
25. Mok A, Khaw KT, Luben R, Wareham N, Brage S. Physical activity trajectories and mortality: population based cohort study. BMJ. 2019;365:l2323. https://doi.org/10.1136/bmj.l2323.
26. Myers J, Prakash M, Froelicher V, Do D, Partington S, Atwood JE. Exercise capacity and mortality among men referred for exercise testing. N Engl J Med. 2002;346(11):793–801. https://doi.org/10.1056/NEJMoa011858.
27. Streckmann F, Zopf EM, Lehmann HC, May K, Rizza J, Zimmer P, et al. Exercise intervention studies in patients with peripheral neuropathy: a systematic review. Sports Med. 2014;44(9):1289–304. https://doi.org/10.1007/s40279-014-0207-5.
28. Wadén J, Tikkanen HK, Forsblom C, Harjutsalo V, Thorn LM, Saraheimo M, et al.; FinnDiane Study Group. Leisure-time physical activity and development and progression of diabetic nephropathy in type 1 diabetes: the FinnDiane study. Diabetologia. 2015;58(5):929–36. https://doi.org/10.1007/s00125-015-3499-6
29. Bohn B, Herbst A, Pfeifer M, Krakow D, Zimny S, Kopp F, et al.; DPV Initiative. Impact of physical activity on glycemic control and prevalence of cardiovascular risk factors in adults with Type 1 diabetes: a cross-sectional multicenter study of 18,028 patients. Diabetes Care. 2015;38(8):1536–43. https://doi.org/10.2337/dc15-0030
30. Mann S, Beedie C, Jimenez A. Differential effects of aerobic exercise, resistance training and combined exercise modalities on cholesterol and the lipid profile: review, synthesis and recommendations. Sports Med. 2014;44(2):211–21. https://doi.org/10.1007/s40279-013-0110-5.
31. Egger A, Niederseer D, Diem G, Finkenzeller T, Ledl-Kurkowski E, Forstner R, et al. Different types of resistance training in type 2 diabetes mellitus: effects on glycaemic control, muscle mass and strength. Eur J Prev Cardiol. 2013;20(6):1051–60. https://doi.org/10.1177/2047487312450132.
32. Houlder SK, Yardley JE. Continuous glucose monitoring and exercise in type 1 diabetes: past, present and future. Biosensors (Basel). 2018;8(3):73. https://doi.org/10.3390/bios8030073.
33. Edwardson CL, Henson J, Bodicoat DH, Bakrania K, Khunti K, Davies MJ, et al. Associations of reallocating sitting time into standing or stepping with glucose, insulin and insulin sensitivity: a cross-sectional analysis of adults at risk of type 2 diabetes. BMJ Open. 2017;7(1):e014267. https://doi.org/10.1136/bmjopen-2016-014267.

11 Effects of Physical Activity on Hypertension of Youth

Paolo Palatini

11.1 Introduction

A large number of factors leading to obesity and metabolic disturbances are responsible for the rise in the prevalence of hypertension among adolescents and young individuals [1]. Among these a major role is played by sedentary activities like watching TV or working on a computer which imply a noticeable reduction in time spent in physical activities. Thus, physical training would represent an ideal way to counter this unfavorable trend in youth to prevent development of hypertension and to decrease blood pressure (BP) in people with hypertension [2–4]. Particular attention should be addressed to young people with peculiar phenotypes, especially to subjects with isolated systolic hypertension (ISH) and hyperkinetic circulation whose pathogenetic and prognostic significance are still debated. These individuals are often characterized by abnormalities of the autonomic nervous system with elevation of heart rate, systolic BP, and cardiac output [5–10]. Training in endurance sports may counteract autonomic nervous system abnormalities and should thus be particularly beneficial in these patients [11, 12]. Indeed, regular physical activity is recommended for reducing BP in subjects with stage 1 hypertension before initiating drug therapy [13]. However, evidence that aerobic exercise may prevent cardiovascular complications in young hypertensive individuals is still scanty.

Another problem in young hypertensive people, chiefly in subjects with ISH, is that a pronounced white-coat effect is often present at BP measurement by the doctor [14]. To assess whether BP is really elevated, out-of-office measurement should always be performed in these individuals especially using ambulatory BP

P. Palatini (✉)
Department of Medicine, Studium Patavinum, University of Padova, Padova, Italy
e-mail: palatini@unipd.it

P. Palatini et al. (eds.), *Exercise, Sports and Hypertension*, Updates in Hypertension and Cardiovascular Protection,
https://doi.org/10.1007/978-3-031-07958-0_11

monitoring (ABPM). The prevalence of white-coat hypertension in adolescents and young individuals has been reported to be very high [15] and ABPM is very helpful for deciding whether eligibility to competitive athletics can be granted.

The main purpose of this chapter is to examine the effects of regular physical activity on resting BP, BP reactivity to stress, autonomic nervous system function, and subclinical organ damage in young subjects in the early stage of hypertension. Another purpose of this chapter is to highlight the mechanisms by which physical training can be beneficial in these subjects and to provide recommendations on the assessment of young people who wish to participate in competitive athletics.

11.2 Autonomic Nervous System Activity in Hypertension of the Young

A wealth of studies has documented that a high sympathetic tone may be present early in life in a large portion of the hypertensive population. This was observed long ago by Julius et al. [16, 17] who in the Tecumseh study found that a large portion of the hypertensive population had high heart rate, cardiac output and plasma norepinephrine. These findings were later confirmed in the young subjects from the Tecumseh Offspring Study, in which about 30% of the participants had sympathetic predominance on the basis of low-frequency (LF) and high-frequency (HF) components of heart rate variability [9]. Similar results were found in an analysis of the HARVEST Study, in which over one-third of the young participants had reduced heart rate variability and signs of sympathetic predominance [18]. Subjects with sympathetic predominance were more likely to develop obesity, hypertension and metabolic abnormalities during a 6-year follow-up compared to participants with normal sympathetic activity. Several different lines of research confirmed the above findings. Subjects with white-coat hypertension have abnormal autonomic cardiac regulation as shown by Fagard et al. [19] who found a greater LF–HF ratio in a group of white-coat hypertensives than in a group of normotensive subjects of control. Similar results were found by Mancia and Grassi [20] and by Grassi et al. [21] in studies performed with microneurographic assessment of sympathetic nerve traffic to skeletal muscle circulation. Also cardiovascular reactivity to stress has been found to be increased in young subjects with hypertension [22, 23]. To compare the BP response to doctor's visit with the BP reaction to a psychosocial challenge (public speaking) we studied 64 young stage-1 hypertensive subjects and 33 normotensive controls [24, 25]. The responses to BP measurement by a doctor and to public speaking were assessed with beat-to-beat Finapres recording. The hypertensive subjects hyperreactive to doctor's visit showed increased reactivity also to public speaking, while those with normal white-coat response had a response to the psychosocial challenge similar to that of the normotensive controls. Epinephrine urinary output was greater in the hyperreactive than the normoreactive subjects. In summary, an abnormal autonomic nervous system activity in the young is often associated with other cardiovascular risk factors, for example, fast heart rate, high total cholesterol, insulin resistance, and obesity [26], and may lead to development of cardiovascular complications.

11.3 Regular Physical Activity Improves Autonomic Nervous System Regulation

One of the main effects of endurance exercise on the cardiovascular system regulation is a reduction of the sympathetic tone accompanied by an increase in vagal activity [4]. These autonomic nervous system changes cause a beneficial effect on heart rate, BP, and metabolic syndrome components (see below) [4]. In addition, a reduction of BP reactivity to stressors has been described in physically active individuals [27]. Further evidence was provided in our laboratory in 75 sedentary and 44 active participants screened for stage 1 hypertension with consistent activity habits assessed with beat-to-beat noninvasive recording [28]. In agreement with previous observations, the BP response to public speaking was greater in the hypertensive than in 63 normotensive individuals of control. Sedentary hypertensive participants showed increased BP reactivity to the speech test (45/22 mmHg, $P < 0.01/<0.001$ versus controls), whereas physically active subjects had a response similar to that of normotensive controls (35/18 mmHg). During a median follow-up of 71 months, average 24-h BP did not virtually change in the active participants (−0.9/0.0 mmHg) whereas it increased significantly in their sedentary peers (2.8/3.2 mmHg, $P = 0.08/0.003$ versus active subjects). Active participants were less likely to develop incident hypertension than sedentary ones with a hazard ratio of 0.53 (95% confidence interval (CI), 0.31–0.94) for clinic hypertension and of 0.60 (95% CI, 0.37–0.99) for ambulatory hypertension. Admittedly, some studies showed no effect of physical activity on BP reactivity using other types of stress tests [27]. Inconsistencies among previous studies are likely to be due to the type of stressor employed by the investigators. BP reactivity in the laboratory is usually tested with mental arithmetic, Stroop color test, or mirror tracing, which elicit much weaker hemodynamic and sympathoadrenal medullary responses compared to psychosocial stressors [29].

The reason why regular aerobic exercise decreases reactivity to stressors is not obvious. According to the "cross-stressor adaptation" theory, adaptations to repeated bouts of exercise can also lead to adaptations to daily life stressors [11]. During mental stress, the increase in BP is primarily due to elevation in cardiac output suggesting that the BP response to stress is mediated by central neural modulation of the beta-adrenergic system [30]. Regular physical activity has been shown to modulate autonomic responses to stressors and to enhance baroreceptor sensitivity [30]. These changes can occur even after short periods of moderate-intensity aerobic exercise training [31]. Thus, to retard or even prevent hypertension and its complications, a program of physical activity should be implemented in young hypertensive subjects especially when signs of sympathetic predominance and/or increased reactivity to stressors is present.

11.4 Isolated Systolic Hypertension in the Athlete

Although ISH is the dominant form of hypertension in the elderly, in the last few decades there has been an increasing interest for ISH in the youth (ISHY). The prevalence of this subtype of hypertension is increasing within the last decades especially in young males [14, 15]. Whether ISHY is innocent or not has been the subject of much debate in recent years and two main hypotheses have been forwarded to explain its pathogenesis. According to some authors ISHY is a "spurious condition" caused by an elevated pulse pressure amplification and low wave arterial reflection from peripheral sites, due to increased arterial elasticity peculiar to young individuals [32–34]. ISHY is common in young athletes as a consequence of the progressive decrease in arterial diameter from the heart to the arm and the corresponding increase in arterial impedance [32, 33]. This results in central systolic BP being normal and much lower than brachial systolic BP and it is known that central BP is more strongly related to vascular and left ventricular hypertrophy (LVH) than is peripheral BP [35]. Another hemodynamic feature peculiar to athletes is a high resting stroke volume with low peripheral resistance and heart rate [36, 37]. This hemodynamic pattern is thus accompanied by a higher pulse pressure with a frequent presence of ISHY. Within the frame of the HARVEST study we found that the 6-year risk of hypertension in ISHY subjects with low central BP was similar to that in a group of normotensive controls [38]. ISHY subjects with high central BP had reduced large artery and small artery compliance, and increased total peripheral resistance compared to both the normotensive subjects of control and the ISHY subjects with low central BP. In a more recent analysis we found that young subjects with high pulse pressure had even a lower risk of developing cardiovascular complications than subjects with low pulse pressure [39]. The level of mean BP was crucial to predict the cardiovascular risk in this population.

In a recent unpublished analysis of our cohort (unpublished observations), we divided the HARVEST participants into four groups: normotensive subjects (NT), sedentary ISHY, physically active ISHY, and subjects with systolic-diastolic hypertension (SDH). Active ISHY had a higher stroke volume than the other three groups and lower peripheral resistance (Fig. 11.1). The hemodynamic characteristics of the sedentary ISHY did not differ from those of the SDH participants. After 8 years of follow-up, they had a marginal increase in body weight, lower than in the NT group, even though the difference was barely significant.

Overall, these findings suggest that in physically active people ISHY may be an innocent clinical condition and assessment of central systolic BP can be of help for distinguishing between truly hypertensive subjects and subjects with spurious hypertension. However, according to other authors ISHY is an abnormal condition characterized not only by increased stroke volume but also by early aortic stiffness [40, 41]. In some of the individuals with ISHY enrolled in the Enigma Study, aortic pulse wave velocity was found to be elevated, suggesting that ISHY may also be associated with premature aortic stiffening [41]. This led the Enigma investigators to conclude that ISHY has the same pathophysiological mechanism as ISH in older subjects and that young subjects with elevated pulse pressure and aortic stiffening

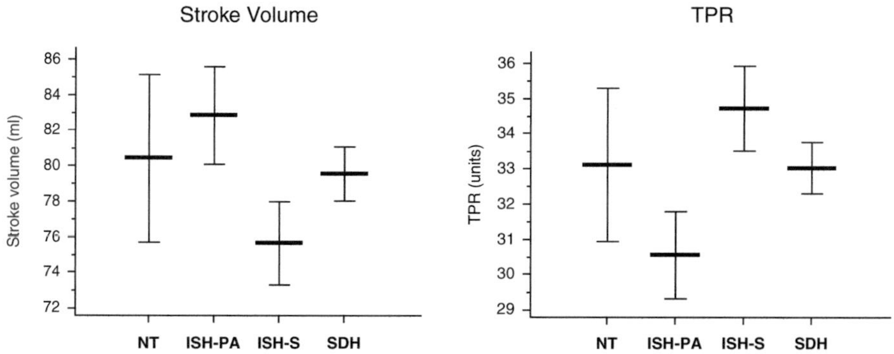

Fig. 11.1 Stroke volume and total peripheral resistance (TPR) in 829 young-to-middle-age stage 1 hypertensive subjects stratified according to hypertension subtype. The subjects with isolated systolic hypertension were further subdivided according to whether they were physically active (ISH-PA) or sedentary (ISH-S). Data are mean and 95% confidence interval. Stroke volume was higher (age-and-sex-adjusted p-value = 0.009) and TPR was lower (age-and-sex-adjusted p-value < 0.001) in ISH-PA than in the other three groups. *NT* indicates normotensive subjects, *SDH* subjects with systolic-diastolic hypertension

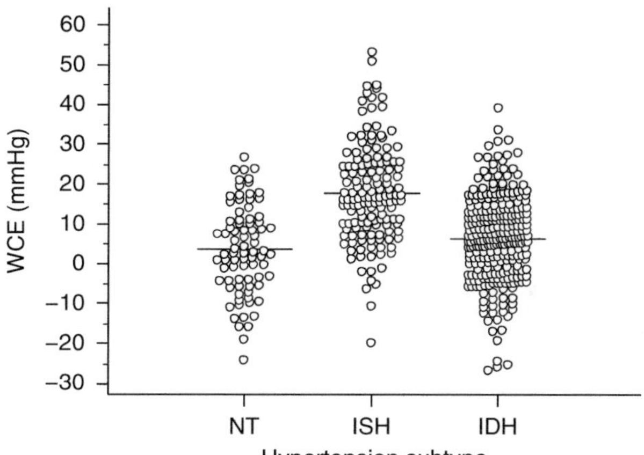

Fig. 11.2 White-coat effect (WCE) in three groups of young subjects with different hypertension subtype from the HARVEST study. The white-coat effect was calculated as the difference between systolic office blood pressure and average 24-h systolic blood pressure and was greater in the participants with isolated systolic hypertension (ISH) than in those with normotension (NT) or isolated diastolic hypertension (IDH) ($p < 0.001$ vs NT and IDH). Adapted from Ref 42

may be predisposed to sustained ISH in later life. In addition, obesity and metabolic disturbances have often been documented to be associated with ISHY both in children and young adults [14, 15]. According to a recent Consensus document endorsed by the European Society of Hypertension, ISHY is a heterogeneous condition [14]. One main confounding factor when assessing the predictive value of ISHY is the presence of a pronounced white-coat effect (Fig. 11.2) and the main prognostic

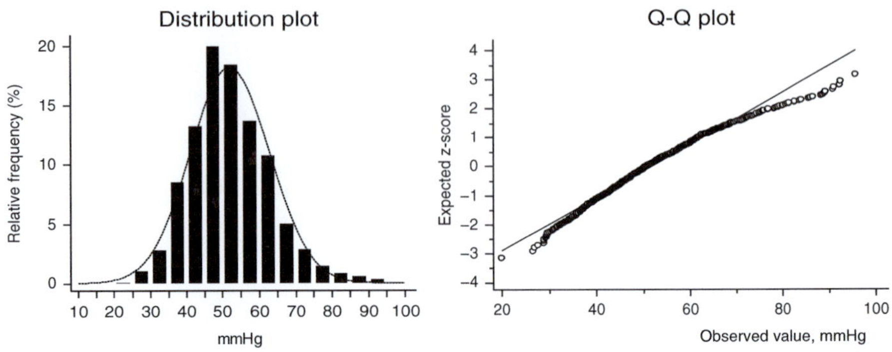

Fig. 11.3 Distribution plot (left panel) and Q-Q plot (right panel) for pulse pressure in 1206 participants from the HARVEST cohort. The distribution plot shows a clear asymmetry with a positive index of skewness (coefficient = 0.61, $p < 0.0001$). A clear departure from the comparison line occurs in the upper tail of the Q-Q plot. These features are typical for the existence of a subpopulation with high pulse pressure likely due to a pronounced white-coat effect

factor in the young-to-middle-age range is the level of ambulatory mean BP [42]. Indeed, the distribution of pulse pressure in the whole HARVEST population was clearly asymmetrical with a positive skewness probably due to the effect of a large alerting reaction in the participants with ISHY (Fig. 11.3).

11.5 Effects of Exercise on Blood Pressure and Metabolic Variables

The beneficial effect of physical activity on resting BP has been shown by a large number of studies [2, 4] and has been thoroughly reviewed in a chapter of this book. With a few exceptions, these studies have shown that physical training is effective in lowering BP levels. However, there is still debate on whether the BP decrease caused by regular physical activity is proportional to exercise intensity during training. A meta-analysis of previous studies suggests that optimal benefits can be achieved at moderate exercise intensities and some studies indicate that there is a U-shaped relationship between training and its BP lowering action [2]. Previous results from our laboratory have shown that in young hypertensive subjects performing light physical activities, ambulatory BP did not differ from that in sedentary subjects suggesting that the BP lowering effect of training does not occur in young hypertensive subjects for light physical activities [43]. Shedding light on this issue is not easy because in no study was there an equal distribution of the participants into different exercise intensity groups. In addition, the effect of age has been overlooked in most studies. In elderly subjects, who more often lead a totally sedentary life, implementing a program of light physical activity might well be more beneficial than in younger individuals [44].

A large number of studies have shown that aerobic physical activity can also reduce body weight and improve the metabolic profile [2, 4]. Regular exercise training can counterbalance the detrimental effects of the metabolic syndrome by reducing sympathetic activity and improving endothelial function. Thus, special attention should be paid by clinicians to people with metabolic syndrome in whom the adverse effect of metabolic disturbances on arterial structure and function can be offset by a program of physical training.

Elevated uric acid has often been found in hypertension in association with obesity and metabolic abnormalities and is considered an important predictor of cardiovascular events and mortality [45–47]. Recent results from the HARVEST have shown that exercise may counteract the pathophysiological mechanisms involved in the association between hyperuricemia and future hypertension [48]. The study was conducted in 1156 young to middle-age participants screened for stage 1 hypertension and followed for a median of 11.4 years. In the whole group, uric acid was an independent predictor of future hypertension. Participants in the upper uric acid tertile had a 31% increase in risk compared with those of the bottom tertile. However, the risk of hypertension was increased only among the sedentary participants with a hazard ratio of 1.44 (95% CI, 1.11–1.88) for the participants of the top uric acid tertile. In contrast, among the active participants no association was found between uric acid and risk of hypertension. Plasma renin activity was 33% lower in our active participants compared to their sedentary counterparts, and this effect could prevent one of the mechanisms for the uric acid–hypertension relationship. A greater insulin sensitivity, improvement of endothelial function, reduction of oxidative stress, and a lower sympathetic activity may have led to the prevention of hypertension in our active participants with hyperuricemia [4, 48, 49].

11.6 Effect of Regular Physical Activity on Hypertension-Mediated Organ Damage

11.6.1 Effect on the Heart

Increased left ventricular mass (LVM) has been shown to be an important predictor of cardiovascular events in hypertension [50]. There was thus concern that exercise in hypertensive individuals could facilitate the development of LVH as a result of the well-known association between physical training and LVM. However, a paradoxical effect of exercise on the heart, with a reduction of LVM, has been documented by Baglivo et al. in a group of middle-aged hypertensive subjects after 16 months of endurance exercise training [51]. In keeping with those results, Kokkinos et al. [52] in a group of African American men and Zanettini et al. [53] in patients with mildly elevated diastolic BP observed a reduction in LVM and wall thickness after a period of aerobic exercise. In contrast, no reduction of LVM was observed in overweight or obese individuals by Hinderliter et al. [54] and by Reid et al. [55].

In a cohort of young-to-middle-age hypertensive subjects we investigated the long-term association of regular physical activity with LVM during a median follow-up of 8.3 years [56]. Physically active subjects were less likely to develop LVH

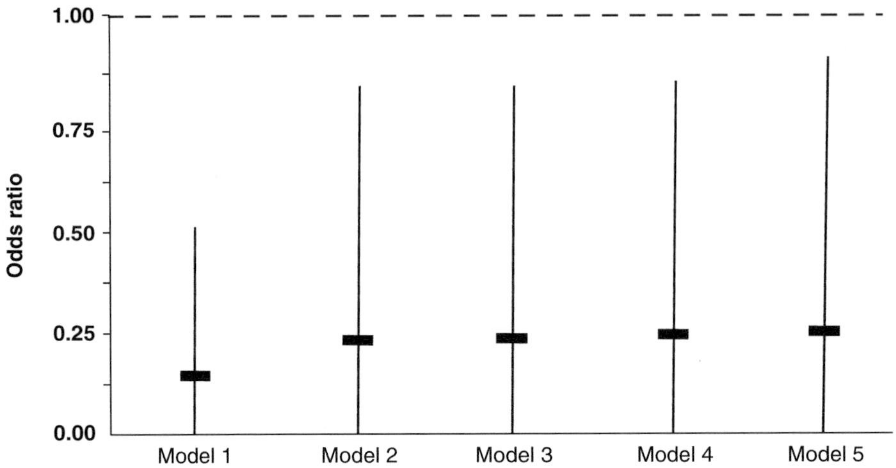

Fig. 11.4 Odds ratios and 95% confidence interval for development of left ventricular hypertrophy according to physical activity status in 454 HARVEST participants (active vs. sedentary). Results of different logistic models. Model 1. Unadjusted. Odds ratio, 0.15 (95%CI, 0.05–0.52), $p = 0.002$; Model 2. Adjusted for age, sex, BMI, systolic and diastolic blood pressure, hypertension duration, parental hypertension, follow-up length, smoking, alcohol, and coffee use. Odds ratio, 0.24 (95%CI, 0.07–0.85), $p = 0.027$; Model 3. Model 2 + baseline left ventricular mass index. Odds ratio, 0.24 (95%CI, 0.07–0.85), $p = 0.026$; Model 4. Model 3 + follow-up change in systolic and diastolic blood pressure. Odds ratio, 0.25 (95%CI, 0.07–0.87), $p = 0.029$; Model 5. Model 4 + follow-up change in body weight. Odds ratio, 0.26 (95%CI, 0.07–0.90), $p = 0.033$. Adapted from Ref 56

than their sedentary peers with an adjusted odds ratio of 0.24 (95%CI, 0.07–0.85). This difference remained significant after multiple adjustments including follow-up changes in BP and body weight (Fig. 11.4). In particular, no athlete developed LVH during the period of observation. Several mechanisms may account for the prevention of LVM growth in hypertensive patients performing aerobic sports. Among the hemodynamic factors, reductions in heart rate, BP, peripheral vascular resistance, blood volume and cardiac output may play a major role. Improved arterial elasticity, enhanced endothelial vasodilator function, suppression of the activity of the renin–angiotensin–aldosterone system, and reduction of insulin resistance are other factors known to occur after a program of physical activity and may be implicated in the cardiac effects [2, 4, 49]. The reduction of sympathetic nervous system activity is likely to be responsible for at least part of these changes. Cardioprotective effects of physical training have been documented also by animal studies [57].

From a diagnostic point of view, it is sometimes difficult for the clinician to establish whether LVH in a hypertensive athlete reflects the increased hemodynamic load or is a benign adaptation to physical training. Echocardiographic assessment of left ventricular structure and function is of great help for distinguishing between the two entities. Detection of left ventricular concentric remodeling, increased left atrial size, and left ventricular diastolic dysfunction suggests a hypertension-related LVH [58].

11.6.2 Effect on Carotid Intima–Media Thickness

Carotid intima–media thickness (IMT) is a good marker of atherosclerotic disease and a predictor of cardiovascular and cerebrovascular events in the general population and in hypertensive people [59]. This increase in risk has been detected also in young persons [60]. Indeed, subclinical atherosclerosis has been found in young subjects in the early stage of hypertension as shown by increased IMT in the common carotid artery, in the bulb, and in the internal carotid artery [60]. Data from the HARVEST have documented that mean-IMT and mean of maximum IMT increase to a greater degree in white-coat hypertensives and sustained hypertensives than in normotensives indicating that white-coat hypertension in the young is not an innocent condition [61].

Only a few studies did examine the effects of regular physical activity on carotid IMT providing conflicting results [62, 63]. Some investigators observed a reduced progression of carotid IMT after a program of physical activity whereas some others did not observe any beneficial effect. Lakka et al. did not find any relation between leisure physical activity and IMT progression in middle-aged Finnish men, though VO_2 max was found to have an inverse association with the increase in maximal IMT and mean IMT [64]. In contrast, other authors found an inverse relation between physical activity and progression of carotid IMT in middle-age people during a 3-year follow-up [65]. Accordingly, results from the HARVEST showed that cumulative maximum IMT of common carotid artery, carotid bulb, and internal carotid artery and cumulative mean IMT of the three segments increased to a greater degree in the sedentary than the active subjects during a 6.5 year follow-up, confirming that regular physical activity is inversely associated with the progression of subclinical atherosclerosis [66]. A favorable effect of exercise on the cardiovascular risk profile and carotid IMT has been found even in obese children [67].

Exercise training causes a greater BP reduction in hypertensive than normotensive individuals [2, 4] and thus physical activity may have a greater impact on the progression of subclinical atherosclerosis in hypertensive people. In the above mentioned HARVEST study [66] BP reduction and decrease in cholesterol explained 35% and 45%, respectively, of the effect of exercise on mean IMT progression. Reduction of heart rate accounted for 20% of its effect [66]. Also in the CARDIA study performed in young adults [68] the beneficial effects of exercise on IMT was mainly mediated by improvement of traditional risk factors.

11.6.3 Effect on Arterial Elasticity

Aerobic exercise has been found to reduce arterial stiffness not only in older adults but also in young and middle-age subjects [69, 70]. The association of physical activity with small artery elasticity in the early stage of hypertension was examined by our group in 366 young-to-middle-age stage 1 hypertensives divided into two categories of physical activity, sedentary (n = 264) and active (n = 102) subjects [71]. After 6 years of follow-up, arterial distensibility assessment was repeated in

151 subjects. After adjusting for age, sex, heart rate, smoking, and BP, small artery compliance was higher in active than in sedentary patients ($p = 0.008$). After 6 years of follow-up, an improvement in the augmentation index accompanied by a decline in total peripheral resistance was found in the active subjects. This association was independent of changes in BP and heart rate. Though not all studies provided consistent results, there is general agreement that regular aerobic exercise attenuates the age-related increase in arterial stiffness not only in older subjects but also in young and middle-age individuals.

11.7 Assessment of BP Response to Exercise

Although an increase in BP is a normal physiologic response during physical effort, an exaggerated BP response during exercise testing can be found also in normotensive subjects and is of difficult interpretation [72]. The exaggerated rise in exercise BP in normotensive subjects is thought to be due to a failure to reduce total peripheral resistance adequately during exercise, and be a marker of initial structural vascular changes which would predate the tonic elevation in BP [72]. Several prospective studies have demonstrated that excessive increases in BP during exercise may be a marker of future sustained hypertension and of increased risk of cardiovascular mortality [73–75]. Different diagnostic criteria have been used in the literature to define an exaggerated BP response to stress testing. Methodological differences between the various studies can account for these discrepancies, depending on whether the test was performed on a treadmill [76] or a bicycle ergometer [77], and the BP was measured at a moderate or a maximum level of exercise [78, 79]. In a study by Izaguirre et al., a maximum diastolic BP above 95 mmHg and systolic BP above 180 mmHg during an exercise test of up to 100 W were the best predictors of new-onset hypertension after 20 years of follow-up in healthy young individuals [80]. However, other authors identified cutoff points of more than 210/110 mmHg (men) or more than 190/110 mmHg (women) [81]. Age differences in the study populations could at least partially be responsible for these different cutoffs. A recent meta-analysis including 16 studies found an association of different categorical systolic BP cutoff points with new onset hypertension and mortality [79]. Another debated issue is the predictive capacity of exercise diastolic and systolic BP. Previous observations have shown that diastolic BP is a more useful predictor when BP is measured at peak exercise, whereas systolic BP is better related to future hypertension when measured during the early stages of effort irrespective of whether exercise was performed on a treadmill [82] or a bicycle [77]. One of the potential risks related to an exaggerated BP response to stress testing is that in the long run repetitive BP peaks triggered by physical activity may determine chronic target organ damage or favor the occurrence of an acute cardiovascular event. That is why special attention should be addressed by clinicians to athletes involved in competitions [72]. However, studies performed in young borderline hypertensive subjects have demonstrated that BP level during strenuous long-lasting exercise cannot be predicted by the maximum BP attained during a short-lasting incremental effort. In our laboratory we investigated two groups of normotensive and hypertensive young athletes during prolonged exercise to exhaustion [83]. A parallel rise in systolic BP was observed in the two groups only during the initial phase of exercise. Thereafter, there was a progressive BP decline throughout the rest of the test and the BP drop was larger among the hypertensive than the normotensive subjects. A weak relationship was found between BP at baseline and BP at peak exercise. Thus, our study showed that during a type of exercise simulating a true sport activity a smaller BP increase occurs in hypertensive than in normotensive subjects at peak exercise and that the BP level reached by a subject at peak exercise is not proportional to BP measured in resting conditions.

11.8 Eligibility for Competitive Athletics

The above findings underscore the beneficial effects of regular exercise in young to middle age subjects for the treatment of hypertension and prevention of its complications. However, caution should be used in subjects with hypertension especially in stages 2 and 3 of the disease. Identification of hypertension in athletes is important especially in the setting of preparticipation to competitions in order to implement appropriate nonpharmacological as well as pharmacological management and follow-up [84]. Recent recommendations for participation in competitive sports in athletes with arterial hypertension have been published by the European Association of Preventive Cardiology, representing the consensus of an international panel of experts [58]. Clinical history, physical examination, and subsequent diagnostic tests should be performed in order to exclude secondary causes, especially in young individuals. In addition, every hypertensive athlete should be thoroughly investigated to exclude target organ damage and coronary artery disease through a detailed examination. According to the European guidelines, in the athletic population the same procedures should be applied as in the general population [58]. In addition, echocardiography should be routinely performed to rule out myocardial hypertrophy or dysfunction or valvular disease. With this technique, increased left ventricular wall thickness and mass, concentric left ventricular hypertrophy, signs of impaired relaxation, and subclinical reduction in systolic function may be found, which may help to distinguish between hypertensive heart disease and the physiologic adaptations leading to athlete's heart. Concentric hypertrophy and/or impaired diastolic function are highly indicative of LV changes induced by hypertension. Also, recently published pediatric hypertension guidelines recommend that all youth with persistently elevated BP undergo echocardiography prior to athletic participation [85]. If LVH is detected youth should be restricted from heavy-resistance sports and have limited athletic participation until the BP has normalized. The American Academy of Pediatrics has recommended that hypertensive youth avoid all physical activities with a high isometric component, especially if the youth has LVH [86].

Exercise stress testing should also be performed in all young athletes to exclude coronary artery disease and excessive exercise hypertension (see above section). As mentioned above, unfortunately an abnormal BP response to exercise has not been clearly defined in the general population [78, 79]. In young elite athletes, a recent study has proposed limits of 220 mmHg in males and 200 mmHg in females [87]. However, according to the European guidelines in asymptomatic athletes with normal BP at rest, the BP values obtained during exercise cannot be used from a diagnostic or a therapeutic standpoint [58]. These subjects should perform periodical follow-ups without restriction from competitive sports [58]. A more restrictive approach to the hypertensive athlete is recommended by the Italian Society of Sports Cardiology [88]. A systolic BP > 240 mmHg during exercise should be considered abnormal and thus eligibility to competitive athletics may be granted if exercise systolic BP is <240 mmHg. If exercise systolic BP is equal to or higher than 240 mmHg, the practice of competitive sports will be allowed only after good BP control is achieved with pharmacological treatment both at rest and during exercise.

Both the European and the Italian Societies stress the importance of performing ABPM in athletes with high BP at rest and/or during exercise. Eligibility to competitions will be subject to the achievement of good BP pressure control verified with ambulatory monitoring [58, 88]. Current thresholds for an elevated ambulatory BP are 130/80 mmHg for average 24-h BP and 135/85 mmHg for daytime BP [13].

All athletes and sportsmen with hypertension, need to be followed up regularly. During the annual precompetition medical examination BP needs to be measured at rest, out of office, and during exercise testing. The overall risk evaluation including routine blood tests has to be updated. Adjustments of medication should be made if needed and competitions should be postponed until BP measurements return within the normal range.

11.9 Conclusion

A number of studies have shown that aerobic exercise can have favorable effects on the cardiovascular system of young adults and can attenuate the BP reaction to stressors. Thus, exercise training together with other nonpharmacological measures should always be considered as the initial approach in the management of young sedentary patients in the early stages of hypertension chiefly in subjects hyperreactive to stressors and with poor cardiovascular risk profile. For prevention and treatment of uncomplicated hypertension 3–5 sessions/week of aerobic exercise for 30–60 min, at 40–60% of maximum working capacity should be performed [4, 13, 37]. Sports such as brisk walking, jogging, running, cycling, swimming, or other aerobic activities should be privileged, which may be supplemented by resistance activities [4, 13, 37]. In both hypertensive adolescents and young adults, already active people should be encouraged to continue aerobic physical activities after thorough clinical assessment has excluded hypertension-mediated organ damage or coronary artery disease.

Acknowledgments None.

Funding None.

Author Contributions P.P. performed the design of the study, data collection and analysis, manuscript writing and revision.

Conflict of Interest None.

Statement All human studies whose data have been used for the present chapter have been reviewed by the appropriate ethics committees and have been performed in accordance with the ethical standards of the 1964 Declaration of Helsinki.

References

1. Fields LE, Burt VL, Cutler JA, Hughes J, Roccella EJ, Sorlie P. The burden of adult hypertension in the United States 1999 to 2000: a rising tide. Hypertension. 2004;44:398–404.
2. Cornelissen VA, Fagard RH. Effects of endurance training on blood pressure, blood pressure-regulating mechanisms, and cardiovascular risk factors. Hypertension. 2005;46:667–75.
3. Hamer M. Sports and psychological processes. Implications for the primary prevention of coronary heart disease. Sports Med. 2006;36:829–38.
4. Fagard RH. Exercise therapy in hypertensive cardiovascular disease. Prog Cardiovasc Dis. 2011;53:404–11.
5. Julius S. The hemodynamic link between insulin resistance and hypertension. J Hypertens. 1991;9:983–6.
6. Kjeldsen SE, Zweifler AJ, Petrin J, Weder AB, Julius S. Sympathetic nervous system involvement in essential hypertension: increased platelet noradrenaline coincides with decreased ß-adrenoreceptor responsiveness. Blood Press. 1994;3:164–71.
7. Mancia G, Grassi G, Giannattasio C, Seravalle G. Sympathetic activation in the pathogenesis of hypertension and progression of organ damage. Hypertension. 1999;34:724–8.
8. Maver J, Strucl M, Accetto R. Autonomic nervous system activity in normotensive subjects with a family history of hypertension. Clin Auton Res. 2004;14:358–9.
9. Palatini P, Majahalme S, Amerena J, Nesbitt S, Vriz O, Michieletto M, et al. Determinants of left ventricular structure and mass in young subjects with sympathetic over-activity. The Tecumseh Offspring Study. J Hypertens. 2000;18:769–75.
10. Palatini P, Julius S. The role of cardiac autonomic function in hypertension and cardiovascular disease. Curr Ther Rep. 2009;11:199–205.
11. Salmon P. Effects of physical exercise on anxiety, depression, and sensitivity to stress: a unifying theory. Clin Psychol Rev. 2001;21:33–61.
12. Hull EM, Young SH, Ziegler MG. Aerobic fitness affects cardiovascular and catecholamine responses to stressors. Psychophysiology. 1984;21:353–60.
13. Mancia G, Fagard R, Narkiewicz K, Redon J, Zanchetti A, Bohm M, et al. 2013 ESH/ESC guidelines for the management of arterial hypertension: the task force for the Management of Arterial Hypertension of the European Society of Hypertension (ESH) and of the European Society of Cardiology (ESC). Eur Heart J. 2013;34:2159–219.
14. Palatini P, Rosei EA, Avolio A, Bilo G, Casiglia E, Ghiadoni L, et al. Isolated systolic hypertension in the young: a position paper endorsed by the European Society of Hypertension. J Hypertens. 2018;36:1222–36.
15. Grebla RG, Rodriguez CJ, Borrell LN, Pickering TG. Prevalence and determinants of isolated systolic hypertension among young adults: the 1999-2004 US National Health and nutrition examination survey. J Hypertens. 2010;28:15–23.
16. Julius S, Jamerson K, Mejia A, Krause L, Schork N, Jones K. The association of borderline hypertension with target organ damage and higher coronary risk. JAMA. 1990;264:354–8.
17. Julius S, Krause L, Schork NJ, Mejia A, Jones KA, Van den Ven C, et al. Hyperkinetic borderline hypertension in Tecumseh, Michigan. J Hypertension. 1991;9:77–84.
18. Palatini P, Longo D, Zaetta V, Perkovic D, Garbelotto R, Pessina AC. Evolution of blood pressure and cholesterol in stage 1 hypertension: role of autonomic nervous system activity. J Hypertens. 2006;24:1375–81.
19. Fagard RH, Stolarz K, Kuznetsova T, Kawecka-Jaszcz K. Sympathetic activity, assessed by power spectral analysis of HR variability, in white-coat, masked and sustained hypertension versus true normotension. J Hypertens. 2007;25:2280–5.

20. Mancia G, Grassi G. The autonomic nervous system and hypertension. Circ Res. 2014;114:1804–14.
21. Grassi G, Mark AL, Esler M. The sympathetic nervous system alterations in human hypertension. Circ Res. 2015;116:976–90.
22. Matthews KA, Katholi CR, McCreath H, Whooley MA, Williams DR, Zhu S, et al. Blood pressure reactivity to psychological stress predicts hypertension in the CARDIA study. Circulation. 2004;110:74–8.
23. Steptoe A. Psychophysiological stress reactivity and hypertension. Hypertension. 2008;52:220–1.
24. Palatini P, Palomba D, Bertolo O, Minghetti R, Longo L, Sarlo M, et al. The white-coat effect is unrelated to the difference between clinic and daytime blood pressure and is associated with greater reactivity to public speaking. J Hypertens. 2003;21:545–53.
25. Palatini P, Bratti P, Palomba D, Bonso E, Saladini F, Benetti E, et al. BP reactivity to public speaking in stage 1 hypertension: influence of different task scenarios. Blood Press. 2011;20:290–5.
26. Palatini P. Role of elevated heart rate in the development of cardiovascular disease in hypertension. Hypertension. 2011;58:745–50.
27. Rimmele U, Zellweger BC, Marti B, Seiler R, Mohiyeddini C, Ehlert U, et al. Trained men show lower cortisol, heart rate and psychological responses to psychosocial stress compared with untrained men. Psychoneuroendocrinology. 2007;32:627–35.
28. Palatini P, Bratti P, Palomba D, Saladini F, Zanatta N, Maraglino G. Regular physical activity attenuates the BP response to public speaking and delays the development of hypertension. J Hypertens. 2010;28:1186–93.
29. Ewart CK, Kolodner KB. Predicting ambulatory blood pressure during school: effectiveness of social and nonsocial reactivity tasks in black and white adolescents. Psychophysiology. 1993;30:30–8.
30. O'Sullivan SE, Bell C. The effects of exercise and training on human cardiovascular reflex control. J Autonom Nerv Syst. 2000;81:16–24.
31. Laterza MC, de Matos LD, Trombetta IC, Braga AM, Roveda F, Alves MJ, et al. Exercise training restores baroreflex sensitivity in never-treated hypertensive patients. Hypertension. 2007;49:1298–306.
32. O'Rourke MF, Vlachopoulos C, Graham RM. Spurious systolic hypertension in youth. Vasc Med. 2000;5:141–5.
33. Mahmud A, Feely J. Spurious systolic hypertension of youth: fit young men with elastic arteries. Am J Hypertens. 2003;16:229–32.
34. Hulsen HT, Nijdam ME, Bos WJ, Uiterwaal CS, Oren A, Grobbee DE, et al. Spurious systolic hypertension in young adults; prevalence of high brachial systolic blood pressure and low central pressure and its determinants. J Hypertens. 2006;24:1027–32.
35. Roman MJ, Okin PM, Kizer JR, Lee ET, Howard BV, Devereux RB. Relation of central and brachial blood pressure to left ventricular hypertrophy and geometry: the strong heart study. J Hypertens. 2010;28:384–8.
36. Pelliccia A. Athlete's heart and hypertrophic cardiomyopathy. Curr Cardiol Rep. 2000;2:166–71.
37. Pescatello LS, Franklin BA, Fagard R, Farquhar WB, Kelley GA, Ray CA, American College of Sports Medicine Position Stand. Exercise and hypertension. Med Sci Sports Exerc. 2004;35:533–53.
38. Saladini F, Santonastaso M, Mos L, Benetti E, Zanatta N, Maraglino G, et al. Isolated systolic hypertension of young to middle-age individuals implies a relatively low risk of developing hypertension needing treatment when central blood pressure is low. J Hypertens. 2011;29:1311–9.
39. Saladini F, Fania C, Mos L, Mazzer A, Casiglia E, Palatini P. Office pulse pressure is a predictor of favourable outcome in young-to-middle-aged subjects with stage 1 hypertension. Hypertension. 2017;70:537–42.

40. McEniery CM, Franklin SS, Wilkinson IB, Cockcroft JR. Isolated systolic hypertension in the young: a need for clarity. J Hypertens. 2013;31:1911–3.
41. McEniery CM, Yasmin, Wallace S, Maki-Petaja K, McDonnell B, Sharman JE, et al. ENIGMA study investigators. Increased stroke volume and aortic stiffness contribute to isolated systolic hypertension in young adults. Hypertension. 2005;46:221–6.
42. Palatini P, Saladini F, Mos L, Fania C, Mazzer A, Casiglia E. Clinical characteristics and risk of hypertension needing treatment in young patients with systolic hypertension identified with ambulatory monitoring. J Hypertens. 2018;36:1810–5.
43. Palatini P, Graniero G, Mormino P, Nicolosi L, Mos L, Visentin P, et al. Relation between physical training and ambulatory blood pressure in stage I hypertensive subjects. Results of the HARVEST trial. Circulation. 1994;90:2870–6.
44. Reaven PD, Barrett-Connor E, Edelstein S. Relation between leisure-time physical activity and blood pressure in older women. Circulation. 1991;83:559–65.
45. Meisinger C, Koenig W, Baumert J, Doring A. Uric acid levels are associated with all cause and cardiovascular disease mortality independent of systemic inflammation in men from the general population: the MONICA/KORA cohort study. Arterioscler Thromb Vasc Biol. 2008;28:1186–92.
46. Fang J, Alderman MH. Serum uric acid and cardiovascular mortality the NHANES I epidemiologic follow-up study, 1971-1992. National Health and Nutrition Examination Survey. JAMA. 2000;283:2404–10.
47. Palatini P, Parati G, Virdis A, Reboldi G, Masi S, Mengozzi A, et al. High heart rate amplifies the risk of cardiovascular mortality associated with elevated uric acid. Eur J Prev Cardiol. 2021.
48. Saladini F, Mos L, Fania C, Garavelli G, Casiglia E, Palatini P. Regular physical activity prevents development of hypertension in young people with hyperuricemia. J Hypertens. 2017;35(5):994–1001.
49. Palatini P, Canali C, Graniero GR, Rossi G, de Toni R, Santonastaso M. Relationship of plasma renin activity with caffeine intake and physical training in mild hypertensive men. HARVEST Study Group. Eur J Epidemiol. 1996;12:485–91.
50. Casale PN, Devereux RB, Milner M, Zullo G, Harshfield GA, Pickering TG, et al. Value of echocardiographic measurement of left ventricular mass in predicting cardiovascular morbid events in hypertensive men. Ann Intern Med. 1986;105:173–8.
51. Baglivo HP, Fabregues G, Burrieza H, Esper RC, Talarico M, Esper RJ. Effect of moderate physical training on left ventricular mass in mild hypertensive persons. Hypertension. 1990;15(suppl 1):I-153–6.
52. Kokkinos PF, Narayan P, Colleran JA, Pittares A, Notargiacomo A, Reda D. Effects of regular exercise on blood pressure and left ventricular hypertrophy in African-American men with severe hypertension. N Engl J Med. 1995;333:1462–7.
53. Zanettini R, Bettega D, Agostoni O, Ballestra B, del Rosso G, di Michele R, et al. Exercise training in mild hypertension: effects on blood pressure, left ventricular mass and coagulation factor VII and fibrinogen. Cardiology. 1997;88:468–73.
54. Hinderliter A, Sherwood A, Gullette EC, Babyak M, Waugh R, Georgiades A, et al. Reduction of left ventricular hypertrophy after exercise and weight loss in overweight patients with mild hypertension. Arch Intern Med. 2002;162:1333–9.
55. Reid CM, Dart AM, Dewar EM, Jennings GL. Interactions between the effects of exercise and weight loss on risk factors, cardiovascular haemodynamics and left ventricular structure in overweight subjects. J Hypertens. 1994;12:291–301.
56. Palatini P, Visentin P, Dorigatti F, Guarnieri C, Santonastaso M, Cozzio S, et al. Regular physical activity prevents development of left ventricular hypertrophy in hypertension. Eur Heart J. 2009;30:225–32.
57. Lee J, Cho HS, Park S, Kim WK. Regular exercise produced cardioprotective effects on rat's heart with hypertension induced by L-NAME administration. Clin Exp Hypertens. 2009;31:364–75.
58. Niebauer J, Börjesson M, Carre F, Caselli S, Palatini P, Quattrini F, et al. Recommendations for participation in competitive sports of athletes with arterial hypertension: a position statement

from the sports cardiology section of the European Association of Preventive Cardiology (EAPC). Eur Heart J. 2018;39:3664–71.

59. O'Leary DH, Polak JF, Kronmal RA, Manolio TA, Burke GL, Wolfson SK Jr. Carotid-artery intima and media thickness as a risk factor for myocardial infarction and stroke in older adults: cardiovascular health study collaborative research group. N Engl J Med. 1999;340:14–22.
60. Pauletto P, Palatini P, Da Ros S, Pagliara V, Santipolo N, Baccillieri S, et al. Factors underlying the increase in carotid intima-media thickness in borderline hypertensives. Arterioscler Thromb Vasc Biol. 1999;19:1231–7.
61. Puato M, Palatini P, Zanardo M, Dorigatti F, Tirrito C, Rattazzi M, et al. Increase in carotid intima-media thickness in grade I hypertensive subjects: white-coat versus sustained hypertension. Hypertension. 2008;51:1300–5.
62. Rauramaa R, Halonen P, Vaisanen SB, Lakka TA, Schmidt-Trucksäss A, Berg A, et al. Effects of aerobic physical exercise on inflammation and atherosclerosis in men: the DNASCO study: a six-year randomized, controlled trial. Ann Intern Med. 2004;140:1007–14.
63. Okada K, Maeda N, Tatsukawa M, Shimizu C, Sawayama Y, Hayashi J. The influence of lifestyle modification on carotid artery intima-media thickness in a suburban Japanese population. Atherosclerosis. 2004;173:329–37.
64. Lakka TA, Laukkanen JA, Rauramaa R, Salonen R, Lakka HM, Kaplan GA, et al. Cardiorespiratory fitness and the progression of carotid atherosclerosis in middle-aged men. Ann Intern Med. 2001;134:12–20.
65. Nordstrom CK, Dwyer KM, Merz CN, Shircore A, Dwyer JH. Leisure time physical activity and early atherosclerosis: the Los Angeles atherosclerosis study. Am J Med. 2003;115:19–25.
66. Palatini P, Puato M, Rattazzi M, Pauletto P. Effect of regular physical activity on carotid intima-media thickness. Results from a 6-year prospective study in the early stage of hypertension. Blood Press. 2011;20:37–44.
67. Meyer AA, Kundt G, Lenschow U, Schuff-Werner P, Kienast W. Improvement of early vascular changes and cardiovascular risk factors in obese children after a six-month exercise program. J Am Coll Cardiol. 2006;48:1865–70.
68. Polak JF, Person SD, Wei GS, Godreau A, Jacobs DR Jr, Harrington A, et al. Segment-specific associations of carotid intima-media thickness with cardiovascular risk factors: the coronary artery risk development in Young adults (CARDIA) study. Stroke. 2010;41:9–15.
69. Hayashi K, Sugawara J, Komine H, Maeda S, Yokoi T. Effects of aerobic exercise training on the stiffness of central and peripheral arteries in middle-aged sedentary men. Jpn J Physiol. 2005;55:235–9.
70. Otsuki T, Maeda S, Iemitsu M, Saito Y, Tanimura Y, Ajisaka R, et al. Vascular endothelium-derived factors and arterial stiffness in strength- and endurance-trained men. Am J Physiol Heart Circ Physiol. 2007;292:H786–91.
71. Saladini F, Benetti E, Mos L, Mazzer A, Casiglia E, Palatini P. Regular physical activity is associated with improved small artery distensibility in young to middle-age stage 1 hypertensives. Vasc Med. 2014;19:458–64.
72. Palatini P. Exaggerated blood pressure response to exercise: pathophysiologic mechanisms and clinical relevance. J Sports Med Phys Fitness. 1998;38(1):1–9.
73. Manolio TA, Burke GL, Savage PJ, Sidney S, Gardin JM, Oberman A. Exercise blood pressure response and 5 year risk of elevated blood pressure in a cohort of young adults: the CARDIA study. Am J Hypertens. 1994;7:234–41.
74. Matthews CE, Pate RR, Jackson KL, Ward DS, Macera CA, Kohl HW, et al. Exaggerated blood pressure response to dynamic exercise and risk of future hypertension. J Cin Epidemiol. 1998;51:29–35.
75. Allison TG, Cordeiro MA, Miller TD, Daida H, Squires RW, Gau GT. Prognostic significance of exercise-induced systemic hypertension in healthy subjects. Am J Cardiol. 1999;83:371–5.
76. Singh JP, Larson MG, Manolio TA, O'Donnell CJ, Lauer M, Evans JC, et al. Blood pressure response during treadmill testing as a risk factor for new onset hypertension: the Framingham heart study. Circulation. 1999;99:1831–6.

77. Miyai N, Arita M, Miyashita K, Morioka I, Shiraishi T, Nishio I. Blood pressure response to heart rate during exercise test and risk of future hypertension. Hypertension. 2002;39:761–6.
78. Schultz MG, Otahal P, Cleland VJ, Blizzard L, Marwick TH, Sharman JE. Exercise-induced hypertension, cardiovascular events, and mortality in patients undergoing exercise stress testing: a systematic review and meta-analysis. Am J Hypertens. 2013;26:357–66.
79. Schultz MG, Gdipappstat PO, Picone DS, Hons B, Sharman JE. Clinical relevance of exaggerated exercise blood pressure. J Am Coll Cardiol. 2015;66:1843–5.
80. Yzaguirre I, Grazioli G, Domenech M, Vinuesa A, Pi R, Gutierrez J, et al. Exaggerated blood pressure response to exercise and late-onset hypertension in young adults. Blood Press Monit. 2017;22(6):339–44.
81. Lauer MS, Pashkow FJ, Harvey SA, Marwick TH, Thomas JD. Angiographic and prognostic implications of an exaggerated exercise systolic blood pressure response and rest systolic blood pressure in adults undergoing evaluation for suspected coronary artery disease. J Am Coll Cardiol. 1995;26:1630–6.
82. Lewis GD, Gona P, Larson MG, Plehn JF, Benjamin EJ, O'Donnell CJ, et al. Exercise blood pressure and the risk of incident cardiovascular disease (from the Framingham heart study). Am J Cardiol. 2008;101:1614–20.
83. Palatini P, Mos L, Mormino P, Munari L, Del Torre M, Valle F, et al. Intra-arterial blood pressure monitoring in the evaluation of the hypertensive athlete. Eur Heart J. 1990;11:348–54.
84. Hurst RT, Burke RF, Wissner E, Roberts A, Kendall CB, Lester SJ, et al. Incidence of subclinical atherosclerosis as a marker of cardiovascular risk in retired professional football players. Am J Cardiol. 2010;105:1107–11.
85. Raghuveer G, Hartz J, Lubans DR, Takken T, Wiltz JL, Mietus-Snyder M, et al. Cardiorespiratory fitness in youth: an important marker of health: a scientific statement from the American Heart Association. Circulation. 2020;142(7):e101–18.
86. Campbell RM, Douglas PS, Eidem BW, Lai WW, Lopez L, Sachdeva R. ACC/AAP/AHA/ASE/HRS/SCAI/SCCT/SCMR/SOPE 2014 appropriate use criteria for initial transthoracic echocardiography in outpatient pediatric cardiology: a report of the American College of Cardiology Appropriate use Criteria Task Force, American Academy of Pediatrics, American Heart Association, American Society of Echocardiography, Heart Rhythm Society, Society for Cardiovascular Angiography and Interventions, Society of Cardiovascular Computed Tomography, Society for Cardiovascular Magnetic Resonance, and Society of Pediatric Echocardiography. J Am Coll Cardiol. 2014;64(19):2039–60.
87. Caselli S, Vaquer Segui A, Quattrini F, Di Gacinto B, Milan A, Assorgi R, et al. Upper normal values of blood pressure response to exercise in Olympic athletes. Am Heart J. 2016;177:120–8.
88. Delise P, Mos L, Sciarra L, Basso C, Biffi A, Cecchi F, et al. Italian Cardiological guidelines (COCIS) for competitive sport eligibility in athletes with heart disease: update 2020. J Cardiovasc Med. 2021;22(11):874–91.

Exercise and Hypertension in Older Persons

12

Giuseppe Romanelli and Alessandra Marengoni

12.1 Aging and Physical Activity

Population aging is a worldwide phenomenon with the oldest old being the fastest-growing in developed countries. The main reasons rely in environmental changes, rapid progression of medical diagnostic and treatments, and implementation of prevention strategies. Despite the increase in life-expectancy, the health of old and very old persons is often characterized by the co-occurrence of multiple chronic conditions which have become the dominant health care burden. There are evidences that compared to less active men and women, older adults who are physically active have lower rates of several specific conditions, such as coronary heart disease, hypertension, stroke, diabetes, cancer, a higher level of cardiorespiratory and functional health, a lower risk of falling, and better cognitive function [1]. Thus, the World Health Organization recommends that older adults do at least 150 min of moderate-intensity aerobic physical activity throughout the week or at least 75 min of vigorous intensity aerobic physical activity throughout the week or an equivalent combination of moderate- and vigorous-intensity activity [1]. Further, the recommendations apply also to older persons already affected by chronic diseases and functional impairment under the guidance and expertise of a physician and dedicated health care professionals.

At present, most studies on physical activity outcomes in older persons have focused on the effects of exercise on sarcopenia, frailty, disability and risk of falls [2–4] and only some have evaluated the role of exercise in term of risk reduction for specific clinical conditions.

An interesting issue is the influence of age on the association between lifestyle and incident vascular conditions, for instance hypertension. Analyses from the

G. Romanelli · A. Marengoni (✉)
Department of Clinical and Experimental Sciences, University of Brescia, Brescia, Italy
e-mail: giuseppe.romanelli@unibs.it; alessandra.marengoni@unibs.it

P. Palatini et al. (eds.), *Exercise, Sports and Hypertension*, Updates in Hypertension and Cardiovascular Protection,
https://doi.org/10.1007/978-3-031-07958-0_12

Nurses' Health Study shows that healthy lifestyles, including physical activity, account for a smaller hypothetical fraction of hypertension in older compared to younger women; however, due to the much higher incidence of hypertension in older age, the public health benefit still is very high [5].

12.2 Physical Exercise and Hypertension

Among nonpharmacological interventions, structured exercise programs are strongly recommended for adults with elevated blood pressure or hypertension [6, 7]. It is well known that the incidence of hypertension increases with older age and represents a significant burden in term of treatment and risk factor for cardiovascular diseases [8]. In older subjects, exercise interventions are important due to multiple effects that, beyond function, may benefit vascular disease markers too [9]. However, the majority of studies evaluating lifestyle interventions have been carried out in young or adult people and only a few trials have evaluated the role of approaches alternative to medications in order to lower blood pressure in older persons with hypertension [10, 11]. A study carried out in 2010 included 63 men and women 76 ± 8 years of age with stage I isolated systolic hypertension [12]; participants were randomized to 16 weeks of exercise consisting of aerobic training or strength training three times per week or to passive control. Participants in the exercise groups had a significant decrease in diastolic (3 mmHg; $p < 0.05$) but not systolic blood pressure. Another article published in 2012 provided some of the first evidence that aerobic exercise may lower blood pressure even among individuals with resistant hypertension, defined as a blood pressure ≥ 140/90 mmHg on three medications or a blood pressure controlled by more than three medications [13]. Fifty individuals were randomized to participate (or not participate) in an 8- to 12-week treadmill exercise program three times per week. Aerobic activity was carried out with a target lactate concentration of 2.0 ± 0.5 mmol/L in capillary blood slightly above the aerobic threshold, and was considered to be at a moderate level. Compared with individuals in the control group, 24-h systolic and diastolic blood pressure levels were significantly reduced by aerobic training. In another study, 54 persons 60 years of age or older with systolic 24-h ambulatory blood pressure > 140 mmHg and/or antihypertensive treatment and diastolic ambulatory blood pressure ≤90 mmHg were randomly assigned to sedentary activity or a 12-week treadmill exercise program. Exercise significantly decreased systolic and diastolic ambulatory blood pressure by 8.5 ± 8.2 and 5.1 ± 3.7 mmHg, respectively. Arterial compliance remained unchanged, whereas endothelium-dependent vasodilation, measured by flow-mediated dilation, significantly increased independently of pulse pressure. The authors concluded that physical exercise is a helpful adjunct to control blood pressure even in older adults with hypertension with markedly increased arterial stiffness [14]. Finally, in a systematic review and meta-analysis, Herro et al. reported that undertaking aerobic exercise regularly over at least 3 months can lead to 5–6 mmHg reduction in systolic blood pressure and 2–3.5 mmHg reduction in diastolic blood pressure among participants aged over 65 years [14]. There did not appear to be any additional benefit in combining aerobic exercise with resistance exercise but the same review showed that quality of the evidence on resistance or isometric exercise is very low excluding the possibility of any reliable conclusion. Finally, there was no additional benefit seen in exercise programs lasting longer than 3 months and similar reductions in blood pressure were seen in trials including both hypertensive and nonhypertensive individuals. Given the limitations of previous clinical trials, other studies are ongoing. The Hypertension Approaches in the Elderly: a Lifestyle two-arm parallel study (HAEL study) aims to evaluate the efficacy of a pragmatic combined exercise training compared with a health education program on ambulatory blood pressure and other health-related outcomes in older individuals [15]. A total of 184 subjects, ≥60 years of age, are randomized on a 1:1 ratio to 12-week interventions consisting either of a combined exercise (aerobic and strength) training, three times per week, or an active-control group receiving health education, once a week. Ambulatory and office blood pressures, cardiorespiratory fitness and endothelial function, together with quality of life, functional fitness and autonomic control will be assessed before and after intervention.

In the real world, one of the low-cost and most frequently performed physical activities in older age is walking. A randomized controlled trial carried out in a rural area of Taiwan recruited a total of 202 participants aged 60 years and over with mild-to-moderate hypertension. Participants randomized to the intervention group received a 6-month walking intervention. A public health nurse provided both face-to-face and telephone support to assist participants and increase their walking. Control group participants received usual primary health care. At 6-month follow-up the difference in mean change in systolic blood pressure between the two groups was −7.0 mmHg ($p = 0.002$), but no differences were observed in diastolic blood pressure [16]. Another randomized clinical trial, with a physical activity intervention of 9-month duration, comprising a walking group of 120 min/week and sociocultural activities, enrolled 207 hypertensive subjects (mean age 68.2 years). In multivariate models, the physical activity intervention, with no modification of the diet, decreased the systolic blood pressure (−8.68 mmHg), and increased some areas of health-related quality of life. An increase in the percentage of subjects with controlled blood pressure was observed by the physical activity program itself. The authors concluded that the physical intervention increases blood pressure control in primary care users with hypertension [17]. A recent systematic review was performed in order to determine the effect of walking as a physical activity intervention on blood pressure in middle-aged and older persons. The authors found moderate-certainty evidence suggesting that walking reduces systolic blood pressure in participants aged 40 years and under, and low-certainty evidence that walking reduces systolic blood pressure in participants aged 41–60 years, and those aged 60 years and over. As secondary outcome of the review, the authors found moderate-certainty evidence suggesting that walking reduces diastolic blood pressure for participants aged 40 years and under and low-certainty evidence suggesting that walking reduces diastolic blood pressure for participants aged 41–60 years and those aged 60 years and over. The authors concluded that moderate- or low-certainty evidence suggests that walking may reduce systolic blood pressure and diastolic blood pressure in all ages [18]. These findings suggest that walking of moderate-intensity, three to five times per week, of 20–40 min duration, and 150 min per week for about 3 months may lower blood pressure.

12.3 Mechanisms

The mechanisms by which regular physical activity may reduce blood pressure are unclear. Findings from animal studies suggest that aerobic exercise may prevent increases in blood pressure through alterations in insulin sensitivity and autonomic nervous system function, while resistance training may prevent increases in blood pressure through a reduction in systemic vascular resistance via decreased activities of the sympathetic and the renin-angiotensin systems [19]. A reduction of reactive oxygen species, inflammation and arterial stiffness have also been proposed to contribute to this phenomenon. Other factors, including improved endothelium-dependent vasodilatation, enhanced baroreceptor sensitivity, and arterial compliance, may also be involved [20]. Cardiovascular diseases are common with aging and vascular changes are the norm. Arterial stiffness and blood pressure increase with increasing age. In the Baltimore Longitudinal Study on Ageing the authors showed that carotid-femoral pulse wave velocity was inversely related to maximal oxygen consumption, suggesting that aerobic exercise attenuate the age-associated increase in arterial stiffness [21]. Some intervention studies held in healthy middle-aged and older adults have demonstrated a significant reduction in arterial stiffness with aerobic exercise training [22, 23]. However, in the Nurses' Health Study, the authors observed attenuation of the association between physical activity and hypertension risk with aging, suggesting that it may result from an age-related increase in arterial stiffness, elastin fragmentation and increase in collagen [5, 24].

12.4 Limitations

Regarding the effect of physical exercise on hypertension in older persons, at present, there are insufficient data to conclude about specific recommendations in term of dose and duration of possible interventions, especially in the long term. Clinical trials are often multiarms with different type of interventions and physical exercise, as well as a small number of participants included in each arm with large variations in adherence to interventions. Further, there is no evidence of what happens in the months after the intervention ceases, and it is unclear whether the benefits can persist or if extra intervention is needed to maintain the benefits. Finally, very old persons and those with cardiovascular diseases or multimorbidity are usually excluded from clinical trials. Observational studies evaluating physical activity benefits have also several limitations including difficulty in categorizing different physical activities, in terms of aerobic or resistance exercise, timing and adherence as well as the fact that they are often subjected to recall bias. This translates to the conclusion that there are no data that show the best combination of physical exercise doses, frequency, type and intensity able to lower blood pressure both in normotensive and hypertensive older persons. These kind of data could be particularly important in older persons because they are commonly prescribed with polypharmacy with a high risk of drug-drug interactions and adverse drug reactions. Thus, lifestyle interventions could be particularly helpful and safe. Indeed, adverse events in clinical trials based on physical exercise interventions are very few and often limited to mild cases.

Despite the above mentioned limitations, there is some evidence about a possible role of walking as beneficial lifestyle for lowering blood pressure; in general, walking is often recommended by healthcare professionals for preventing several health problems, whereas other specific types of physical exercise are still not fully recommended in geriatric medical practice and physical training is often not included in programs of prevention of aging-related diseases. Recently, expert consensus guidelines on exercise recommendations in older adults has been published with the aim to optimize the use of exercise and physical activity both as a preventative medicine and as a therapeutic agent (Table 12.1) [25].

Table 12.1 Exercise recommendations for optimal ageing and maintenance of functional capacities in older adults. From: *International Exercise Recommendations in Older Adults (ICFSR): Expert Consensus Guidelines* [25]

	Resistance training	Aerobic exercise training	Balance training
Frequency (days per week)	2–3	3–7	1–7
Volume	1–3 sets of 8–12 repetitions, 8–10 major muscle groups	20–60 min/session	1–2 sets of 4–10 different exercises emphasizing static and dynamic postures
Intensity	Start at 30–40% of 1RM and progress to heavier loads of 70–80% 1 RM (15–18 on Borg scale) 1–3 min rest between sets Power training at 40–60% of 1RM	12–14 on Borg Scale[a] (55–70% heart rate reserve or maximum exercise capacity)	Progressive difficulty as tolerated[b] Narrowing the base of support Perturbation of ground support Decrease in proprioceptive sensation Diminished or misleading visual inputs Movement of the center of mass of the body away from the vertical or stationary position Dual tasking: Adding a cognitive distractor or secondary physical task while practicing a balance task
Specific physiological adaptations	• Strength • Power • Hypertrophy • Endurance • Maximal aerobic capacity	• Maximal aerobic capacity • Sub-maximal endurance • Cardiac contractility/ stroke volume • Peripheral oxygen extraction • Arterial stiffness • Heart rate variability	• Dynamic stability

(continued)

Table 12.1 (continued)

	Resistance training	Aerobic exercise training	Balance training
Exercise examples	• Multiple and single joint exercises (free weights and machine) with slow to moderate lifting velocity • Bench press and squat • Knee extensions and knee curls • Exercise selection can be varied through alterations in body posture, grip, hand and foot stance, unilateral vs bilateral exercises • Once body weight no longer serves as a sufficient source of overload, additional resistance can be provided by machines or free weights as needed to ensure progression	• Dancing • Cycling • Hiking • Jogging/long-distance running • Swimming • Walking with change in pace and direction • Treadmill walking • Stair climbing • Step-ups • Seated stepping • Recumbent cycling may start with 5–10 min and progress to 15–30 min. The intensity is proportional to heart rate and/or perceived exertional scales if on B blockers or has pacemaker and can be increased from moderate to vigorous depending on fitness.	• Tai chi • Standing yoga or ballet movements • Tandem walking • Standing on one leg, stepping over objects, climbing slowly up and down steps • Turning • Standing on heels and toes, walking on a compliant surface such as foam mattresses • Maintaining balance on a moving vehicle, such as a bus or train • Dual-tasking: Adding cognitive distractor while maintaining balance Many conditions in older adults require balance training before aerobic exercise/gait retraining

[a] Original Borg Scale of Perceived Exertion from 6 (easy) to 20 (maximal)

[b] Intensity is increased by decreasing the base of support [e.g., progressing from standing on two feet while holding on to the back of a chair to standing on one foot with no hand support); by decreasing other sensory input (e.g., closing eyes or standing on a foam pillow); by perturbing the center of mass (e.g., holding a heavy object out to one side while maintaining balance, standing on one leg while lifting the other leg out behind the body, or leaning forward as far as possible without falling or moving feet); or by dual-tasking (adding a secondary cognitive [e.g., naming animals] or physical (e.g., juggling) task while tandem walking]

References

1. https://www.who.int/dietphysicalactivity/physical-activity-recommendations-65years.pdf. Accessed 28 July 2021.
2. Lee S-Y, Tung H-H, Liu C-Y, Chen L-K. Physical activity and sarcopenia in the geriatric population: a systematic review. JAMDA. 2018;19(5):378–83.
3. Pereira CLN, Vogelaere P, Baptista F. Role of physical activity in the prevention of falls and their consequences in the elderly. Eur Rev Aging Phys Act. 2008;5:51–8.
4. Pahor M, Guralnik JM, Ambrosius WT, Blair S, Bonds DE, Church TS, et al. Effect of structured physical activity on prevention of major mobility disability in older adults: the LIFE study randomized clinical trial. JAMA. 2014;311(23):2387–96.
5. Cohen L, Curhan GC, Forman JP. Influence of age on the association between lifestyle factors and risk of hypertension. J Am Soc Hypertens. 2012;6(4):284–90.

6. Whelton PK, Carey RM, Aronow WS, Casey DE Jr, Collins KJ, Dennison Himmelfarb C, et al. ACC/AHA/AAPA/ABC/ACPM/AGS/APhA/ASH/ASPC/NMA/PCNA guideline for the prevention, detection, evaluation, and management of high blood pressure in adults: executive summary: a report of the American College of Cardiology/American Heart Association task force on clinical practice guidelines. Hypertension. 2018;71(6):1269–324.
7. James PA, Oparil S, Carter BL, Cushman WC, Dennison-Himmelfarb C, Handler J, et al. 2014 evidence-based guideline for the management of high blood pressure in adults: report from the panel members appointed to the eighth joint National Committee (JNC 8). JAMA. 2014;311(5):507–20.
8. Psaty BM, Furberg CD, Kuller LH, Cushman M, Savage PJ, Levine D, et al. Association between blood pressure level and the risk of myocardial infarction, stroke, and total mortality: the cardiovascular health study. Arch Intern Med. 2001;161(9):1183–92.
9. Nowak KL, Rossman MJ, Chonchol M, Seals DR. Strategies for achieving healthy vascular aging. Hypertension. 2018;71(3):389–402.
10. Brook RD, Appel LJ, Rubenfire M, Ogedegbe G, Bisognano JD, Elliott WJ, et al. Beyond medications and diet: alternative approaches to lowering blood pressure: a scientific statement from the American heart association. Hypertension. 2013;61(6):1360–83.
11. Corso LML, Macdonald HV, Johnson BT, Farinatti P, Livingston J, Zaleski AL, et al. Is concurrent training efficacious antihypertensive therapy? A meta-analysis. Med Sci Sports Exerc. 2016;48(12):2398–406.
12. Martins RA, Veríssimo MT, Coelho e Silva MJ, Cumming SP, Teixeira AM. Effects of aerobic and strength-based training on metabolic health indicators in older adults. Lipids Health Dis. 2010;9:76.
13. Dimeo F, Pagonas N, Seibert F, Arndt R, Zidek W, Westhoff TH. Aerobic exercise reduces blood pressure in resistant hypertension. Hypertension. 2012;60:653–8.
14. Westhoff TH, Franke N, Schmidt S, Vallbracht-Israng K, Meissner R, Yildirim H, et al. Too old to benefit from sports? The cardiovascular effects of exercise training in elderly subjects treated for isolated systolic hypertension. Kidney Blood Press Res. 2007;30(4):240–7.
15. Umpierre D, Santos LP, Botton CE, Wilhelm EN, Helal L, Schaun GZ, et al.; The HAEL Study Group. The "Hypertension approaches in the elderly: a lifestyle study" multicenter, randomized trial (HAEL study): rationale and methodological protocol. BMC Public Health. 2019;19(1):657.
16. Lee L-L, Arthur A, Avis M. Evaluating a community-based walking intervention for hypertensive older people in Taiwan: a randomized controlled trial. Prev Med. 2007;44(2):160–6.
17. Arija V, Villalobos F, Pedret R, Vinuesa A, Jovani D, Pascual G, Basora J. Physical activity, cardiovascular health, quality of life and blood pressure control in hypertensive subjects: randomized clinical trial. Health Qual Life Outcomes. 2018;16(1):184.
18. Lee L-L, Mulvaney CA, Wong YKY, Chan ES, Watson MC, Lin H-H. Walking for hypertension. Cochrane Database Syst Rev. 2021;2(2):CD008823.
19. Diaz KM, Shimbo D. Physical activity and the prevention of hypertension. Curr Hypertens Rep. 2013;15(6):659–68.
20. Fagard RH, Cornelissen VA. Effect of exercise on blood pressure control in hypertensive patients. Eur J Cardiovasc Prev Rehabil. 2007;14:12–7.
21. Vaitkevicius PV, Fleg JL, Engel JH, O'Connor FC, Wright JG, Lakatta LE, et al. Effects of age and aerobic capacity on arterial stiffness in healthy adults. Circulation. 1993;88:1456–62.
22. Tanaka H, Dinenno FA, Monahan KD, Clevenger CM, DeSouza CA, Seals DR. Aging, habitual exercise, and dynamic arterial compliance. Circulation. 2000;102:1270–5.
23. Moreau KL, Donato AJ, Seals DR, DeSouza CA, Tanaka H. Regular exercise, hormone replacement therapy and the age-related decline in carotid arterial compliance in healthy women. Cardiovasc Res. 2003;57:861–8.
24. Lakatta EG, Levy D. Arterial and cardiac aging: major shareholders in cardiovascular disease enterprises: part I: aging arteries: a "set up" for vascular disease. Circulation. 2003;107(1):139–46.
25. Izquierdo M, Merchant RA, Morley JE, Anker SD, Aprahamian I, Arai H, et al. International exercise recommendations in older adults (ICFSR): expert consensus guidelines. J Nutr Health Aging. 2021;25(7):824–53.

Exercise for Systemic and Pulmonary Arterial Hypertension: Killing Two Birds with One Stone

13

Olga Vriz

Abbreviations

6MWD	6-min walking distance
CO	Cardiac output
CPET	Cardiopulmonary exercise testing
DPG	Diastolic pressure gradient
ET	Exercise training
LAP	Left atrial pressure
LV	Left ventricle
PAH	Pulmonary artery hypertension
PAP	Pulmonary artery pressure
PASP	Pulmonary artery systolic pressure
PAWP	Pulmonary arterial wedge pressure
PH	Pulmonary hypertension
PVR	Pulmonary vascular resistance
QoL	Quality of life
RV	Right ventricle
SV	Stroke volume
TPR	Total pulmonary resistance
TRV	Tricuspid velocity regurgitation
TTE	Transthoracic echocardiography
VCO_2	Carbon dioxide
VO_2	Oxygen uptake

O. Vriz (✉)
Heart Centre, King Faisal Specialist Hospital and Research Centre, Riyadh, Saudi Arabia

P. Palatini et al. (eds.), *Exercise, Sports and Hypertension*, Updates in Hypertension and Cardiovascular Protection,
https://doi.org/10.1007/978-3-031-07958-0_13

13.1 Introduction

A wealth of evidence has shown that regular physical activity has a favorable effect on the prevention of systemic hypertension and, as such, is considered a fundamental component of its treatment [1]. Exercise can be easily incorporated into a patient's lifestyle and can be an effective treatment for low-risk patients or, if combined with pharmacological treatments, in patients with an increased cardiovascular risk profile [2, 3]. Pulmonary hypertension is characterized by an increase in pulmonary artery pressure (PAH) and increased pulmonary vascular resistance (PVR), which leads to pulmonary artery remodeling and, if left untreated, into right ventricular (RV) maladaptation and failure, before developing into high, long-standing afterload and eventually death [4]. Treatment of PH is based on multidrug therapy which improves symptoms dramatically, increases exercise capacity and improves survival, but still leaves patients with poor functional capacity, RV function, and quality of life (QoL) [5]. On the other hand, excess physical activity has historically been thought to cause stress symptoms and it was only in 2009 that PH guidelines were updated to suggested that physical activity (within symptom limits) can improve functional capacity and QoL [6, 7]. Although exercise intolerance is commonly reported across all types of PH based on the complex interaction between pulmonary, cardiovascular, and musculoskeletal systems, little is known about the effect of physical exercise on PH.

13.2 Definition of Pulmonary Hypertension

Pulmonary hypertension is a disorder that can complicate a wide variety of cardiovascular and pulmonary diseases [8–12] and is characterized by progressive vascular remodeling with concurrently increased pulmonary vascular resistance and RV overload that may lead to RV failure and death [6]. PH, as systemic hypertension, is characterized with high levels of pulmonary artery pressure (PAP). PH is classified into five groups according to clinical presentation, pathological findings, hemodynamic characteristics and treatment strategy [6] (Table 13.1). The cutoff value is a mean pulmonary artery pressure (mPAP) higher than 25 mmHg as measured by right heart catheterization. Usually, mPAP in normal subjects at rest is 14 ± 4 mmHg, reaching approximately 20 mmHg. The term "PAH" includes patients with a pre-capillary pulmonary pressure (PAWP) ≤ 15 mmHg and PVR > 3 Wood units (WU) in the absence of lung disease or other rare diseases [6]. Since right heart catheterization is not an exam that can be used routinely, transthoracic echocardiography (TTE) can be used in everyday clinical practice to estimate pulmonary artery systolic pressure (PASP), derived from tricuspid valve regurgitation (TRV) plus the estimated right atrial pressure. Normal resting values determined by TTE are usually defined as a peak TRV of ≤2.8–2.9 m/s or a PASP of 35 or 36 mmHg, assuming an RA pressure of 3–5 mmHg [13], but up to 40 mmHg in old and obese patients. During exercise, PASP should not change significantly and 40 mmHg is considered the upper limit of normal [14], but higher values have been

Table 13.1 Classification of pulmonary hypertension [6]

Definition	Hemodynamic characteristics	Clinical groups
PH	PAPm ≥25 mmHg	All
Pre-capillary PH	PAPm ≥25 mmHg PAWP ≤15 mmHg	• Pulmonary arterial hypertension. • PH due to lung disease. • Chronic thromboembolic PH. • PH with unclear and/or multifactorial mechanisms.
Post-capillary PH	PAPm ≥25 mmHg PAWP >15 mmHg	• PH due to left heart disease. • PH with unclear and/or multifactorial mechanisms.
Isolated post-capillary PH	DPG <7 mmHg and/or PVR ≤3 WU	
Combined pre- and post-capillary PH	DPG ≥7 mmHg and/or PVR >3 WU	

DPG diastolic pressure gradient (diastolic PAP – mean PAWP), *PAPm* mean pulmonary arterial pressure, *PAWP* pulmonary arterial wedge pressure, *PH* pulmonary hypertension, *PVR* pulmonary vascular resistance, *WU* wood units. PAPm measured by right heart catheterization

reported by Argiento et al. [15]. PASP levels can be much higher in athletes, such as 51 mmHg at 240 W and a stroke volume of 91 mL [16].

13.2.1 Physiopathology of PAH

Pulmonary arterial hypertension is a complex, multifactorial disorder characterized by vasoconstriction, imbalanced vasoactive mediator levels, excessive cell proliferation, and impaired apoptosis in pulmonary vessels, which all lead to structural remodeling [17, 18]. The disorder is first characterized by endothelial dysfunction and vasoconstriction (stage 1), progressing to medial hypertrophy, mitogen and cytokine release, and inflammatory cell recruitment (stage 2). Up to this point, symptoms are still reversible, but once extracellular matrix remodeling with medial hyperplasia occurs (stage 3), symptoms are irreversible. The last step is characterized by intimal lesions, plexiform lesions, arterial thrombosis, and adventitia fibrosis with final RV involvement (stage 4) (Fig. 13.1).

13.2.2 Normal Pulmonary Hemodynamics in Response to Exercise

The pulmonary circulation is a low-pressure, high-flow circuit. Low pressure prevents fluid moving out of the pulmonary vessels into the interstitial space, and allows the RV to operate at minimal energy cost [19]. Physical exercise causes an increase in oxygen uptake (VO_2) and carbon dioxide (VCO_2) output up to 20-fold above resting values with an increase in CO up to 30–40 L/min in well trained athletes [15, 20]. Exercise may thus be considered a stressful condition for the

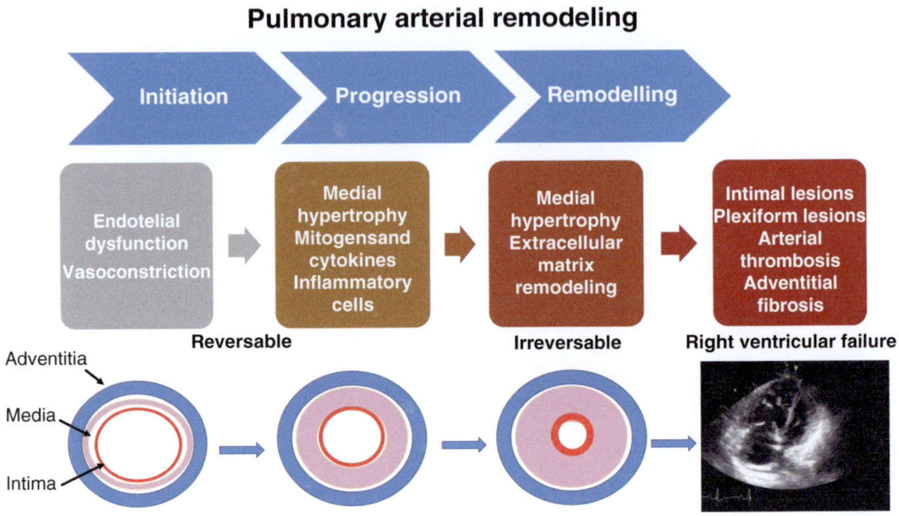

Fig. 13.1 Arterial vessel remodeling in pulmonary arterial hypertension

pulmonary circulation, which must receive the entire CO while keeping the lungs dry and the right ventricle compensated. In normal conditions, pulmonary pressure is related to both CO and other factors [21] such as PVR (determined by the resistance of the pre-capillary pulmonary arteries), total pulmonary resistance (TPR) (composed of PVR plus left ventricular filling resistance), arterial compliance (or distensibility of the resistive pulmonary arteries, α index) [22], and left atrial pressure (LAP, transmitting the pressure upstream in a close to 1:1 manner in the fully recruited pulmonary circulation also affecting pulmonary capillary wedge pressure) [15, 23–25]. During exercise in normal subjects, PAP increases proportionally to CO and the RV end systolic volume decreases as physical effort increases. On the other hand, in PH, PAP increases disproportionally to the increase in CO and RV end diastolic volume [26]. For example, an increase in PAP > 30 mmHg for CO < 10 L/min is associated with dyspnea and fatigue among those individuals at risk of developing PH.

This is true for dynamic exercise; static exercise has completely different hemodynamics characterized by increased systemic vascular resistance but limited increase in cardiac output and VO2 uptake, with a limited intrathoracic pressure change [27].

13.2.3 Exercise Limitation in PAH

13.2.3.1 RV Implications

During physical exercise in normal conditions, the pulmonary artery system is characterized by a drop in PVR due to the recruitment of the vascular bed, pulmonary vascular distensibility, and distention of the pre-capillary vessels and capillaries from flat to more circular to accommodate the three– to fourfold increase in CO [28]. In PH, pulmonary vascular distensibility is reduced, causing significant increase in PAP, resulting in limited exercise capacity. Since the RV has a thin wall chamber that adapts to volume overload but not to pressure overload, increased PAP leads to progressive RV dilation, dysfunction, RV-pulmonary artery uncoupling, decreased RV-CO, and inadequate delivery of oxygen to tissues [29]. Moreover, due to ventricular dependence, as both ventricles are nested within the pericardium [30], increase in pressure and volume in the RV accompanies a paradoxical leftward shift of the inter-ventricular septum, causing the left ventricle (LV) to compress and shrink, such that it is unable to fill up properly in diastole, leading to additional reduction in LV SV [31, 32].

Another effect of PAH on exercise limitation seems to be related to chronotropic incompetence associated with low oxygen pulse (VO_2/heart rate) [29]. A downregulation of ß-adrenoreceptor activity in the RV myocardial mass has been described [33] and is associated with disease severity [34]. Furthermore, impaired chronotropic capacity impairs the ability to increase CO during exercise, leading to decreased muscular oxygen availability (Fig. 13.2).

13.2.3.2 Ventilation-Perfusion Mismatch

PAH is characterized by arterial hypoxemia and arterial hypocapnia due to low alveolar–arterial diffusion, low mixed venous oxygen saturation, and high physiologic dead space. Hypoxemia stimulants increase ventilation during rest and exercise, and are associated with reduced perfusion of well-ventilated alveoli and can ultimately increase dead space. Overdrive of the sympathetic pathway could also play a role in hyperventilation due to the increased sensitivity of chemoreceptors [35, 36]. The

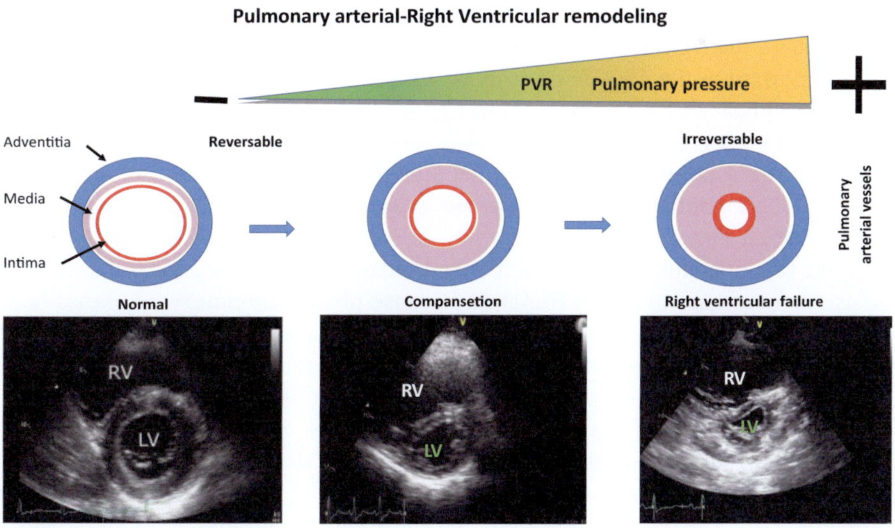

Fig. 13.2 Effect of pulmonary arterial remodeling on the right ventricle. *PVR* pulmonary vascular resistances, *LV* left ventricle, *RV* right ventricle

pulmonary circulation is rich in sympathetic nerve endings which play a role in vascular growth, differentiation and, in susceptible subjects, in vascular remodeling. The role of sympathetic activation was indirectly supported by the epidemic explosion of PAH after the release on the market of amphetamine derivative anorexigens [37, 38]. Furthermore, sympathetic activation is an adaptive response to low CO. Autonomic imbalance, sympathetic activation, and decreased parasympathetic activity, attributed to baroreflex sensitivity impairment, are associated with exercise intolerance and ventilatory inefficiency in PAH.

13.2.3.3 Muscle Dysfunction

Both peripheral and respiratory muscle dysfunction further contribute to exercise intolerance. Peripheral muscle dysfunction is related to low CO, vasoconstriction with poor oxygen delivery in addition to deconditioning. Furthermore, altered skeletal muscle microcirculation contributes to muscle dysfunction due to a reduced capillary–fiber ratio. In PAH, it has been noted that morphological and functional changes occur, such as the reduction in voluntary and involuntary skeletal muscle power, a lower proportion of type I fibers (fatigue resistance and postural control fibers), the increased proportion of type II fibers (quicker to fatigue and highly inefficient based on ATPase activity), and an enzyme shift toward anaerobic metabolism with reduced exercise capacity [39]. Hyperventilation, either during physical activity or at rest, contributes to respiratory muscle dysfunction because the increased work is not combined with increased CO and blood supply; in fact, 15% of the CO is requested by respiratory muscles in normal conditions [40]. Overstimulation of the diaphragm, the most important inspiratory muscle, causes contractile dysfunction which, combined with expiratory and inspiratory muscle impairment, reduces the thoracic pump function, thereby reducing its capacity to generate a pressure gradient to draw blood from the periphery to the right atrium and increase RV-SV. Such pump suction is particularly important in the context of increased PVR and/or RV impairment. Potential causes of muscle dysfunction might be hypoperfusion and low CO [41], decreased size and number of mitochondria [42], decreased oxidative enzymes [43], a decrease in muscle fiber cross-sectional area [44] and modification of actin [45], or a reduced number of actin–myosin cross-bridges in the diaphragm [46]. Moreover, an altered microvascular O_2 delivery-to-utilization rate will in turn slow the rate of adaptation to aerobic metabolism [47, 48]. Systemic inflammation is also involved in muscle dysfunction because pro-inflammatory cytokines have a detrimental effect on striated muscle, damaging the functional of contractile proteins and stimulating proteolysis [48]. Moreover, muscle dysfunction might be associated with early anaerobic metabolism which could exaggerate early peripheral muscle fatigue and limit exercise capacity.

The role of nutrition and its relationship with physical exercise and QoL is not yet explored in PAH, but some similarities are shared with left ventricular heart failure where more data are available. Malnutrition, weight loss and muscle waste are often found in PAH and are co-actors in the etiology of muscle dysfunction and fatigue. The underlying mechanisms of malnutrition are low CO, intestinal edema,

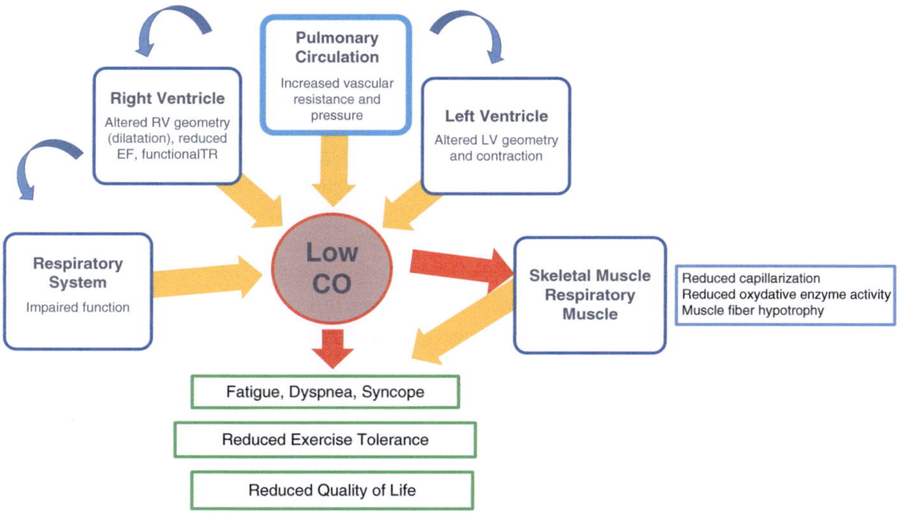

Fig. 13.3 Factors responsible for reduced CO in PH, along with reduced exercise tolerance and quality of life. *CO* cardiac output, *EF* ejection fraction, *TR* tricuspid regurgitation

inflammation, abnormal kidney function, changes in the microbiome and side effects of PAH-specific medication and diuretics, and deficiencies in iron and vitamin D absorption [49].

13.2.3.4 Inflammation

The relationship between cytokines and the initiation and progression of PAH has been demonstrated, and is typically characterized by a chronic increase in tumor necrosis factor (TNF)-α, interleukin (IL)-6, and IL-10 [50]. For example, overexpression of IL-6 induces PAH and vascular remodeling in animal models and further increases hypoxia-driven PH, and has also been shown to reduce apoptotic cell death. TNF-α augments pulmonary vasoconstriction and increases pulmonary vascular reactivity; its deficiency has shown to have a protective effect against PH development in murine models. Moreover, TNF-α seems to be related to the increased production of reactive oxygen species (ROS), which plays direct and indirect roles in vascular remodeling [51] (Fig. 13.3).

13.3 Exercise Training in PH

Historically, exercise training has not been recommended for patients with PAH due to the risk of sudden right heart failure and death. However, an increasing number of trials, including randomized controlled trials (RCT), and cohort studies have demonstrated the benefit of exercise on exercise capacity, peak oxygen consumption, and QoL. Physical exercise was described as a potential nonpharmacological approach for the management of PH by the European Society of Cardiology

Guidelines in 2009 [6]. These recommendations were based on the findings of Mereles et al. who were the first to demonstrate that exercise training (ET) was a promising intervention as an adjunct to medical therapy by improving 6 min walking distance (6MWD), peak VO_2, and QoL [7]. Supervised exercise training in physically deconditioned patients is classed as medical therapy by the European Guidelines 2015 (class IIa level of evidence: B), which however suggest that excessive physical activity leading to stress symptoms should be avoided (class III, level of evidence: C). However, the 2015 guidelines lack clarity in drawing a causative link between ET and the improvement of symptoms, patient functional capacity and outcomes. Furthermore, information is lacking on the types of exercise therapy or exercise modality (e.g., endurance or resistance training), frequency, duration, and intensity [52].

Nowadays, the evidence in favor of ET programs as an adjunct to the best standard of care is becoming more robust [53]. Typically, ET programs comprise exercises involving low cardiocirculatory stress, resistance training (e.g., with 500–1000 g dumbbells), respiratory training, body perception, yoga, and respiratory muscle-strengthening exercises. In general, the rehabilitation programs start in hospital and, once the patients are discharged, they continue at home following customized instructions. This approach seems to induce a positive effect on many targets, such as RV function, pulmonary circulation, musculature of the limbs, respiratory muscles, chemoreceptors, and baroreceptors. Indeed, in 2019 the European Respiratory Society published a state of the art on the clinical effects and mechanisms of action induced by exercise training and modalities [54]; these guidelines, alongside with systematic reviews [55, 56], agreed on the beneficial effect of ET in moderate PH (New York Heart Association (NYHA)/World Health Organization (WHO) Functional Class, class II and III) (Table 13.2).

13.3.1 Possible Effects of Exercise Training on PH

ET seems to feature all the credentials required to improve endothelial dysfunction, muscular blood supply, peripheral O2 extraction, muscular strength, ventilatory efficiency, ventricular contractility, reduce adrenergic tone and inflammatory response, increase vagal modulation, and restore baroreflex arterial sensitivity [57] (Fig. 13.4).

13.3.2 Inflammation

Several studies have demonstrated that both acute and chronic ET reduce systemic and local inflammation by reducing numbers of monocytes and macrophages, downregulating the expression of inflammatory genes in the pulmonary circulation and reducing systemic C-reactive protein and TNF-α levels [58]. In idiopathic PAH patients, exercise induces an immediate relative decrease in Th17 lymphocytes and a sustained reduction of IL-1-ß and IL-6 cytokines [50, 59]. A further effect of

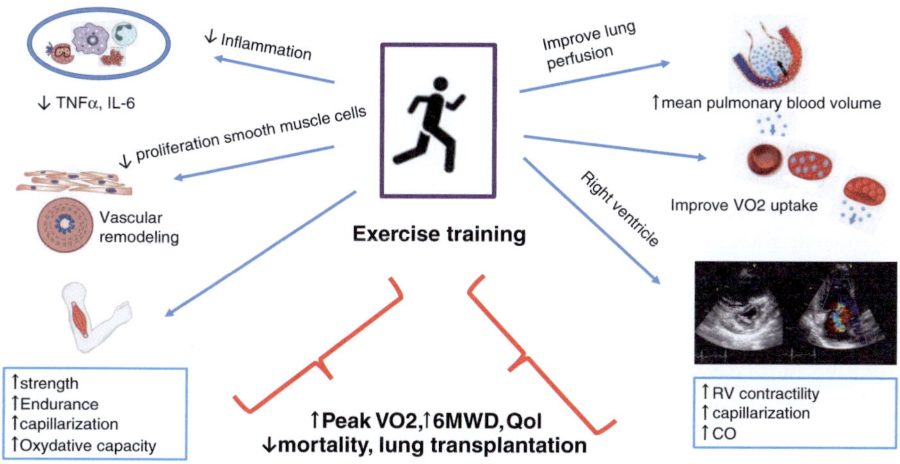

Fig. 13.4 Effects of exercise training in PH patients. *CO* cardiac output, *RV* right ventricle, *6MWD* 6-min walking distance, *QoL* quality of life

exercise is the impact on adrenal hormones via the hypothalamic-pituitary adrenal axis and the sympathetic nervous system, resulting in increased cortisol, norepinephrine and epinephrine. Cortisol has an anti-inflammatory effect while catecholamines have been shown to reduce cytokines such as TNF and IL-1ß; both hormones contribute to the anti-inflammatory effect of exercise [60].

13.3.3 Antioxidative Effects

Exercise training seems to induce an antioxidant effect: during acute exercise, exercise-induced reactive oxygen species and free radicals are created, mediating the upregulation of antioxidant molecules through an increase in glutathione reductase or superoxide dismutase levels [61].

13.3.4 Vascular and Right Ventricular Effect

In a study in rats where stable PH was achieved by monocrotaline (MCT), it was demonstrated that exercise rehabilitation training induced tolerance to increasing levels of exercise, which was related to a significant increase in the capillary density of RV myocardial tissue [62]. Indeed, in mild MCT-induced PAH, physical exercise has been shown to attenuate RV fibrosis and improve RV systolic pressure [63]. Indeed, Colombo et al. compared rats with MCT-induced PH to healthy controls, and divided both cohorts into sedentary and "exercised" subgroups. RV end-systolic pressure was decreased by 45% in the exercised PH group, with an 86% increase in the total volume of intramyocardial capillaries and 46% reduction in pulmonary artery thickness compared with the sedentary PH groups [64]. It has also been shown that chronic physical exercise increases pulmonary endogenous nitric oxide (NO) synthase expression in PAH rats, which in turn enhances NO production and vasodilatation [63]. The effect of physical exercise can also prevent vascular remodeling; in a hypoxia-induced PH model in mice, it was shown that the combination of training plus sildenafil had a more significant inhibitory effect on small pulmonary vessel muscularization than pharmacological treatment alone [63]. Similar results were found in an MCT-induced PAH rat model which found reduced pulmonary wall thickness in small and middle-diameter vessels compared with controls [64].

In PAH patients, physical training was found to be associated with improved cardiorespiratory function, decreased type II(x) fibers in the skeletal muscles and relative increase in type II(a) and type I fibers as less fatigable muscle profile [65], capillarization of the quadricep muscles and oxidative enzyme activity [66], and a significant increase in 6MWD (from 67 ± 59 m to 96 ± 61 m) [7, 48]. Ley et al. [67] used magnetic resonance to demonstrate a significant increase in 6MWD after 3 weeks of training, with improved lung blood volume and diminished peak flow velocity in the pulmonary artery circulation, suggestive of vasodilation in the pulmonary vessels. Exercise training may have beneficial effects on the right ventricle, since Ehlken et al. [68] found it was associated with decreased mean pulmonary pressure (−5 mmHg) and PVR (−1.3 Wood Units) and increased cardiac index (+0.4 L/min/m^2). The effects may also be beneficial in the long-term, since a group of patients in one study who received exercise training as an add-on to optimized medical therapy had better survival and fewer worsening events (lung transplantation, hospitalization, new PAH-targeted medication) at 1 and 3 year follow-ups, compared with the control group [69]. In a small group of patients wearing an actigraph placed on the wrist able to record the movements during the usual everyday home activities, it was demonstrated that daytime activity of less than 15 h/day was related to shorter survival [70] (Table 13.2).

Table 13.2 Effect of exercise training from Yuan et al. [55]. 2 randomized trials, 4 observational controlled studies, 6 observational studies, 449 patients

	Heart rate	6MWD	CPET	Work load
3 weeks	−2.9 beats/min	Increase Δ6MWD of 64.6 m	Increase in peak VO_2 per kg of 1.3 mL/min/kg.	Increase of 13.1 W
12 weeks exercise	No change	Increase in Δ6MWD of 62.2 m	Increase in peak VO_2 per kg of 1.7 mL/min/kg.	
12 or 15 weeks	No change	Increase in Δ6MWD of 63.7 m		Increase of 17.0 W
After 15 weeks training		Total improvement in QoL	The improvement in QoL in observational studies indicates that not only physical activity is involved but also other factors	

Exercise training is safe in stable PH patients with optimized medical treatment for at least 2 months. The Heidelberg group [71] reported side effects in 13.6% of their population that were not directly related to exercise. The most frequent adverse event was respiratory infection that required antibiotic therapy, followed by fatigue, dizziness, and hypotension that required training adjustment. Supraventricular arrhythmia, syncope, and pre-syncope were reported in less than 1% of the cases [71, 72] (Table 13.3).

Table 13.3 Exercise modality and monitoring [48, 54, 55, 73, 74]

Patients with moderate PH, clinically stable and received optimized PH-targeted medical treatment over at least 2 months				
Randomized trials controls	Patients/controls 71/66	Follow-up: 3 weeks in hospital + 12 weeks at home		
Observational studies	390/41	Follow-up: 3 weeks in hospital + 12 weeks at home or 4–12 weeks in an outpatient rehabilitation clinic		
Etiology	Miscellaneous			
Training modalities	In hospital start ET	Outpatient program/ rehabilitation clinic	Home-based exercise program	
Duration (examples) Frequency	3 weeks 2–5 times/week	12 weeks 2–5 session/ week in room hospital	Long term 2–5 times/week 15–30 min × session	Supervised by phone calls 2/week
Efficacy	General improvement. Only 30% of the studies did not show any improvement in 6MWD but other parameters improved such as exercise capacity, QoL			
Training modalities	Bicycle ergometer	Resistance exercise; low-weight dumbbell training or strength training	Respiratory muscle training	Breathing exercise
	Brisk treadmill walking	Resistance exercise/ moderate endurance training of leg muscle		
Monitoring/ supervision	Oxygen saturation (>85–90%)	Heart rate (<120–130 beats/min)	Perception of exertion by Borg dyspnea score	
Multidisciplinary lessons	Educational lesson "panic control"	Relaxation techniques	Educational lessons	Yoga
Physical monitoring improvement	6MWD		Cardiopulmonary exercise testing (CPET)	
Quality of life monitoring improvement	Physical functioning, general health perception, vitality, social functioning, role emotional, mental health. (short form health survey, SF-36)			
Contraindications	Unstable PH, RV decompensation, recent chest pain, light-headedness, dizziness, pre-syncope or syncope on exertion			

Although there is a consensus on the beneficial effect of ET in stable PAH, some points require further investigation such as the beneficial effect of ET on survival and RV remodeling and function. Randomized controlled trials are needed as well as a larger number of observations.

13.4 Conclusion

The effect of physical activity on systemic hypertension is well known, even if medical therapy is the mainstay of hypertension management. Systemic hypertension is often complicated by other conditions such as dyslipidemia, hyperinsulinemia, glucose intolerance, obesity, sympathetic overactivity, and arterial stiffness. Lifestyle changes improve multiple risk factors, and among those physical activity is a useful tool in the prevention and management of hypertension; constant training is recommended and may even negate the need for medical therapy in some patients. Exercise training has also been shown to be a safe and useful add-on therapy for PH patients with a majority of trials and metanalyses demonstrating a significant improvement in exercise capacity and QoL. Nonetheless, much less is known about PH compared with systemic hypertension, and findings for the latter condition cannot be applied to PH. Nonetheless, physical activity seems to improve muscle function, pulmonary perfusion, blood gas exchange, right ventricular function, and inhibition of inflammatory activation and smooth muscle cell proliferation. On the other hand, there are still some unclear effects that still need clarification in randomized trials, such as the effect of ET on RV function and hemodynamics, and indeed the role of ET in the prognosis and potential worsening of PH. Moreover, the optimal type of ET, and its modality, frequency, and intensity, along with the optimal lengths of the program, still need to be determined.

References

1. Williams B, Mancia G, Spiering W, Agabiti Rosei E, Azizi M, Burnier M, et al. 2018 practice guidelines for the management of arterial hypertension of the European Society of Cardiology and the European Society of Hypertension. Blood Press. 2018;27(6):314–40.
2. Palatini P, Visentin P, Dorigatti F, Guarnieri C, Santonastaso M, Cozzio S, et al. Regular physical activity prevents development of left ventricular hypertrophy in hypertension. Eur Heart J. 2008;30(2):225–32.
3. Wasfy MM, Baggish AL. Exercise dose in clinical practice. Circulation. 2016;133(23):2297–313.
4. Richter MJ, Grimminger J, Krüger B, Ghofrani HA, Mooren FC, Gall H, et al. Effects of exercise training on pulmonary hemodynamics, functional capacity and inflammation in pulmonary hypertension. Pulm Circ. 2017;7(1):20–37.
5. Kim NH, Fisher M, Poch D, Zhao C, Shah M, Bartolome S. Long-term outcomes in pulmonary arterial hypertension by functional class: a meta-analysis of randomized controlled trials and observational registries. Pulm Circ. 2020;10(4):2045894020935291.

6. Galiè N, Hoeper MM, Humbert M, Torbicki A, Vachiery J-L, Barbera JA, et al. Guidelines for the diagnosis and treatment of pulmonary hypertension: the task force for the diagnosis and treatment of pulmonary hypertension of the European Society of Cardiology (ESC) and the European Respiratory Society (ERS), endorsed by the International Society of Heart and Lung Transplantation (ISHLT). Eur Heart J. 2009;30(20):2493–537.
7. Mereles D, Ehlken N, Kreuscher S, Ghofrani S, Hoeper MM, Halank M, et al. Exercise and respiratory training improve exercise capacity and quality of life in patients with severe chronic pulmonary hypertension. Circulation. 2006;114(14):1482–9.
8. Garbi M, Chambers J, Vannan MA, Lancellotti P. Valve stress echocardiography. JACC Cardiovasc Imaging. 2015;8(6):724–36.
9. D'Andrea A, Stanziola AA, Saggar R, Saggar R, Sperlongano S, Conte M, et al. Right ventricular functional reserve in early-stage idiopathic pulmonary fibrosis: an exercise two-dimensional speckle tracking Doppler echocardiography study. Chest. 2019;155(2):297–306.
10. Serra W, Chetta A, Santilli D, Mozzani F, Dall'Aglio PP, Olivieri D, et al. Echocardiography may help detect pulmonary vasculopathy in the early stages of pulmonary artery hypertension associated with systemic sclerosis. Cardiovasc Ultrasound. 2010;8:25.
11. Nathan SD, Barbera JA, Gaine SP, Harari S, Martinez FJ, Olschewski H, et al. Pulmonary hypertension in chronic lung disease and hypoxia. Eur Respir J. 2019;53(1):1801914. [cited 2021 May 21]. Available from: https://www.ncbi.nlm.nih.gov/pmc/articles/PMC6351338/.
12. Mair KM, Gaw R, MacLean MR. Obesity, estrogens and adipose tissue dysfunction—implications for pulmonary arterial hypertension. Pulm Circ. 2020;10(3):2045894020952019. [cited 2021 May 21]. Available from: https://www.ncbi.nlm.nih.gov/pmc/articles/PMC7506791/.
13. Rudski LG, Lai WW, Afilalo J, Hua L, Handschumacher MD, Chandrasekaran K, et al. Guidelines for the echocardiographic assessment of the right heart in adults: a report from the American Society of Echocardiography endorsed by the European Association of Echocardiography, a registered branch of the European Society of Cardiology, and the Canadian Society of Echocardiography. J Am Soc Echocardiogr. 2010;23(7):685–713; quiz 786–8.
14. Grünig E, Weissmann S, Ehlken N, Fijalkowska A, Fischer C, Fourme T, et al. Stress Doppler echocardiography in relatives of patients with idiopathic and familial pulmonary arterial hypertension: results of a multicenter European analysis of pulmonary artery pressure response to exercise and hypoxia. Circulation. 2009;119(13):1747–57.
15. Argiento P, Chesler N, Mulè M, D'Alto M, Bossone E, Unger P, et al. Exercise stress echocardiography for the study of the pulmonary circulation. Eur Respir J. 2010;35(6):1273–8.
16. Bossone E, Vriz O, Bodini BD, Rubenfire M. Cardiovascular response to exercise in elite ice hockey players. Can J Cardiol. 2004;20(9):893–7.
17. Wilkins MR. Pulmonary hypertension: the science behind the disease spectrum. Eur Respir Rev. 2012;21(123):19–26.
18. Humbert M, Guignabert C, Bonnet S, Dorfmüller P, Klinger JR, Nicolls MR, et al. Pathology and pathobiology of pulmonary hypertension: state of the art and research perspectives. Eur Respir J. 2019;53(1):1801887.
19. Vonk Noordegraaf A, Westerhof BE, Westerhof N. The relationship between the right ventricle and its load in pulmonary hypertension. J Am Coll Cardiol. 2017;69(2):236–43.
20. Gerche AL, Claessen G, Van de Bruaene A, Pattyn N, Van Cleemput J, Gewillig M, et al. Cardiac MRI. Circ Cardiovasc Imaging. 2013;6(2):329–38.
21. Coffman KE, Curry TB, Dietz NM, Chase SC, Carlson AR, Ziegler BL, et al. The influence of pulmonary vascular pressures on lung diffusing capacity during incremental exercise in healthy aging. Physiol Rep. 2018;6(2):e13565. Available from: https://www.ncbi.nlm.nih.gov/pmc/articles/PMC5789722/.
22. Reeves JT, Linehan JH, Stenmark KR. Distensibility of the normal human lung circulation during exercise. Am J Physiol Lung Cell Mol Physiol. 2005;288(3):L419–25.
23. Wachter R, Schmidt-Schweda S, Westermann D, Post H, Edelmann F, Kasner M, et al. Blunted frequency-dependent upregulation of cardiac output is related to impaired relaxation in diastolic heart failure. Eur Heart J. 2009;30(24):3027–36.

24. Burgess MI, Jenkins C, Sharman JE, Marwick TH. Diastolic stress echocardiography: hemodynamic validation and clinical significance of estimation of ventricular filling pressure with exercise. J Am Coll Cardiol. 2006;47(9):1891–900.
25. Maeder MT, Thompson BR, Brunner-La Rocca H-P, Kaye DM. Hemodynamic basis of exercise limitation in patients with heart failure and Normal ejection fraction. J Am Coll Cardiol. 2010;56(11):855–63.
26. Wierzbowska-Drabik K, Kasprzak JD, D Alto M, Ágoston G, Varga A, Ferrara F, et al. Reduced pulmonary vascular reserve during stress echocardiography in confirmed pulmonary hypertension and patients at risk of overt pulmonary hypertension. Int J Cardiovasc Imaging. 2020;36(10):1831–43.
27. Motoji Y, Forton K, Pezzuto B, Faoro V, Naeije R. Resistive or dynamic exercise stress testing of the pulmonary circulation and the right heart. Eur Respir J. 2017;50(1):1700151.
28. Waxman AB. Exercise physiology and pulmonary arterial hypertension. Prog Cardiovasc Dis. 2012;55(2):172–9.
29. Sun X-G, Hansen JE, Oudiz RJ, Wasserman K. Exercise pathophysiology in patients with primary pulmonary hypertension. Circulation. 2001;104(4):429–35.
30. Kroeker CAG, Shrive NG, Belenkie I, Tyberg JV. Pericardium modulates left and right ventricular stroke volumes to compensate for sudden changes in atrial volume. Am J Physiol Heart Circ Physiol. 2003;284(6):H2247–54.
31. Friedberg MK, Redington AN. Right versus left ventricular failure: differences, similarities, and interactions. Circulation. 2014;129(9):1033–44.
32. Naeije R, Badagliacca R. The overloaded right heart and ventricular interdependence. Cardiovasc Res. 2017;113(12):1474–85.
33. Bristow MR, Minobe W, Rasmussen R, Larrabee P, Skerl L, Klein JW, et al. Beta-adrenergic neuroeffector abnormalities in the failing human heart are produced by local rather than systemic mechanisms. J Clin Invest. 1992;89(3):803–15.
34. Wensel R, Jilek C, Dörr M, Francis DP, Stadler H, Lange T, et al. Impaired cardiac autonomic control relates to disease severity in pulmonary hypertension. Eur Respir J. 2009;34(4):895–901.
35. Velez-Roa S, Ciarka A, Najem B, Vachiery J-L, Naeije R, van de Borne P. Increased sympathetic nerve activity in pulmonary artery hypertension. Circulation. 2004;110(10):1308–12.
36. Alberto Neder J, O'Donnell DE. Heart, lungs, and muscle interplay in worsening activity-related breathlessness in advanced cardiopulmonary disease. Curr Opin Support Palliat Care. 2020;14(3):157–66.
37. Abenhaim L, Moride Y, Brenot F, Rich S, Benichou J, Kurz X, et al. Appetite-suppressant drugs and the risk of primary pulmonary hypertension. International primary pulmonary hypertension study group. N Engl J Med. 1996;335(9):609–16.
38. Gurtner HP. Aminorex and pulmonary hypertension. A review. Cor Vasa. 1985;27(2–3):160–71.
39. Batt J, Ahmed SS, Correa J, Bain A, Granton J. Skeletal muscle dysfunction in idiopathic pulmonary arterial hypertension. Am J Respir Cell Mol Biol. 2014;50(1):74–86.
40. Meyer FJ, Lossnitzer D, Kristen AV, Schoene AM, Kübler W, Katus HA, et al. Respiratory muscle dysfunction in idiopathic pulmonary arterial hypertension. Eur Respir J. 2005;25(1):125–30.
41. Hambrecht R, Niebauer J, Fiehn E, Kälberer B, Offner B, Hauer K, et al. Physical training in patients with stable chronic heart failure: effects on cardiorespiratory fitness and ultrastructural abnormalities of leg muscles. J Am Coll Cardiol. 1995;25(6):1239–49.
42. Enache I, Charles A-L, Bouitbir J, Favret F, Zoll J, Metzger D, et al. Skeletal muscle mitochondrial dysfunction precedes right ventricular impairment in experimental pulmonary hypertension. Mol Cell Biochem. 2013;373(1–2):161–70.
43. Malenfant S, Potus F, Fournier F, Breuils-Bonnet S, Pflieger A, Bourassa S, et al. Skeletal muscle proteomic signature and metabolic impairment in pulmonary hypertension. J Mol Med. 2015;93(5):573–84.
44. Breda AP, Pereira-de-Albuquerque AL, Jardim C, Morinaga LK, Suesada MM, CJC F, et al. Skeletal muscle abnormalities in pulmonary arterial hypertension. PLoS One. 2014;9(12):e114101.

45. Himori K, Abe M, Tatebayashi D, Lee J, Westerblad H, Lanner JT, et al. Superoxide dismutase/catalase mimetic EUK-134 prevents diaphragm muscle weakness in monocrotalin-induced pulmonary hypertension. PLoS One. 2017;12(2):e0169146.
46. Lecarpentier Y, Coirault C, Lerebours G, Desche P, Scalbert E, Lambert F, et al. Effects of angiotensin converting enzyme inhibition on crossbridge properties of diaphragm in cardiomyopathic hamsters of the dilated bio 53-58 strain. Am J Respir Crit Care Med. 1997;155(2):630–6.
47. Barbosa PB, Ferreira EMV, Arakaki JSO, Takara LS, Moura J, Nascimento RB, et al. Kinetics of skeletal muscle O2 delivery and utilization at the onset of heavy-intensity exercise in pulmonary arterial hypertension. Eur J Appl Physiol. 2011;111(8):1851–61.
48. Marra AM, Arcopinto M, Bossone E, Ehlken N, Cittadini A, Grünig E. Pulmonary arterial hypertension-related myopathy: an overview of current data and future perspectives. Nutr Metab Cardiovasc Dis. 2015;25(2):131–9.
49. Kwant CT, Ruiter G, Noordegraaf AV. Malnutrition in pulmonary arterial hypertension: a possible role for dietary intervention. Curr Opin Pulm Med. 2019;25(5):405–9.
50. Harbaum L, Renk E, Yousef S, Glatzel A, Lüneburg N, Hennigs JK, et al. Acute effects of exercise on the inflammatory state in patients with idiopathic pulmonary arterial hypertension. BMC Pulm Med. 2016;16(1):145.
51. Cai H. NAD(P)H oxidase-dependent self-propagation of hydrogen peroxide and vascular disease. Circ Res. 2005;96(8):818–22.
52. Galiè N, Humbert M, Vachiery J-L, Gibbs S, Lang I, Torbicki A, et al. 2015 ESC/ERS Guidelines for the diagnosis and treatment of pulmonary hypertension: The Joint Task Force for the Diagnosis and Treatment of Pulmonary Hypertension of the European Society of Cardiology (ESC) and the European Respiratory Society (ERS): Endorsed by: Association for European Paediatric and Congenital Cardiology (AEPC), International Society for Heart and Lung Transplantation (ISHLT). Eur Heart J. 2016;37(1):67–119.
53. Buys R, Avila A, Cornelissen VA. Exercise training improves physical fitness in patients with pulmonary arterial hypertension: a systematic review and meta-analysis of controlled trials. BMC Pulm Med. 2015;15:40.
54. Grünig E, Eichstaedt C, Barberà J-A, Benjamin N, Blanco I, Bossone E, et al. ERS statement on exercise training and rehabilitation in patients with severe chronic pulmonary hypertension. Eur Respir J. 2019;53(2):1800332.
55. Yuan P, Yuan X-T, Sun X-Y, Pudasaini B, Liu J-M, Hu Q-H. Exercise training for pulmonary hypertension: a systematic review and meta-analysis. Int J Cardiol. 2015;178:142–6.
56. Morris NR, Kermeen FD, Holland AE. Exercise-based rehabilitation programmes for pulmonary hypertension. Cochrane Database Syst Rev. 2017;1:CD011285.
57. Zhang X, Xu D. Effects of exercise rehabilitation training on patients with pulmonary hypertension. Pulm Circ. 2020;10(3):2045894020937129.
58. Mattusch F, Dufaux B, Heine O, Mertens I, Rost R. Reduction of the plasma concentration of C-reactive protein following nine months of endurance training. Int J Sports Med. 2000;21(1):21–4.
59. Peake JM, Della Gatta P, Suzuki K, Nieman DC. Cytokine expression and secretion by skeletal muscle cells: regulatory mechanisms and exercise effects. Exerc Immunol Rev. 2015;21:8–25.
60. Walsh NP, Gleeson M, Pyne DB, Nieman DC, Dhabhar FS, Shephard RJ, et al. Position statement. Part two: maintaining immune health. Exerc Immunol Rev. 2011;17:64–103.
61. de Sousa CV, Sales MM, Rosa TS, Lewis JE, de Andrade RV, Simões HG. The antioxidant effect of exercise: a systematic review and meta-analysis. Sports Med. 2017;47(2):277–93.
62. Handoko ML, de Man FS, Happé CM, Schalij I, Musters RJP, Westerhof N, et al. Opposite effects of training in rats with stable and progressive pulmonary hypertension. Circulation. 2009;120(1):42–9.
63. Brown MB, Neves E, Long G, Graber J, Gladish B, Wiseman A, et al. High-intensity interval training, but not continuous training, reverses right ventricular hypertrophy and dysfunction in a rat model of pulmonary hypertension. Am J Physiol Regul Integr Comp Physiol. 2017;312(2):R197–210.

64. Colombo R, Siqueira R, Becker CU, Fernandes TG, Pires KM, Valença SS, et al. Effects of exercise on monocrotaline-induced changes in right heart function and pulmonary artery remodeling in rats. Can J Physiol Pharmacol. 2013;91(1):38–44.
65. Mainguy V, Maltais F, Saey D, Gagnon P, Martel S, Simon M, et al. Effects of a rehabilitation program on skeletal muscle function in idiopathic pulmonary arterial hypertension. J Cardiopulm Rehabil Prev. 2010;30(5):319–23.
66. de Man FS, Handoko ML, Groepenhoff H, van 't Hul AJ, Abbink J, Koppers RJH, et al. Effects of exercise training in patients with idiopathic pulmonary arterial hypertension. Eur Respir J. 2009;34(3):669–75.
67. Ley S, Fink C, Risse F, Ehlken N, Fischer C, Ley-Zaporozhan J, et al. Magnetic resonance imaging to assess the effect of exercise training on pulmonary perfusion and blood flow in patients with pulmonary hypertension. Eur Radiol. 2013;23(2):324–31.
68. Ehlken N, Lichtblau M, Klose H, Weidenhammer J, Fischer C, Nechwatal R, et al. Exercise training improves peak oxygen consumption and haemodynamics in patients with severe pulmonary arterial hypertension and inoperable chronic thrombo-embolic pulmonary hypertension: a prospective, randomized, controlled trial. Eur Heart J. 2016;37(1):35–44.
69. Ehlken N, Verduyn C, Tiede H, Staehler G, Karger G, Nechwatal R, et al. Economic evaluation of exercise training in patients with pulmonary hypertension. Lung. 2014;192(3):359–66.
70. Ulrich S, Fischler M, Speich R, Bloch KE. Wrist actigraphy predicts outcome in patients with pulmonary hypertension. Respir Int Rev Thorac Dis. 2013;86(1):45–51.
71. Grünig E, Lichtblau M, Ehlken N, Ghofrani HA, Reichenberger F, Staehler G, et al. Safety and efficacy of exercise training in various forms of pulmonary hypertension. Eur Respir J. 2012;40(1):84–92.
72. Nagel C, Prange F, Guth S, Herb J, Ehlken N, Fischer C, et al. Exercise training improves exercise capacity and quality of life in patients with inoperable or residual chronic thromboembolic pulmonary hypertension. PLoS One. 2012;7(7):e41603.
73. Pandey A, Garg S, Khunger M, Garg S, Kumbhani DJ, Chin KM, et al. Efficacy and safety of exercise training in chronic pulmonary hypertension: systematic review and meta-analysis. Circ Heart Fail. 2015;8(6):1032–43.
74. Dalla Vecchia LA, Bussotti M. Exercise training in pulmonary arterial hypertension. J Thorac Dis. 2018;10(1):508–21.

High Altitude and Blood Pressure: Clinical Implications

14

Grzegorz Bilo, Martino Pengo, Camilla Torlasco, Sergio Caravita, and Gianfranco Parati

14.1 What Is High Altitude?

High altitude (HA) is an extreme environment, in which human body is exposed to several challenging conditions factors including low temperatures, low air humidity and high UV radiation levels. The foremost factor determining physiological responses to HA is, however, the low atmospheric pressure. Although the relative oxygen concentration remains about 21%, regardless of the altitude, the proportional reduction of oxygen partial pressure in the inspired air leads to an absolute reduction of oxygen availability for the organism (hypobaric hypoxia, Fig. 14.1) and, in consequence, to hypoxemia and tissue hypoxia [1, 3]. Human body is

G. Bilo · G. Parati (✉)
Department of Medicine and Surgery, University of Milano-Bicocca, Milan, Italy

Department of Cardiology, San Luca Hospital, Istituto Auxologico Italiano, IRCCS, Milan, Italy

University of Milano-Bicocca, Milan, Italy
e-mail: g.bilo@auxologico.it; gianfranco.parati@unimib.it

M. Pengo · C. Torlasco
Department of Cardiology, San Luca Hospital, Istituto Auxologico Italiano, IRCCS, Milan, Italy

University of Milano-Bicocca, Milan, Italy
e-mail: m.pengo@auxologico.it; c.torlasco@auxologico.it

S. Caravita
Department of Cardiology, San Luca Hospital, Istituto Auxologico Italiano, IRCCS, Milan, Italy

University of Milano-Bicocca, Milan, Italy

Department of Management Information and Production Engineering, University of Bergamo, Dalmine, BG, Italy
e-mail: s.caravita@auxologico.it

P. Palatini et al. (eds.), *Exercise, Sports and Hypertension*, Updates in Hypertension and Cardiovascular Protection,
https://doi.org/10.1007/978-3-031-07958-0_14

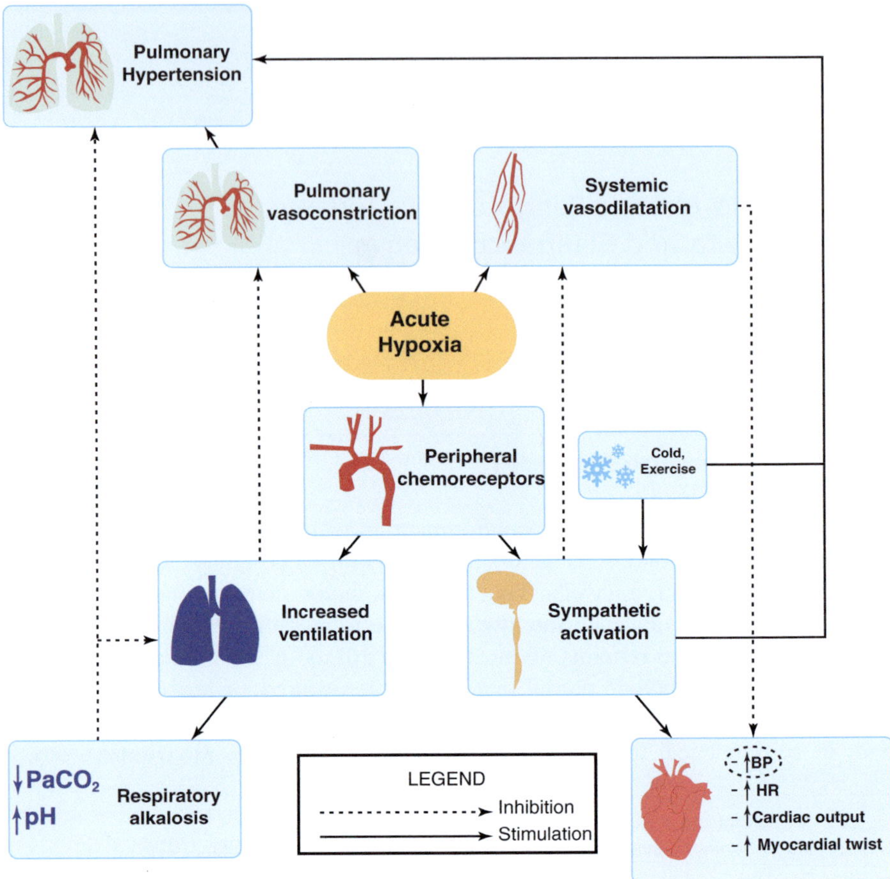

Fig. 14.1 Principal mechanisms underlying circulatory and respiratory response to acute HA exposure. From Parati et al. [1, 2]

equipped with a number of physiological responses which counteract the decreased oxygen supply to the tissues and their activation generally allows to adapt rapidly to hypoxic challenge. Sometimes, however, there responses may become maladaptive and lead to pathological conditions such as acute mountain sickness (AMS) or chronic mountain sickness (CMS or Monge's disease) [4].

From medical point of view, HA is defined as an altitude at which physiological responses of the organism to hypoxia become relevant. Since atmospheric pressure decreases in a continuous manner with altitude and there is a considerable interindividual variability in response to hypoxia, there is no real threshold level for HA. However, conventionally an altitude above 2500 m above sea level (where the PaO_2 is about 60 mmHg) is considered as the lower limit of HA. Another important limit is that of about 8000 m—above this altitude the "death zone" starts, where the mechanisms of adaptation to hypoxia cannot maintain the homeostasis making survival impossible in the long term [5].

14.2 How HA Affects Circulation

Traditionally, the research on HA physiology and pathophysiology focused mainly on pulmonary circulation, considering that alveolar hypoxia exerts direct effect on pulmonary vessels. In fact, hypoxic pulmonary vasoconstriction is a physiological response aimed at maintaining adequate ventilation–perfusion matching. This response normally redirects blood flow from hypoventilated lung areas to those with adequate ventilation but, in a condition of generalized hypoxia at HA it commonly induces pulmonary hypertension and may lead to high altitude pulmonary oedema (HAPE) [3]. On the other hand, the responses of peripheral circulation to HA and, in particular, changes in systemic arterial blood pressure (BP) were less extensively studied and are less understood. Nonetheless, this issue merits attention, considering that millions of people are exposed to elevated altitudes either acutely, or chronically, including a relevant proportion of those with cardiovascular risk factors or diseases, such as arterial hypertension [6, 7]. Short-lasting HA exposure is common in the setting of mountain tourism and of high-altitude industries (e.g. mining). Furthermore, millions of people permanently live at HAs, mainly in Asia, South America and Ethiopia.

14.2.1 Effects of Acute HA Exposure on BP in Healthy Individuals at Rest and During Exercise

The net effect of hypoxia on BP depends on an interplay of multiple factors and regulatory mechanisms and is determined by the degree of hypoxia, duration and time course of the exposure, the presence of other factors (physical and mental stress, nutrition/hydration, pharmacological treatment) and individual characteristics. Because of this complexity, considerable differences regarding BP behaviour were reported, depending on study setting and design.

Several studies in physiology laboratories addressed the impact of hypoxia on BP in animals and humans in a controlled setting of simulated HA (hypobaric chamber or breathing normobaric hypoxic gas mixture), typically during a relatively short exposure to hypoxia. Generally, modest to no changes in mean arterial pressure during short-lasting (up to several hours) hypoxia exposure were observed, despite important changes in systemic haemodynamics [8]. On the other hand, a number of field studies were performed in order to explore longer lasting HA exposures in "real life" conditions where other relevant factors such as cold, physical exertion, emotional stress and changes in food and water intake are also involved.

Most (but not all) studies in which BP was measured conventionally (typically two to three measurements in a short sequence performed with a manual or oscillometric device) showed a possible pressor effect of acute HA exposure, starting 4–6 h since HA was reached [3, 8–10]. More consistent information was obtained in studies making use of a method allowing for more reproducible and extensive evaluation of BP, that is 24-h ambulatory BP monitoring (ABPM). This technique has allowed to assess BP at HA under daily life conditions, including daytime challenges and night-time sleep.

Early studies in small groups of healthy volunteers provided initial evidence of ambulatory BP increase during acute HA exposure [9, 11, 12]. More solid evidence was provided by HIGHCARE (*HIGH* altitude *CA*rdiovascular *RE*search)-Himalaya study performed in Nepal. Forty-seven healthy volunteers were evaluated at sea level, after short (2–3 days) exposure to 3400 m altitude, then immediately after reaching 5400 m (Mt. Everest Base Camp) and after 12 days of permanence at this altitude. Already at 3400 m 24-h, daytime and night-time BP clearly increased, and a further increment in BP was observed after arrival at 5400 m with no clear evidence of BP reduction after 12 days of permanence at this altitude (Fig. 14.2) [13]. More recently these findings were extended to healthy volunteers exposed to an altitude of 2000 m (e.g. moderate altitude), in whom a modest but significant 24-h BP increase was observed [14]. Taken together these observations clearly indicate a

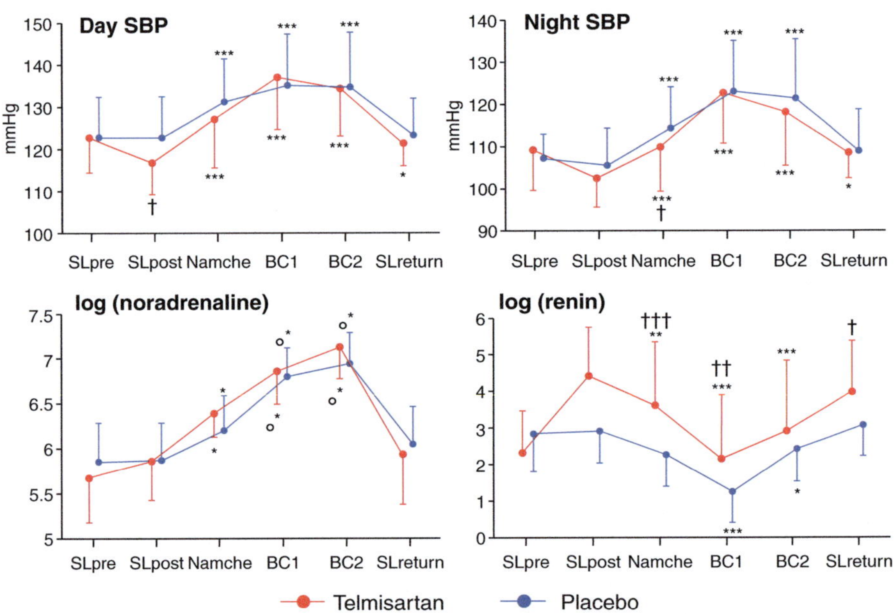

Fig. 14.2 Changes in systolic blood pressure during daytime (upper left) and night-time (upper right) in healthy participants of HIGHCARE-Himalaya Study randomized to placebo (blue lines) or telmisartan 80 mg od (red lines). Lower panels show parallel changes occurring in the levels of noradrenaline (left) and renin (right). Data obtained at sea level pre-treatment (SLpre), at sea level post treatment (SLpost), at 3400 m (Namche), at Mt. Everest base camp, 5400 m, during first 3 days (BC1) and after 11–12 days (BC2), and immediately after return to sea level (SLreturn). Different symbols indicate statistical significance of differences between groups (cross symbols) and of differences between altitudes considering SLpost as reference (circles and asterisks). From Parati et al. [13], modified, by permission

significant pressor effect of short-term HA exposure, the size of BP increase being proportional to the altitude reached.

The results of several studies performed with ABPM indicate that BP increase at HA may be particularly pronounced during sleep, leading to a reduction in physiological nocturnal BP fall (dipping) [9, 12, 15]. In HIGHCARE-Himalaya this phenomenon was observed at very high altitude (5400 m) but not at 3400 m [13]. Conversely, no change in nocturnal dipping was found in subjects exposed to an altitude of 2000 m [14].

Little is known about evolution of BP changes during HA sojourn longer than 2 weeks. Although some data indicate that after months of HA permanence BP does not significantly differ from pre-exposure values [16], in a study in young army recruits BP increase tended to persist even after 12 months at HA [17].

A very particular model of HA exposure is that of chronic intermittent hypoxia (CIH), where relatively brief periods of HA permanence are alternated with stay at low altitude. This model is commonly found among workers of mines in South America located at HAs, especially in Chile. These workers typically spend 4 or 7 days working at HA and 3 or 7 days, respectively, at their homes. The aim is to minimize the likelihood of complications of living permanently at HA (in particular, chronic mountain sickness) and to ensure an acceptable quality of life of the workers. This model was shown to induce acclimatization process, albeit not as complete as in permanent HA inhabitants [18]. As shown in a recent study, workers following such schedule for at least 2 years still displayed a significant, acute BP increase on arrival at altitude of 3870 m (by about 15 mmHg for systolic and 9 mmHg for diastolic 24-h BP). However, normalization of conventional BP was observed at the end of 7 days' HA stay, suggesting an accelerated cardiovascular adaptation to hypoxia in these subjects [19].

Considering that HA exposure is frequently associated with physical effort (sport, physical work) it is interesting to know how BP behaves during exercise at HA. Winkler et al. performed a study in subjects acutely exposed to simulated altitude and reported that BP was higher at a given workload than during normoxic exercise. This difference was no longer evident when hypoxic and normoxic exercise BP was compared at the same heart rate (HR). This suggests that higher BP observed in hypoxic exercise was largely explained by an increase in HR [20]. Few field studies at HA in healthy untreated individuals focused on BP behaviour during exercise. Valentini et al. reported similar peak exercise SBP at sea level (SL) but at HA the achieved VO2 and HR were significantly lower than at SL, indicating lower peak exercise intensity in the former condition [21]. In fact, HA hypoxia reduces exercise capacity mainly because of limited muscle oxygen delivery [22] and this appears to limit BP increase at peak exercise to values observed also at SL [23]. Accordingly, in the HIGHCARE-ANDES study, lowlanders exposed to HA achieved BP values at peak exercise which were similar to those attained at sea level [24]. However, VO_2, as an objective measure for exercise intensity and as a surrogate for cardiac output, was expectedly reduced at HA as compared to SL. Thus, after BP was normalized for VO_2, it was definitely higher at HA than at SL [24]. Furthermore, when BP trajectories were plotted as a function of VO_2, BP increase during exercise resulted both upward-shifted and steepened at HA as compared to SL [23, 24].

14.2.2 Mechanisms of BP Changes

A number of physiological responses are activated (or suppressed) at HA, which may have opposing effects on BP and their net effect depends heavily on the duration of exposure.

Most data on the initial (first hours) phase of exposure to hypobaric hypoxia come from laboratory studies in simulated hypoxia and indicate a major role of direct hypoxic vasodilatation with a decrease in peripheral vascular resistances. This is counterbalanced by an increase in heart rate (due to parasympathetic withdrawal and sympathetic activation mediated foremostly by arterial chemoreflex), which, together with unchanged stroke volume, leads to an increase in cardiac output. As the result, BP remains typically unchanged in this phase [8].

If HA permanence continues, the situation changes and after several hours BP starts to increase (see above) and remains elevated for at least 2–3 weeks. Interestingly, this occurs despite a progressive decrease in plasma volume, due to increased diuresis typically observed during HA permanence, with a consequent reduction in stroke volume (contractility of the left ventricle remains unchanged). The principal factor underlying this hypertensive response appears to be an important increase in sympathetic activity, causing an increase both in HR and in peripheral resistances. This response is mainly mediated by the activation of peripheral chemoreflex by low pO_2 (Fig. 14.1) and was confirmed by increased plasma levels of noradrenalin and by direct microneurographic studies [13, 25, 26]. It was shown that an increase in blood oxygenation induced by slow, deep breathing is accompanied by an immediate decrease of BP values, supporting the role of chemoreflex activation [27]. Changes in arterial baroreflex also occur; in fact, resetting to higher operating BP and/or reduced baroreflex sensitivity was reported [25, 28].

The involvement of endocrine mechanisms of BP regulation during HA exposure appears to be secondary to the above changes in autonomic control. In particular, renin–angiotensin–aldosterone (RAAS) system activity is suppressed at very high altitude (above 3400 m) [13], possibly because of the activation of kidney baroreceptors secondary to BP increase or due to a direct inhibition of renin secretion by hypoxia (Fig. 14.2) [29]. Other mechanisms relevant in determining BP level at HA, include modulation of large arteries elastic properties by sympathetic activation (an increase in aortic stiffness was observed), impaired endothelial function and increase in blood viscosity, the latter due to haemoconcentration (loss of plasma volume followed by increased erythropoiesis) [30–33].

As previously mentioned, HA may have a larger hypertensive effect during sleep, leading to a reduced BP dipping. The underlying mechanisms are not clear but the following factors may be involved: (1) decrease of blood oxygenation, particularly pronounced during sleep at HA, responsible for stimulation of peripheral chemoreceptors. This stimulation may sustain abnormally high sympathetic tone during sleep and wake; (2) the occurrence of central apnoeas during sleep is common at HA and, although the association of central apnoeas with BP increase is not documented, it may not be fully ruled out [34]; (3) impaired arterial baroreflex function (with consequently reduced response to hydrostatic effects on BP); (4) poor sleep quality (due to AMS symptoms, low air humidity, psychological stress).

14.3 Clinical Implications

The clinical implications of BP response to HA exposure are related to several aspects: (1) whether BP increase during acute HA exposure may by itself lead to cardiovascular complications, in particular in individuals already characterized by an increased cardiovascular risk; (2) whether HA permanence modifies the effects of antihypertensive drugs; (3) whether permanent living at HA may affect BP and hypertension prevalence.

14.3.1 HA and Cardiovascular Pathological Conditions

In healthy individuals BP elevations during acute HA exposure are, on average, moderate and the BP values reached in this condition are unlikely to cause direct harm. The situation might be different in patients with cardiovascular diseases, more susceptible to BP related complications. Several studies were performed in patients with hypertension acutely exposed to HA. In our study, carried out on the Peruvian Andes, untreated patients with mild hypertension displayed a significant increase in ambulatory BP values on the second day after the arrival at 3200 m as compared to their sea level values, but this brief permanence was not associated with clinically relevant problems [15]. Also, Savonitto et al. found higher pre-exercise BP at HA compared to lower altitude in hypertensive patients [35]. Acute pressor response to acute HA exposure was also manifest in well controlled hypertensive miners, working according to a CIH exposure model (7 days at HA and 7 days at SL), upon arrival at the mine. This increase however was of modest magnitude, and BP returned to SL level after 7 days pf permanence at HA [19]. In this last study BP increase tended to be more pronounced in hypertensive than in normotensive participants, especially during the night, with a marked reduction in nocturnal BP dipping. Interestingly, 24-h ABPM revealed that in an elevated proportion of individuals ambulatory BP exceeded normality thresholds, while conventional BP remained within normal limits (masked hypertension phenotype; Fig. 14.3). Again, this BP increase was not associated with any acute cardiovascular complication [19].

Even if the HA-induced short-lasting increase in resting BP appears to be devoid of immediate clinical importance in most hypertensive individuals, the possibility that exercise might induce very pronounced BP elevations in this setting may raise some concern. Apparently, though, even if the curve of BP increase with increasing workload is shifted upwards in hypertensive individuals acutely exposed to HA (compared to either SL condition and to normotensive counterparts) [20, 23, 35] and appears steeper than in normotensives when normalized for oxygen

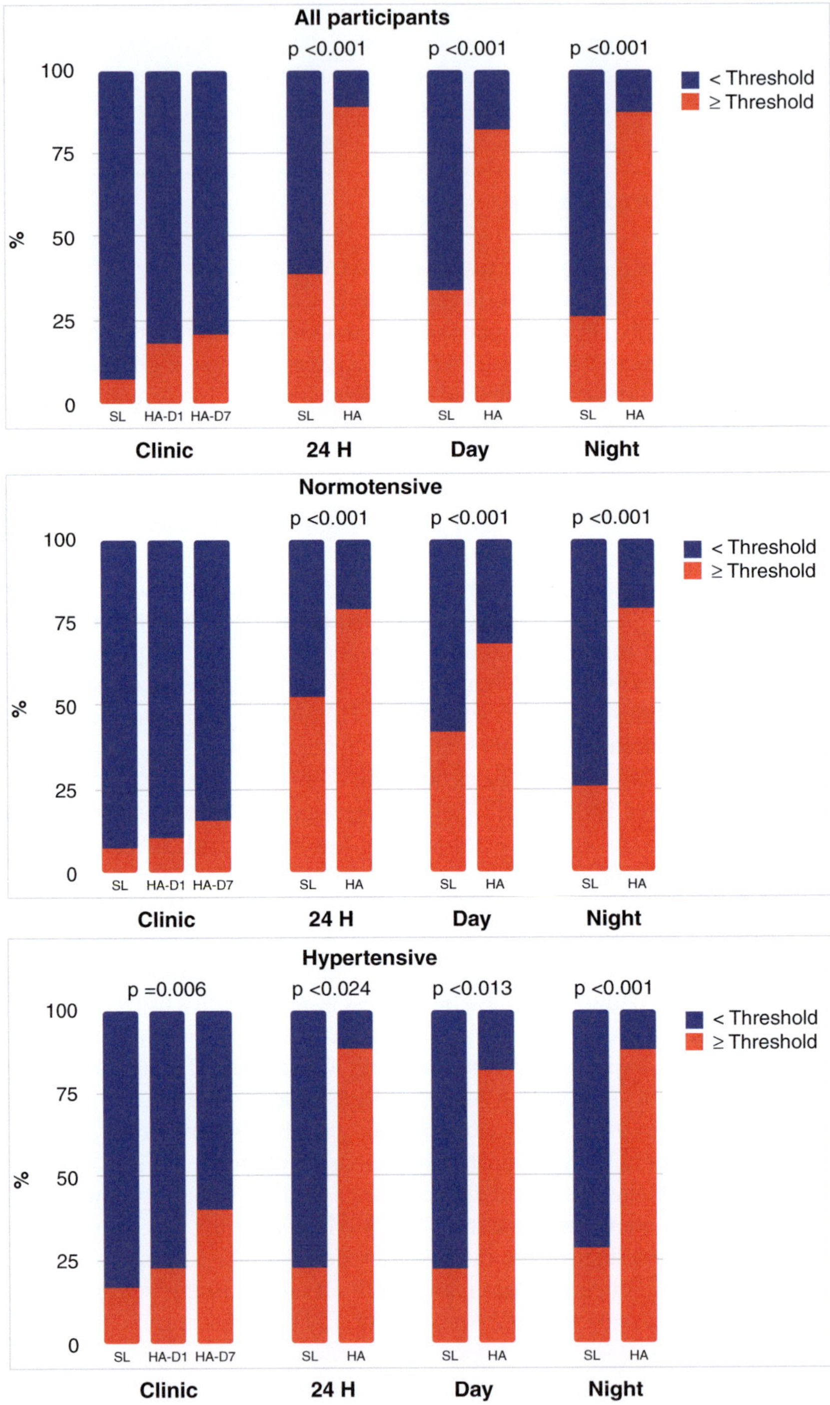

Fig. 14.3 Relative prevalence of participants exceeding clinic, mean 24-h, daytime, and night HT threshold at SL and HA in miners working in chronic intermittent hypoxia model. From Lang et al. [19]

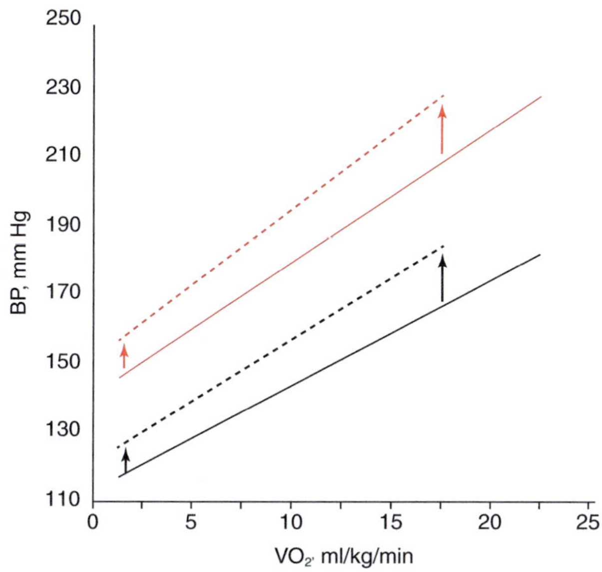

Fig. 14.4 Schematic representation of changes in systolic blood pressure (BP) during exercise at high altitude. With increasing workload and oxygen consumption (VO_2, *x* axis) at altitude BP increases more steeply (dotted lines) than at sea level (continuous line). However, peak exercise BP is similar in both conditions because the achieved peak VO2 is lower at altitude. In individuals under antihypertensive treatment (blue lines), the pattern is similar but BP is shifted towards lower values. Modified from Caravita et al. [2, 23]

consumption [23, 24], the limitation of peak exercise capacity which characterizes a HA condition again limits the BP increase to values comparable to those achieved at SL (while remaining higher than in normotensives, Fig. 14.4) [20, 23, 24].

Arguably, although the available evidence does not indicate the presence of immediate risks in hypertensive patients acutely exposed to HA, it comes from small studies performed with different aims and therefore the authors of a European position statement on HA exposure of individuals with cardiovascular conditions remained cautious in this regard and recommended that patients with uncontrolled or severe hypertension should avoid HA exposure (Table 14.1) [1].

Acute BP rise in general increases left ventricle afterload and thereby also cardiac work. At HA this is combined with a higher HR and a reduced blood oxygenation. This triad creates unfavourable condition for maintaining adequate balance between myocardial oxygen supply and demand, as documented by the observed reduction in the subendocardial viability ratio (SEVR, an index characterizing aortic pressure waveform, reflecting the ratio between diastolic coronary perfusion and systolic energy requirements in the coronary circulation) [36]. Such an imbalance between myocardial oxygen supply and demand at HA may be of particular concern in individuals with coronary artery disease and, in fact, several cases of myocardial ischemia onset during acute HA exposure were described [37–40]. Nonetheless, studies in patients with revascularized coronary artery disease did not show any

Table 14.1 Main practical recommendations for patients with hypertension who are planning high-altitude stay and evidence on antihypertensive drugs use in this condition. Adapted from Parati et al. [1, 2]

Recommendations		
• Patients with moderate–severe hypertension and hypertensive patients with moderate–high cardiovascular risk should check BP values before and during HA sojourn.		
• Well-controlled hypertensive patients/mild hypertensive patients may reach very HA (>4000 m) with adequate medical therapy.		
• Uncontrolled/severe hypertensive patients should avoid HA exposure in order to prevent risk of organ damage.		
• When moderate–severe hypertensive patients and hypertensive patients at moderate–high cardiovascular risk plan exposure to HA, adequate modification of their antihypertensive therapy should be considered in co-operation with their physician.		
Evidence on antihypertensive drugs effects at HA		
Drugs	*Pros*	*Cons*
Angiotensin II receptor blockers (telmisartan 80 mg)	Safely lowered BP in healthy subjects during short exposure to 3400 m	Ineffective during prolonged stay at very HA (5400 m)
Acetazolamide	May lower BP, prevent/improve mountain sickness symptoms and increase oxygen saturation	Limited BP data, adverse effects with prolonged use
Other diuretics	No data	Not recommended (may worsen fluid depletion caused by HA permanence)
Calcium antagonists (nifedipine)	Reduces pulmonary pressure, used in HAPE treatment. In combination with telmisartan 80 mg, slow release nifedipine 30 mg effectively lowered BP in hypertensive patients at an altitude of 3300 m	Side effects typical for this group (headache, flushing, leg oedema). No data on BP effects in monotherapy
Beta-blockers (carvedilol, nebivolol)	Vasodilatory beta-blockers maintained their BP-lowering effects in healthy subjects during acute exposure to 4500 m	Reduced exercise performance and blood oxygenation (less so with beta 1-selective compound, nebivolol)
ACE inhibitors	No data	Possibly the same as for angiotensin receptor blockers, due to RAAS suppression

BP blood pressure, *HA* high altitude, *HAPE* high-altitude pulmonary oedema, *RAAS* renin–angiotensin–aldosterone system

evidence of acute ischemia either at rest or while exercising at HA [39, 41, 42] and therefore it appears that patients with stable coronary artery disease and no or little symptoms can safely go to HA [1, 43]. Similarly, the limited available information indicates that stable heart failure patients at NYHA II functional class tolerate well short-term exposure to 3500 m altitude [44].

It is not known if acute BP increase due to HA exposure may trigger cardiovascular events. Some insight comes from a recent study by Niebauer and Burtscher who found a strong association between hypertension and sudden cardiac death during skiing (but not hiking) in the mountains. This suggests that protection from the consequences of a dramatic increase in myocardial work induced by high-intensity effort during skiing might require maintaining adequate BP control in this condition [45].

14.3.2 HA and Antihypertensive Treatment

Several studies investigated the effects of antihypertensive drugs at HA (Table 14.1). Overall, the investigated molecules maintained their BP-lowering efficacy at HA with a notable exception of angiotensin receptor blockers, which, during the first week of exposure to altitudes of 4000 m or higher were shown to lose their efficacy, likely because of RAAS suppression [13, 46]. Tolerability issues of different drug classes have to be considered in this regard. In fact, beta-blockers (especially non-selective ones) appear to have poorer tolerability profile, their use being associated with reduced exercise capacity, generally impaired well-being and lower oxygen saturation during acute HA exposure. This may partly depend on the limitation of compensatory increase in heart rate but also on a negative impact on the ventilatory control and alveolar oxygen diffusion, the latter due to blockade of alveolar beta-2 adrenergic receptors [21]. Conversely, telmisartan–nifedipine GITS combination not only effectively controlled BP increase (at rest and during exercise) in mildly hypertensive patients exposed to 3100 m altitude but also improved blood oxygen saturation and muscle oxygen delivery (possibly due to vasodilating effect of calcium antagonist in pulmonary arterial bed) [24, 47, 48]. Although no studies investigated the effects of diuretics, these drugs are generally not indicated as plasma volume normally decreases during HA permanence and diuretics might induce hypovolemia. An exception in this regard is represented by acetazolamide, a mild diuretic frequently prescribed for the prevention of HA illnesses because of its ability to counter respiratory alkalosis. This drug has BP-lowering capabilities at HA, both at rest and during exercise, that may depend on increased diuresis as well as on improved oxygenation at altitude [48–50]. Unfortunately, numerous and frequent side effects limit its clinical usefulness.

14.3.3 BP and Hypertension in Highlanders

Short-term BP effects of HA cannot be readily extrapolated to permanent HA inhabitants. This is because long-term individual adaptation to this environment will inevitably lead to different cardiovascular homeostasis. Moreover, population specific factors such as genetic and epigenetic adaptations and lifestyle differences will differently affect BP in different highland areas. The understanding of epidemiology and determinants of hypertension in these populations is, however, of interest considering that a sizeable part of humanity lives at altitudes above 2500 m (over 140 million people according to some estimates).

Historical studies in Peruvian highlanders suggested very low prevalence of hypertension in the town of Cerro de Pasco at about 4500 m [51]. It has to be considered that in the past highland populations were very young and had relatively healthy lifestyle from the cardiovascular point of view. However, the socioeconomic changes characterized by the increased life span and obesity prevalence, together with less active lifestyle, not accompanied by adequate health education, inevitably changed this scenario. In fact, studies in Asia indicate that, in highlander communities, hypertension prevalence is overall similar or higher compared with lowlanders. Considering the relationship with the altitude of residence, inconsistent results were obtained, although meta-analyses of studies in Asian highlanders suggests a direct linear association between altitude and BP [52, 53].

Among distinct features characterizing highlanders and possibly involved in determining BP levels, a special mention must go to erythrocytosis with haematocrit levels frequently exceeding 50%. This phenomenon characterizes especially Andean populations and may be associated with a clinical syndrome known as chronic mountain sickness. Recent observations indicate that excessive erythrocytosis may be independently associated with hypertension and other metabolic alterations, potentially influencing long term cardiovascular risk [54, 55].

Of note, hypertension prevalence may be significantly underestimated in highland populations in studies relying on conventional BP measurements only. Our recent report indicated that in Peruvian highlanders hypertension prevalence tripled when BP was assessed by means of 24-h ABPM, largely due to nocturnal hypertension. Consequently, there was a considerable group of highlander individuals with masked hypertension, a condition known to have adverse prognostic relevance [54]. It has to be acknowledged, though, that data on cardiovascular outcomes in these populations are very limited. More solid information comes from studies in Swiss and Austrian populations, indicating possible benefits of living at moderately elevated altitudes (between 1000 and 2000 m) in terms of cardiac and cardiovascular mortality, even after adjusting for other environmental factors [56, 57]. It remains to be seen whether these benefits are confirmed in other populations and at even higher altitudes.

14.4 Conclusions

Acute HA exposure leads to significant increase in BP both in normotensive and hypertensive individuals, mediated foremostly by chemoreflex-driven sympathetic activation. In the short term this may constitute a potentially hazardous condition, especially in high-risk individuals who perform high-intensity exercise, although direct evidence in this regard is missing. Several well-known antihypertensive drugs are safe and effective in controlling BP in this setting. The prevalence of hypertension in people permanently living at high altitude requires further investigation also through use of 24h ambulatory BP monitoring.

References

1. Parati G, Agostoni P, Basnyat B, Bilo G, Brugger H, Coca A, et al. Clinical recommendations for high altitude exposure of individuals with pre-existing cardiovascular conditions. Eur Heart J. 2018;39:1546–54.
2. Bilo G, Caravita S, Torlasco C, Parati G. Blood pressure at high altitude: physiology and clinical implications. Kardiol Pol. 2019;77:596–603.
3. Bärtsch P, Gibbs JSR. Effect of altitude on the heart and the lungs. Circulation. 2007;116:2191–202.
4. Erik R, Swenson PB. Human adaptation to hypoxia. New York: Springer; 2014. https://doi.org/10.1097/00000542-195909000-00076.
5. Imray C, Booth A, Wright A, Bradwell A. Acute altitude illnesses. BMJ. 2011;343:1–10.
6. Williams B, Mancia G, Spiering W, Agabiti Rosei E, Azizi M, Burnier M, et al. 2018 ESC/ESH guidelines for the management of arterial hypertension. Eur Heart J. 2018;39:3021–104.
7. Keyes LE, Mather L, Duke C, Regmi N, Phelan B, Pant S, et al. Older age, chronic medical conditions and polypharmacy in Himalayan trekkers in Nepal: an epidemiologic survey and case series. J Travel Med. 2016;23:taw052.
8. Vogel JR, Harris CW, Vogel JA, Harris CW. Cardiopulmonary responses of resting man during early exposure to high altitude. J Appl Physiol. 1967;22:1124–8.
9. Bilo G, Caldara G, Styczkiewicz K, Revera M, Lombardi C, Giglio A, et al. Effects of selective and nonselective beta-blockade on 24-h ambulatory blood pressure under hypobaric hypoxia at altitude. J Hypertens. 2011;29:380–7.
10. Liu Y, Zhang J-H, Gao X-B, Wu X-J, Yu J, Chen J-F, et al. Correlation between blood pressure changes and AMS, sleeping quality and exercise upon high-altitude exposure in young Chinese men. Mil Med Res. 2014;1:19.
11. Wolfel EE, Selland MA, Mazzeo RS, Reeves JT. Systemic hypertension at 4,300 m is related to sympathoadrenal activity. J Appl Physiol. 1994;76:1643–50.
12. Veglio M, Maule S, Cametti G, Cogo A, Lussiana L, Madrigale G, et al. The effects of exposure to moderate altitude on cardiovascular autonomic function in normal subjects. Clin Auton Res. 1999;9:123–7.
13. Parati G, Bilo G, Faini A, Bilo B, Revera M, Giuliano A, et al. Changes in 24 h ambulatory blood pressure and effects of angiotensin II receptor blockade during acute and prolonged high-altitude exposure: a randomized clinical trial. Eur Heart J. 2014;35:3113–22.
14. Torlasco C, Bilo G, Giuliano A, Soranna D, Ravaro S, Oliverio G, et al. Effects of acute exposure to moderate altitude on blood pressure and sleep breathing patterns. Int J Cardiol. 2020;301:173–9.
15. Bilo G, Villafuerte FC, Faini A, Anza-Ramírez C, Revera M, Giuliano A, et al. Ambulatory blood pressure in untreated and treated hypertensive patients at high altitude. Hypertension. 2015;65:1266–72.
16. Dhar P, Sharma VK, Hota KB, Das SK, Hota SK, Srivastava RB, et al. Autonomic cardiovascular responses in acclimatized lowlanders on prolonged stay at high altitude: a longitudinal follow up study. PLoS One. 2014;9:84274.
17. Siques P, Brito J, Banegas JR, Leon-Velarde F, de la Cruz-Troca JJ, Lopez V, et al. Blood pressure responses in young adults first exposed to high altitude for 12 months at 3550 m. High Alt Med Biol. 2009;10:329–35.
18. Richalet J-P, Donoso MV, Jimenez D, Antezana A-M, Hudson C, Cortes G, et al. Chilean miners commuting from sea level to 4500 m: a prospective study. High Alt Med Biol. 2002;3:159–66.
19. Lang M, Paéz V, Maj G, Silva-Urra J, Labarca-Valenzuela C, Caravita S, et al. Blood pressure response in miners exposed to chronic intermittent hypoxia in Chile. Front Cardiovasc Med. 2021;8. https://doi.org/10.3389/fcvm.2021.701961.
20. Winkler L, Lhuissier FJ, Richalet J-P. Systemic blood pressure at exercise in hypoxia in hypertensive and normotensive patients. J Hypertens. 2017;35:2402–10.

21. Valentini M, Revera M, Bilo G, Caldara G, Savia G, Styczkiewicz K, et al. Effects of beta-blockade on exercise performance at high altitude: a randomized, placebo-controlled trial comparing the efficacy of nebivolol versus carvedilol in healthy subjects. Cardiovasc Ther. 2012;30:240–8.
22. Naeije R. Physiological adaptation of the cardiovascular system to high altitude. Prog Cardiovasc Dis. 2010;52:456–66.
23. Caravita S, Faini A, Baratto C, Bilo G, Macarlupu JL, Lang M, et al. Upward shift and steepening of the blood pressure response to exercise in hypertensive subjects at high altitude. J Am Heart Assoc. 2018;7:e008506.
24. Caravita S, Faini A, Bilo G, Villafuerte FC, Macarlupu JL, Lang M, et al. Blood pressure response to exercise in hypertensive subjects exposed to high altitude and treatment effects. J Am Coll Cardiol. 2015;66:2806–7.
25. Halliwill JR, Minson CT. Effect of hypoxia on arterial baroreflex control of heart rate and muscle sympathetic nerve activity in humans. J Appl Physiol. 2002;93:857–64.
26. Simpson LL, Steinback CD, Stembridge M, Moore JP. A sympathetic view of blood pressure control at high altitude: new insights from microneurographic studies. Exp Physiol. 2021;106:377–84.
27. Bilo G, Revera M, Bussotti M, Bonacina D, Styczkiewicz K, Caldara G, et al. Effects of slow deep breathing at high altitude on oxygen saturation, pulmonary and systemic hemodynamics. PLoS One. 2012;7:e49074.
28. Bourdillon N, Yazdani S, Subudhi AW, Lovering AT, Roach RC, Vesin J-M, et al. AltitudeOmics: baroreflex sensitivity during acclimatization to 5,260 m. Front Physiol. 2018;9:767.
29. Zaccaria M, Rocco S, Noventa D, Varnier M, Opocher G. Sodium regulating hormones at high altitude: basal and post-exercise levels. J Clin Endocrinol Metab. 1998;83:570–4.
30. Bruno RM, Ghiadoni L, Pratali L. Vascular adaptation to extreme conditions: the role of hypoxia. Artery Res. 2016;14:15–21.
31. Yanamandra U, Singh SSP, Yanamandra S, Mulajkar D, Grewal RS, Singh SSP, et al. Endothelial markers in high altitude induced systemic hypertension (HASH) at moderate high altitude. Med J Armed Forces India. 2017;73:363–9.
32. Lewis NCS, Bailey DM, Dumanoir GR, Messinger L, Lucas SJE, Cotter JD, et al. Conduit artery structure and function in lowlanders and native highlanders: relationships with oxidative stress and role of sympathoexcitation. J Physiol. 2014;592:1009–24.
33. Revera M, Salvi P, Faini A, Giuliano A, Gregorini F, Bilo G, et al. Renin–angiotensin–aldosterone system is not involved in the arterial stiffening induced by acute and prolonged exposure to high altitude novelty and significance. Hypertension. 2017;70:75–84.
34. Insalaco G, Romano S, Salvaggio A, Braghiroli A, Lanfranchi P, Patruno V, et al. Blood pressure and heart rate during periodic breathing while asleep at high altitude. J Appl Physiol. 2000;89:947–55.
35. Savonitto S, Cardellino G, Sardina M, Chebat E, Baldi G, Beun-Garbe D, et al. Effects of a cable car trip on blood pressure and cardiovascular hormones in lowlander and highlander normotensives. Cardiologia. 1991;36:385–90.
36. Salvi P, Revera M, Faini A, Giuliano A, Gregorini F, Agostoni P, et al. Changes in subendocardial viability ratio with acute high-altitude exposure and protective role of acetazolamide. Hypertension. 2013;61:793–9.
37. Caravita S, Faini A, Bilo G, Revera M, Giuliano A, Gregorini F, et al. Ischemic changes in exercise ECG in a hypertensive subject acutely exposed to high altitude. Possible role of a high-altitude induced imbalance in myocardial oxygen supply-demand. Int J Cardiol. 2014;171:e100–2.
38. Wyss CA, Koepfli P, Fretz G, Seebauer M, Schirlo C, Kaufmann PA, et al. Influence of altitude exposure on coronary flow reserve. Circulation. 2003;108:1202–7.
39. Schmid J-P, Noveanu M, Gaillet R, Hellige G, Wahl A, Saner H. Safety and exercise tolerance of acute high altitude exposure (3454 m) among patients with coronary artery disease. Heart. 2006;92:921–5.

40. Levine BD, Zuckerman JH, DeFilippi CR. Effect of high-altitude exposure in the elderly: the Tenth Mountain division study. Circulation. 1997;96:1224–32.
41. De Vries ST, Kleijn SA, van 't Hof AWJ, Snaak H, van Enst GC, et al. Impact of high altitude on echocardiographically determined cardiac morphology and function in patients with coronary artery disease and healthy controls. Eur J Echocardiogr. 2010;11:446–50.
42. De Vries ST, Komdeur P, Aalbersberg S, Van Enst GC, Breeman A. Effects of altitude on exercise level and heart rate in patients with coronary artery disease and healthy controls. Neth Heart J. 2010;18:118–21.
43. Dehnert C, Bärtsch P. Can patients with coronary heart disease go to high altitude? High Alt Med Biol. 2010;11:183–8.
44. Schmid JP, Nobel D, Brugger N, Novak J, Palau P, Trepp A, et al. Short-term high altitude exposure at 3454 m is well tolerated in patients with stable heart failure. Eur J Heart Fail. 2015;17:182–6.
45. Niebauer J, Burtscher M. Sudden cardiac death risk in downhill skiers and mountain hikers and specific prevention strategies. Int J Environ Res Public Health. 2021;18:1621.
46. Lucas SJE, Malein WL, Thomas OD, Ashdown KM, Rue CA, Joyce KE, et al. Effect of losartan on performance and physiological responses to exercise at high altitude (5035 m). BMJ Open Sport Exerc Med. 2021;7:e000982.
47. Lang M, Faini A, Caravita S, Bilo G, Anza-Ramìrez C, Villafuerte FC, et al. Blood pressure response to six-minute walk test in hypertensive subjects exposed to high altitude: effects of antihypertensive combination treatment. Int J Cardiol. 2016;219:27–32.
48. Caravita S, Faini A, Bilo G, Lang M, Parati G. Role of acetazolamide and telmisartan/nifedipine-GITS combination in antagonizing the blood pressure rise induced by high altitude exposure. Int J Cardiol. 2016;225:324–6.
49. Caravita S, Faini A, Lombardi C, Valentini M, Gregorini F, Rossi J, et al. Sex and acetazolamide effects on chemoreflex and periodic breathing during sleep at altitude. Chest. 2015;147:120–31.
50. Burtscher J, Gatterer H, Faulhaber M, Burtscher M. Acetazolamide pre-treatment before ascending to high altitudes: sustained effect on systemic blood pressure during submaximal exercise. Int J Clin Exp Med. 2016;9:6656–62.
51. Ruiz L, Peñaloza D. Altitude and hypertension. Mayo Clin Proc. 1977;52:442–5.
52. Aryal N, Weatherall M, Bhatta YKD, Mann S. Blood pressure and hypertension in adults permanently living at high altitude: a systematic review and meta-analysis. High Alt Med Biol. 2016;17:185–93.
53. Mingji C, Onakpoya IJ, Perera R, Ward AM, Heneghan CJ, et al. Relationship between altitude and the prevalence of hypertension in Tibet: a systematic review. Heart. 2015;101:1054–60.
54. Bilo G, Acone L, Anza-Ramírez C, Macarlupú JL, Soranna D, Zambon A, et al. Office and ambulatory arterial hypertension in highlanders. Hypertension. 2020;76:1962–70.
55. Corante N, Anza-Ramírez C, Figueroa-Mujíca R, Macarlupú JL, Vizcardo-Galindo G, Bilo G, et al. Excessive erythrocytosis and cardiovascular risk in Andean highlanders. High Alt Med Biol. 2018;19:221–31.
56. Faeh D, Moser A, Panczak R, Bopp M, Röösli M, Spoerri A, et al. Independent at heart: persistent association of altitude with ischaemic heart disease mortality after consideration of climate, topography and built environment. J Epidemiol Community Health. 2016;70:798–806.
57. Burtscher J, Millet GP, Burtscher M. Does living at moderate altitudes in Austria affect mortality rates of various causes? An ecological study. BMJ Open. 2021;11:e048520.

15 Antihypertensive Therapy in Athletes

L. Mos, G. Plett, and C. Degano

15.1 Introduction

Hypertension is the most common condition to be identified in health checks for athletes, particularly in the category of master athletes.

The Italian guidelines relating to medical fitness for sport have permitted the use of antihypertensive drugs for competitive athletes since 1995, and since then antihypertensive therapy has played a fundamental role in managing the condition of athletes suffering from arterial hypertension.

The recent guidelines set out by the European Association of Preventive Cardiology (EAPC) also address the issue of sporting activity in hypertensive subjects receiving drug therapy [1].

If the subject is classified as "low cardiovascular risk" the ESC (European Society of Cardiology) guidelines recommend an initial non-pharmacological therapeutic approach, with lifestyle changes for a period of at least 3 months (lowering salt intake, reducing body weight, avoiding alcohol and stopping smoking, together with a suitable exercise program). In case of grade 3 hypertension and/or "high cardiovascular risk" or "very high" it is advisable to start medical therapy promptly.

15.2 Choice of Medication

For athletes with hypertension it is also important to be able to control blood pressure levels, both at rest and during exercise, without affecting performance and only using drugs approved by the World Anti-Doping Agency (WADA) (Table 15.1).

L. Mos (✉) · G. Plett · C. Degano
SOS Cardiologia—Ospedale Sant'Antonio, San Daniele del Friuli, UD, Italy
e-mail: lucio.mos@libero.it; gloriaplett@libero.it

P. Palatini et al. (eds.), *Exercise, Sports and Hypertension*, Updates in Hypertension and Cardiovascular Protection,
https://doi.org/10.1007/978-3-031-07958-0_15

Table 15.1 Characteristics of the ideal drug for hypertensive athletes

The drug must do the following.
• Control BP both at rest and during exertion.
• Not reduce the cardiac response to exercise.
• Have no arrhythmogenic effect.
• Not cause interference with the distribution of blood to the muscle.
• Not cause interference with energy substrates.
• Not be a substance prohibited by doping regulations.
• Not cause orthostatic hypotension (already physiologically present at the end of exercise).
• Must not cause electrolyte imbalance.
• Cover 24 h with a single dose.
• Have no significant side effects.

Many classes of antihypertensive drugs can interfere with athletic performance, as they act on physiological mechanisms that affect sporting performance and have significant impacts on metabolism and muscle function.

15.2.1 ACE Inhibitors

ACE inhibitors have shown good efficacy in controlling BP, and compared to angiotensin II receptor blockers have a higher rate of therapy being suspended due to side effects [2].

In the athlete they are the first-line drug of choice [3].

Some studies have demonstrated a slight reduction in both systolic and diastolic blood pressure during exercise in patients receiving captopril [4], enalapril [5, 6]; heart rate remains unchanged [4] and peripheral vascular resistance is reduced by all ACE inhibitors [4, 6, 7].

These drugs do not affect VO_2 max or exercise tolerance (both sub-maximal and maximal) and this feature makes them particularly suitable for use with patients who undertake physical activity [5]. Some studies also suggest that elderly (non-heart failure) patients taking ACE inhibitors experience a lower reduction in walking speed, hand grip and knee extension strength than patients taking other hypertensive medication or not receiving any therapy [8].

In 2007 Sumukadas et al. found that treatment with perindopril in elderly patients with functional impairment and without heart failure can increase exercise capacity in a way that is similar to a 6-month training program. The pathophysiological mechanism underlying this phenomenon is probably linked to metabolic changes at the muscular level [9, 10].

It is known that ACE inhibitors induce a shift in myosin heavy chains towards slow, aerobic isoforms, which are related to improved physical performance [11].

These drugs also increase insulin sensitivity, glycogen storage and glucose uptake by the muscle; they have a limiting effect on the proinflammatory mechanism triggered by angiotensin and increase the concentration of bradykinin and nitric oxide.

This causes the suppression of the inflammatory cascade and an increase in muscular vascular permeability leading to an increase in the intake of glucose and amino acids, and consequently better muscle metabolic efficiency [10].

However, recent studies by Sumukadas et al. seem to indicate that the addition of these drugs in elderly patients with functional impairment undergoing training, does not lead to any improvement in the ability to perform physical exercise compared to the training program alone [12].

The potential side effects of this class of drug are first dose hypotension (in hypovolemic subjects or those who are taking diuretics at the same time), and a dry cough.

Captopril in particular, at high doses can cause neutropenia and proteinuria in patients with acute renal failure [13] (Table 15.2).

It is currently thought that SARS-CoV-2 uses ACE2, a key component of the RAS (renin–angiotensin system), to penetrate cells, presumably by binding to ACE2 via the viral spike protein. Previous studies have reported the up-regulation of ACE2 by RAS inhibitors and these results have encouraged the hypothesis that ACE inhibitors and angiotensin II receptor blockers (ARBs) could increase the severity of SARS CoV-2 infection due to the up-regulation of ACE2. However, there is no evidence that RAS blockers increase the expression of ACE2, or that increased levels of ACE2 are connected to severe acute respiratory syndrome from SARS-CoV-2. Furthermore, there is ample experimental evidence that shows that increased ACE2 levels can actually help protect against lung lesions, with the beneficial effect of RAS inhibition in SARS-CoV-2 infections, although it has not yet been demonstrated whether supporting the protective mechanism of the RAS through this therapeutic approach is effective in tackling COVID-19.

A recent observational multi-centre study in Italy and a meta-analysis of 19 studies [14] has provided some answers in this regard, demonstrating that the intake of RAAS (renin–angiotensin–aldosterone system) inhibitors is not associated with increased mortality or greater severity of the disease.

The review by the European Society of Hypertension (ESH) task force concludes that current evidence does not indicate that RAS blockers have any harmful effect on COVID-19 infections and RAS blockers should not be suspended or discontinued in patients who are stable [15].

Table 15.2 Ace inhibitors

Ace inhibitors Indications: First-line choice		
Contraindications	Absolute	Previous angioneurotic Oedema; hyperkalemia; bilateral renal artery stenosis; pregnancy.
	Relative	Women of child-bearing potential without reliable contraception
In athletes	For	First-line choice; not banned by doping regulations; no effects on VO_2 max; no effects on exercise tolerance; good metabolic effect; possible control of proinflammatory mechanisms.
	Against	Possible minor functional impairment in the elderly.

15.2.2 Angiotensin II Receptor Blockers

Similarly to ACE inhibitors, Angiotensin II receptor blockers (ARBs) are widely used anti-hypertensive drug, they are often chosen for subjects who have shown an intolerance to the former (e.g. dry cough).

ARBs, as well as ACE inhibitors, are considered the first-line anti-hypertensive drugs of choice for athletes [3]. They both share many of the same metabolic and haemodynamic characteristics, as they act on the same molecular pathway.

In numerous studies, ARBs have also shown beneficial effects on physical performance, especially in the elderly.

A study by Vescovo et al. reports that a 6-month treatment with losartan significantly increases VO_2 max and the ventilatory threshold on the cardiopulmonary test [13]. On the other hand, De Rosa et al. showed how the use of candesartan improves the VO_2 peak in cardiopulmonary tests in hypertensive grade 1 or 2 patients with secondary ventricular hypertrophy, compared to control subjects (placebo) [16].

This class of drugs could also have a beneficial effect on muscle recovery after injury. Indeed, the administration of 30 mg/day of losartan immediately after trauma seems to improve the recovery of muscle strength. This property perhaps depends on an overexpression of follistatin, a positive regulator of skeletal muscle growth [17].

In a study conducted on mice, chronic administration of telmisartan has been shown to cause an increase in slow twitch muscle fibres, prevent body weight loss, improve endurance and post-exercise oxygen consumption. These effects were absent in genetically modified mice lacking peroxisome proliferator activated receptor (PPAR). Consequently, the increase in muscle function and exercise tolerance seems to be due to the activation of PPAR and the AMPK pathway (adenosine monophosphate activated protein kinase) [18].

It is important to remember that high intensity physical exercise can cause negative effects on the cardiovascular system, including platelet activation; these effects are more pronounced in hypertensive patients.

A 2014 study demonstrated a reduction in platelet activation following high-intensity sporting activity in hypertensive patients who were treated with 160 mg of valsartan and who had well controlled blood pressure [19]. From a metabolic point of view, ARBs cause a significant reduction in circulating glucose levels by antagonizing the effect of angiotensin II on the mechanisms of insulin signal transduction.

These drugs therefore reduce insulin resistance and accentuate the uptake and use of glucose by muscles and other tissues in a similar way to ACE inhibitors. In this regard Fujimoto et al. have shown that the administration of Telmisartan increases glucose uptake and the expression of the GLUT4 (glucose transporter type 4) protein on adipocytes [20].

There is also experimental evidence that suggests that angiotensin II promotes osteoclastic activity and bone resorption. Consequently, it has been hypothesized that ARBs and ACE inhibitors may have a protective effect against osteoporosis in the elderly.

Table 15.3 Angiotensin II receptor blockers

Angiotensin II receptor blockers		
Indications: First-line choice if patient cannot take or is intolerant of ACE inhibitors		
Contraindications	Absolute	Hyperkalaemia; bilateral renal artery stenosis; pregnancy.
	Relative	Women of child-bearing potential without reliable contraception
In athletes	For	First-line choice as an alternative to ACE inhibitors; not banned by doping regulations; no effects on VO_2 max, may actually improve it; no effects on exercise tolerance; good metabolic effect; possible beneficial effect of telmisartan on muscle recovery after injury
	Against	

However, contrary to what was expected, a 2012 study in elderly American subjects demonstrated a bone density-reducing effect caused by ACE inhibitors, but not by ARBs. Nonetheless, there was no evidence of a significant increase in fractures in patients receiving this therapy [21]. Although ACE inhibitors and ARBs are considered as the first-line drug of choice for athletes, it should be remembered that they should be avoided in women of childbearing age due to possible teratogenic effects in the case of pregnancy [1] (Table 15.3).

It is likely that direct renin inhibitors can have effects on physical activity similar to ARBs; however, their use by athletes has not yet been adequately researched, and therefore their use is not recommended [3].

15.2.3 Calcium Channel Blockers

CCBs, in particular dihydropyridines, are considered the medicine of choice for athletes who cannot take either ACE inhibitors or ARBs [3]. This class of drugs has shown significant success in reducing systolic–diastolic blood pressure during exercise, probably attributable to the effect of the drug on peripheral arterial resistance [22–25]. In 1996 Gillies et al. found that the treatment with amlodipine 5 mg is effective in lowering resting systolic pressure but does not alter the normal haemodynamic response during exercise in athletic hypertensive individuals; maximal and prolonged submaximal exercise performance and skeletal muscle function are unaltered after the ingestion of amlodipine in these patients [26].

Non-dihydropyridine CCBs, however, have negative inotropic and negative chronotropic effects that can lead to the impairment of sporting performance.

Some studies have shown that verapamil has more pronounced negative inotropic effects than other drugs in the same class, but both verapamil and diltiazem cause a slight decrease in heart rate during exercise [24, 27], without significant changes in cardiac output [28]. During cardiopulmonary tests, diltiazem does not significantly modify VO_2 max [25].

From a metabolic point of view, a lipolysis stimulating effect would be expected (attributable to the stimulation of alpha 2 adrenergic receptors) [29]; however, it has been shown that free fatty acids do not increase during administration of verapamil [30].

For the class of dihydropyridine CCBs, prolonged treatment with nifedipine does not increase heart rate, cardiac output or systolic volume during exercise [24, 31]. Nifedipine also appears capable of increasing the fraction of myocardial shortening during high-intensity exercise, reducing the telediastolic volume due to the action on peripheral resistance [22, 28].

According to a study undertaken in 2001, nifedipine was found to have a good effect on resting blood pressure, but also has an effect on the blood pressure response to exercise when compared to benidipine and placebo. This has been linked to nifedipine being faster acting, which affects the body's ability to implement compensation mechanisms. Furthermore, nifedipine was seen to increase plasma renin activity (PRA), causing the activation of the renin–angiotensin–aldosterone system (RAAS) which could be the cause of cardiovascular events [32]. However, these negative effects were not seen in subjects receiving benidipine [33].

From a metabolic point of view, a significant hyperglycaemia inducing effect was observed during sustained effort (60% VO_2 max). This effect can be attributed to the inhibition of insulin function and the stimulation of catecholaminergic and IGF (insuline-like growth factor action), which result in an increase in hepatic glycogenolysis [34].

In the cardiopulmonary test the anaerobic threshold (AT) was reduced after administration of nifedipine (in a single dose), while VO_2 max and maximum power reached during exercise remained unaltered [35] (Table 15.4).

For these reasons, dihydropyridine CCB are considered the medicine of choice for hypertensive athletes who cannot take ACE inhibitors or ARBs. Nonetheless, their usefulness in controlling pressure during isometric exercise remains controversial.

Verapamil and diltiazem can be used in case of intolerance to dihydropyridines [3].

Table 15.4 Dihydropyridine CCB and non-dihydropyridine CCB

Dihydropyridine CCB Indications: alternative to RAS inhibitors—better effect on stroke prevention		
Contraindications	Absolute	
	Relative	Tachyarrhythmia; heart failure (HFrEF, class III or IV); constipation; pre-existing severe leg oedema;
In athletes	For	Athletes who cannot take RAS system inhibitors; Nifedipine may increase the fraction of myocardial shortening during high intensity exercise; cause hyperglycaemia during exertion
	Against	CPET AT reduced after administration of nifedipine
Non-dihydropyridine CCBs Indications: Only if a simultaneous reduction in HR is desired		
Contraindications	Absolute	Any high-grade AV block; severe left ventricular dysfunction (with LVEF <40%); bradycardia (HR <60).
	Relative	Constipation
In athletes	For	
	Against	Lower HR and negative inotropic effect; impairment of performance

15.2.4 Alpha Agonists/Blockers

Alpha blockers are not recommended for the treatment of arterial hypertension as they have poor tolerability.

In hypertensive patients the administration of clonidine or methyldopa causes a reduction in blood pressure and heart rate during exercise [36, 37].

Clonidine does not affect vascular resistance or induce reduction in cardiac output [38].

In terms of exercise tolerance, this drug does not change VO_2 max during cardiopulmonary tests even though it seems to negatively affect the duration of exercise (decreased by 3.9%) [37].

Prazosin causes a reduction in the increase in blood pressure during exercise and reduces resting pressure, but it does not affect the stroke volume (SV) [39].

For patients who cannot take the drugs mentioned above, an alternative is the use of doxazosin; however, this can lead to orthostatic hypotension at the end of exercise, in particular if exercise is interrupted abruptly.

15.2.5 Beta Blockers

As a class of drugs, beta blockers are particularly unsuitable for the management of hypertensive athletes.

From a haemodynamic point of view they reduce the systolic and diastolic pressure both at rest and during physical exercise [40–49]. This characteristic is typical of selective drugs [41, 45, 47, 49], of non-selective ones [40, 44, 46, 49], of those with intrinsic sympathomimetic action [48, 50] and of those with combined action (alpha and beta blockers) [43].

All drugs in this class cause, during exercise, a reduction in stroke volume, left ventricular function (SV reduced by 18–25%) [51, 52] and peripheral resistance [50].

Furthermore, the known negative chronotropic effect of these molecules causes a reduction in HR (heart rate) during exercise of 20–30% [47, 52, 53].

This bradycardising effect is less pronounced in drugs with intrinsic sympathomimetic actions [48, 50].

Vanhees et al. found that bisoprolol, in healthy young men, reduced endurance exercise capacity of 19.4 ± 6.7% compared with placebo [54].

A randomised placebo-controlled crossover trial of adults with mild or moderate asthma given bisoprolol daily for a minimum of 2 weeks found no difference in exacerbations between the groups [55].

Rescue β-agonist therapy after a controlled bronchoconstriction was also non-inferior with bisoprolol treatment.

Beta blockers also have a significant impact on metabolism, due to the reduction of glycogenolysis and beta oxidation processes normally induced by the sympathetic nervous system [56].

In particular, non-selective drugs cause a more marked reduction in glycogenolysis and lipolysis than selective drugs. This effect is seen particularly in the reduction in endurance time during aerobic exercise. In this sense, the molecule that has shown the greatest negative effect is propranolol [56–58]. In this regard, the use of propanolol leads to a reduction in VO_2 max of 6–14% [59–62] (which it is more pronounced in patients with a good level of fitness) [53] and an 11% reduction in the anaerobic threshold after 3 months of therapy [63].

An early increase in blood lactate during physical activity has also been demonstrated, probably due to a delay in adapting the cardiovascular system to the demands of the muscles. With the use of propanolol, for example, there is an increase in blood lactate in the initial minutes of exercise and then a decrease in them after 25 min of exercise (to 65% of VO_2 max), compared to control subjects [64].

The decrease in lactate after 25 min of exercise is probably linked to the fact that glycogenolysis is stimulated by the activation of beta receptors [65].

Some studies also show that the expected increase in VO_2 max after aerobic training in subjects who took propranolol was not found [66]. However, other studies contradict these findings [67].

In any case, the concentration of muscle mitochondrial enzymes after a period of training does not seem to increase as expected in subjects treated with this drug [68, 69].

For all these reasons, beta blockers are not suitable drugs for anti-hypertensive therapy in athletes.

It should also be remembered that these drugs are not recommended in cases of bradycardia (bpm <50) and second-degree atrioventricular block (characteristics commonly found in athlete's heart), in cases of third-degree atrioventricular block or in skill sports where doping rules prohibit their use.

When it is necessary to use beta blockers, it is preferable to use a combination of alpha-beta blockers as this causes less impairment of muscle vascularization and has less of an effect on maximum oxygen consumption [70].

Separate consideration should be given to nebivolol, a latest generation beta blocker with very high cardioselectivity (B1/B2 > 300) [71] which is associated with a significant effect in reducing peripheral resistance.

The vasodilatory property of the molecule is not expressed by blocking the $\alpha 1$ receptors, as happens with labetalol and carvedilol, but by the direct action of the drug on the enzyme nitric oxide synthetase (eNOS) [72]. Nitric oxide plays a key role in endothelial function by causing vasodilation, reducing the expression of endothelial receptors for proinflammatory and adhesion molecules, as well as the suppression of signalling pathways for the triggering of inflammatory processes [73, 74].

In this regard, a study conducted in obese patients subjected to intense physical exercise highlights how the administration of this active ingredient for 8 weeks at therapeutic doses results in a reduction in pro-inflammatory cytokines and leptin and an increase in adiponectin, exerting a protective effect against the inflammatory stress induced by intense physical exercise [75].

Table 15.5 Beta blockers and nebivolol

Beta blockers Indications: Specific conditions → hypertension + angina; hypertension + post–heart attack; hypertension + HF-rEF; HR control needed; reduced stroke prevention compared to other classes; greater side effects lead to increased suspension of therapy.		
Contraindications	Absolute	Asthma; high-grade AV block; bradycardia (HR <60)
	Relative	Metabolic syndrome; glucose intolcrance
In athletes	For	
	Against	Only in specific conditions; banned as doping agent in some sports; drop in cardiac output and HR during exercise; adverse metabolic effect; drop in VO_2 max and AT
Nebivolol Indications: Greater tolerability; fewer side effects; better effect on endothelial dysfunction and arterial stiffness		
In athletes	For	Protective effect against inflammatory state caused by intense exercise
	Against	Banned as doping agent in some sports

Several studies have also documented a significant improvement in diastolic function. The *SENIORS* study [76] showed that nebivolol is well tolerated in elderly patients with heart failure with both preserved and reduced ejection fraction.

Some studies on patients with heart failure and preserved ejection fraction have found good control of systolic blood pressure and heart rate both at rest and at peak exertion after treatment with nebivolol. However, the expected increase in VO_2 max was not observed [77] (Table 15.5).

15.2.6 Diuretics

Diuretic drugs are banned by the World Anti-Doping Agency, and therefore they cannot be used by athletes who compete.

Diuretics help in the clearance of any illicit substances, affecting the results of anti-doping tests; furthermore, in sports that are divided into weight categories (such as combat and weightlifting sports) they can help athletes qualify for a lower weight category.

Therapy with thiazides reduces systolic blood pressure (BP) at rest and during exercise by about 20–30% and diastolic BP by 15–20%, with a simultaneous reduction in peripheral arterial resistance [78].

These drugs also favour the onset of electrolyte imbalances such as hypokalaemia and hypomagnesaemia, which can be a factor in triggering cardiac arrhythmias. An increase in ventricular premature beats was seen in patients receiving hydrochlorothiazide compared to control subjects [79, 80].

Table 15.6 Diuretics

Diuretics		
Indications: Heart failure prevention; electrolyte imbalance risk; therapy often suspended due to side effects		
Contraindications	Absolute	Gout
	Relative	Metabolic syndrome; glucose intolerance; pregnancy; hypercalcaemia; hypokalaemia;
In athletes	For	
	Against	Always banned by doping regulations; increased risk of electrolyte imbalance and BEV; changes to thermoregulation;

Diuretics can also lead to dehydration in athletes who undertake prolonged aerobic exercise in hot climates and interfere with thermoregulation. According to a 2000 study, dehydration induced by pre-exercise diuretics causes a greater imbalance in thermoregulation during physical exercise. The decrease in plasma volume caused by the diuretic causes the activation of the sympathetic nervous system with a consequent increase in the release of norepinephrine and stroke work and a reduction in cutaneous blood flow with impaired heat dispersion [81].

According to a 2005 study, acute dehydration caused by diuretics (with consequent loss of body mass of 2–2.5%) does not affect the performance of maximum power and sprint, consequently the diuretic would not provide the expected effect of improved athletics performance in these categories of sports [82]. Similarly, the factors that affect aerobic performance in instances of moderate dehydration have no impact on results in sprinting and in activities where explosive strength is required [82] (Table 15.6).

15.3 Pharmacological Combinations

The most recent guidelines have focused on promoting an effective *treatment strategy* in the control of BP, in particular they emphasize the greater efficacy of combination therapy compared to monotherapy. Studies suggest that the combination of two drugs is able to control BP in about 2/3 of patients [83], while the combination of three drugs is effective in over 80% of hypertensive patients [84, 85].

The most effective combinations are those of an ACE inhibitor or an ABR with a calcium channel blocker or a thiazide or thiazide-like diuretic.

These combinations are available in a single preparation at fixed doses, which reduces the number of tablets that need to be taken daily and helps increase adherence to therapy [86, 87] which is generally lower in cases of hypertension, especially in young athletes who are completely asymptomatic.

This approach is facilitated by the availability of different set doses of the two drugs in a range of combinations which makes it possible to independently adjust the dosage of the two molecules.

Combination therapy using a synergy of pharmacological and physiological approaches is more effective in reducing blood pressure for the same dosage and achieves the target blood pressure faster.

Reducing the effective dose of individual molecules limits potentially adverse effects by reducing the risk of diuretic-induced hypokalaemia and the incidence of peripheral oedema due to calcium channel blockers. The recommended combinations also ensure an inhibition of the RAAS, which is important for various groups of patients (diabetics, LVH, proteinuria).

Combinations with beta blockers, on the other hand, are recommended for specific clinical conditions (symptomatic angina, post–heart attack, HFrEF, hyperadrenergic states with need for heart rate control) [88].

Unfortunately, only limited information is currently available about the hemodynamic effects and the implications for physical exercise of combinations of drugs.

A 2011 study was conducted in this regard examining the association of lisinopril (40 mg/day) with a beta blocker (carvedilol 20, then 40 mg/day) and ARBs (valsartan 160 then 320 mg/day).

By adding valsartan or carvedilol to the ACE inhibitor, a reduction in stroke work was observed with different mechanisms (vasodilation and a reduction of preload with ARBs, reduction in heart rate with the beta blockers). During exercise, valsartan maintained the reduction in central systolic pressure and peripheral resistance and the increase in blood pressure; carvedilol did not. Neither drug affected the response to exercise or carotid flow.

Although a greater cardio-depressive effect of the combination with carvedilol was expected, the study revealed a comparable heart rate and stroke work reduction effect with both drug combinations [89].

The combination of telmisartan and nifedipine seems to have a good anti-hypertensive effect in controlling BP during sub-maximal exercise at high altitude, counteracting the excess pressure increase at altitude found in the hypertensive patients [90].

The combination of enalapril and hydrochlorothiazide reduces systolic pressure by 12.6% at peak exercise without changing the VO_2 max and the level of fatigue perceived during maximal and sub-maximal exercise [5].

It is noteworthy to observe that drug combinations including beta blockers or diuretics cannot be used by competitive athletes.

15.4 Nutraceuticals

Nutraceuticals offer clinicians an extra resource for the treatment of hypertension. They can be a first-line choice for athletes who are reluctant to accept starting drug-based therapy.

There is substantial clinical evidence supporting the use of nutraceuticals, which can be found in various meta-analyses. This has led the SIIA (Italian Society of Arterial Hypertension) and subsequently the ESH to systematize the data in the literature, producing a concise document that focuses on a reduced number of active compounds where there is evidence for their use in clinical practice.

The panel of experts has set out precise recommendations, which can be summarized as follows.

- Regarding foods, the most convincing evidence is found for beet juice, followed by pomegranate juice, infusion of hibiscus, sesame and catechins.
- Regarding nutrients, blood pressure levels can be reduced by magnesium, potassium (to be used with caution in patients with advanced renal insufficiency and/or potassium-sparing diuretics/antialdosterones) and vitamin C.
- Regarding non-nutritious nutraceuticals, consideration should be given to soy isoflavones in perimenopausal women, resveratrol in insulin-resistant subjects, and melatonin in subjects suffering from nocturnal hypertension [91, 92].

15.5 Conclusions

When we consider anti-hypertensive therapy for athletes, the choice of active ingredients to be used is complex and must take into account numerous considerations.

For these reasons, the first-line choice of anti-hypertensive drugs for athletes are ACE inhibitors and ARBs.

Alternatively, dihydropyridine CCB and alpha blockers can be used, as they do not affect sporting performance.

Diuretics should always be avoided: apart from being considered to be doping agents in all sports, they also induce haemodynamic and electrolyte alterations that can lead to arrhythmias and reduce the athlete's performance.

Beta blockers reduce heart rate, alter the haemodynamic response to exercise, cause metabolic impairment and reduce exercise tolerance, so their use should be limited to cases where there are no other options, and in these cases nebivolol is to be preferred.

Finally, the possibility of using nutraceuticals in pre-hypertension must also be remembered; however, as highlighted in the documents drawn up by SIIA and ESH, this approach should never be considered as a substitute for a pharmacological approach when this is indicated.

To promote patient compliance, it may be useful for those who have not achieved the desired effect with first-line drugs, to use pre-established antihypertensive combinations (ARBs or ACE inhibitor/calcium channel blocker) as recommended by the ESC/ESH (European Society of Cardiology/European Society of Hypertension) guidelines.

References

1. Niebauer J, Borjesson M, Carre F, et al. Recommendations for participation in competitive sports of athletes with arterial hypertension: a position statement from the sports cardiology section of the European Association of Preventive Cardiology. Eur Heart J. 2018;39:3664–71.
2. Kronish IM, Woodward M, Sergie Z, et al. Meta-analysis: impact of drug class on adherence to antihypertensives. Circulation. 2011;123:1611–21.

3. Mos L, Panno A, Contursi M, Penco M, Abrignani M. Protocolli cardiologici pei il giudizio di idoneità allo sport agonistico. Roma: Casa editrice scientifica internazionale; 2017. p. 121–35.
4. Fagard R, Lijnen P, Amery A. Hemodynamic response to captopril at rest and during exercise in hypertensive subjects. Am J Cardiol. 1982;49:1569–71.
5. Leon AS, McNally C, Casal D, et al. Enalapril alone and in combination with hydroclhlorothiazide in the treatment of hypertension: effect on tradmill exercise performance. J Cardiopulmonary Reabil. 1986;6:251–6.
6. Lund-Johansen P, Omvik P. Long term hemodynamic effects of enalapril at rest and during exercise and essential hypertension. Scand J Urol Nephrol Suppl. 1984;79:87–91.
7. Omvik P, Lund-Johansen P. Combined captopril and hydrochlorothiazidetherapy in severe hypertension. Long-term haemodynamic changes at rest and during exercise. J Hypertens. 1984;2:73–80.
8. Onder G, Penninx BWJH, Balkrishnan R, et al. Relation between use of angiotensin-converting enzyme inhibitors and muscle strength and physical function in older women: an observational study. Lancet. 2002;359:926–30.
9. Sumukadas D, Witham MD, Struthers AD, et al. Effect of perindopril on physical function in ederly people with functional impairment: a randomized controlled trioal. CMAJ. 2007;177:867–74.
10. Coelho V, Probst V, Nogari B, et al. Angiotensin-2 blockage, muscle strength, and exercise capacity in physically independent older adults. J Phys Ther Sci. 2016;28:547–52.
11. Vescovo G, Dalla Libera L, Serafini F, et al. Improved exercise tolerance after losartan and enalapril in heart failure: correlation with changes in skeletal muscle myosin heavy chain composition. Circulation. 1998;98:1742–9.
12. Sumukadas D, Band M, Miller S, et al. Do ACE inhibitors improve the response to exercise training in functionally impaired older adults? A randomized controlled trial. J Gerontol A Biol Sci Med. 2014;69:736–43.
13. Joshi VD, Dahake AP, Suthar AP. Adverse effects associated with the use of antihypertensive drugs: an overview. Int J Pharm Tech Res. 2010;2(1):10–3.
14. THE COVID-19 Risk and Treatments (CORIST) Collaboration. RAAS inhibitors are not associated with mortality in COVID-19 patients: findings from an observational multicenter study in Italy and a meta-analysis of 19 studies. Vascular Pharmacol. 2020;135:106805.
15. Kreutz R, Algharably EAE, Azizi M, et al. Hypertension, the renin-angiotensin system, and the risk of lower respiratory tract infections and lung injury: implications for COVID-19. Cardiovasc Res. 2020;116(10):1688–99.
16. De Rosa ML, Chiariello M. Candesartan improves maximal exercise capacity in hypertensives: results of a randomized placebo-controlled crossover trial. J Clin Hypertens. 2009;11:192–200.
17. Uehara K, Kobayashi T, Ota S, et al. Angiotensin receptor blocker improves skeletal muscle function recovery in a dose dependent manner. 56th Annual Meeting of the Orthopaedic Research Society; Poster 1582.
18. Feng X, Luo Z, Ma L, et al. Angiotensin II receptor blocker telmisartan enhances running endurance of skeletal muscle through activation of the PPAR-δ/AMPK pathway. J Cell Mol Med. 2011;15:1572–81.
19. Gkaliagkousi E, Gavriilaki E, Yiannaki E, et al. Platelet activation in essential hypertension during exercise: pre- and post-treatment changes with an angiotensin II receptor blocker. Am J Hypertens. 2014;16:482–7.
20. Fujimoto M, Masuzaki H, Tanaka I, et al. An angiotensin II AT1 receptor antagonist, telmisartan augments glucose uptake and GLUT4 protein expression in 3T3-L1 adipocytes. FEBS Lett. 2004;576:492–7.
21. Kwok T, Leung J, Zhang YF, et al. Does the use of ACE inhibitors or angiotensin in receptor blockers affect bone loss in older men? Osteoporos Int. 2012;23:2159–67.
22. Andersen K, Vik-Mo H. Increased left ventricular empty at maximal exercise after reduction in afterload. Circulation. 1984;69:492–6.

23. Gould BA, Hornung RS, Mann S, Balasubramanian V, Raftery B. Slow channel inhibitors verapamil and nifedipine in the management of hypertension. J Cardiovasc Pharmacol. 1982;4(Suppl.3):s369–73.
24. Klein W, Brandt D, Vrecko K, Harringer M. Role of calcium antagonists in the treatment of essential hypertension. Circ Res. 1983;52(Suppl I):174–81.
25. Yamakado T, Oonishi N, Kondo S, Noziri A, Nakano T, Takezewa H. Effects of diltiazem on cardiovascular responses during exercise in systemic hypertension and comparison with propranolol. Am J Cardiol. 1983;52:1023–7.
26. Gillies HC, Derman EW, Noakes TD. Effect of amlodipine on exercise performance and cardiovascular and skeletal muscle function in physically active hypertensive patients. Clin Drug Invest. 1996;12:135–45.
27. Stein D, Lowenthal DT, Porter S, et al. Effects of nifedipine and verapamil on isometric and dynamic exercise in normal subjects. Am J Cardiol. 1984;54:386–9.
28. D'agostino HJ, Pritchett ELC, Shond DG, Jones HR. Effect of verapamil on left ventricular function at rest and during exercise in normal men. J Cardiovasc Pharmacol. 1983;5:812–7.
29. Lefkowitz RJ, Carbon MG, Stiles GL. Mechanism of membrane-receptor regulation. Biochemical, physiological, and clinical insight derived from studies of the adrenergic receptors. N Engl J Med. 1984;310:1570–9.
30. Petri H, Arends BG, Van Baak MA. The effect of verapamil on cardiovascular and metabolic responses to exercise. Eur J Appl Physiol. 1986;55:499–502.
31. Lund-Johansen P. Hemodynamic effects of verapamil essential hypertension at rest and during exercise. Acta Med Scand Suppl. 1982;681:109–12.
32. Alderman MH, Madhavan S, Ooi WL, Cohen H, Sealey JE, Laragh JH. Association of the renin-sodium profile with the risk of myocardial infarction in patients with hypertension. N Engl J Med. 1991;324:10.
33. Kakinoki S, Nomura A, Takechi S, Kitabatake A. Effects of short- and long-acting calcium channel blockers on the relationship between blood pressure and physical activity. Am J Hypertens. 2001;14:66–9.
34. Raffestin B, Denjean A, Legrand C, et al. Effects of nifedipine on responses to exercise in normal subjects. J Appl Physiol. 1985;58:702–9.
35. Chick T, Halperin AK, Jackson JE, Van ASA. The effect of nifedipine on cardiopulmonary responses during exercise in normal subject. Chest. 1986;89:641–6.
36. Lowenthal DT, Affrime MB, Rosenthal L, Gould A, Borruso J, Falkner B. Dynamic and biochemical responses to single and repeated doses of clonidine during dynamic physical activity. Clin Pharmacol Ther. 1982;32:18–24.
37. Agre JC, Leon AS, Hunninghake DB, Mc NM, C., Bell C. The effects of methyldopa and propranolol on the response to dynamic and static excercise during treatment of mild hypertension in men. J Cardiopulmonary Rehabil. 1986;6:214–30.
38. Lund-Johansen P. Hemodynamic changes at rest and during exercise in long-term clonidine therapy of essential hypertension. Acta Med Scand. 1974;195:111–5.
39. Scharf S, Lee HB, Wexler JP, Blaufaz D. Cardiovascular consequences of primary antihypertensive therapy with prazosin hydrochloride. Am J Cardiol. 1984;53:32A–6A.
40. Rosenthal L, Affrime MB, Lowenthal DT, et al. Biochemical and dynamic responses to single and repeated doses of methyldopa and propanolol during dynamic physical activity. Clin Pharmacol Ther. 1982;32:701–10.
41. Anderson KL, Ottmann W, Piatkowski W, Green KA. Working ability and exercise tolerance during treatment of mild hypertension. Int Arch Occup Environ Health. 1985;56:49–55.
42. Chobanian AV, Tifft CP. The use of beta-adrenergic blockers in hypertensive patients and their effects on the cardiovascular responses to exercise and stress. Cardiovascular Rev Rep. 1981;2:549–55.
43. Feit A, Holtzman R, Cohen M, El-Sherif N. Effect of labetolol on exercise tolerance and double product in mild to moderate essential hypertension. Am J Med. 1985;78:937–41.
44. Inouye I, Massie B, Benowitz N, et al. Monotherapy in mild to moderate hypertension: comparison of hydrochlorothiazide, propranolol and prazosin. Am J Cardiol. 1984;53:24A–8A.

45. Macdonald IA, Bennett T, Brown AM, et al. The effects of acute or chronic ingestion of propanolol or metoprolol on metabolic and hormonal responses to prolonged submaximal exercise in hypertensive men. Br J Clin Pharmacol. 1984;17:283–93.
46. Pickering TG, Case DB, Sullivan PA, Laragh JH. Comparison of antihypertensive and hormonal effects of captopril and propanolol at rest and during exercise. Am J Cardiol. 1982;49:1566–9.
47. Reybrouck T, Amery A, Billiet L. Hemodynamic response to graded exercise after chronic beta-adrenergic blockade. J Appl Physiol. 1977;42:133–8.
48. White WB, Schulman P, McCabe E, Hager WD. Effects of chronic cetamolol therapy on resting, ambulatory, and exercise blood pressure and heart rate. Clin Pharmacol Ther. 1986;39:664–8.
49. Wilcox RG, Bennett T, Macdonald IA, Herbert M, Skene AM. The effects of acute or chronic ingestion of propranolol or metoprolol on the physiological responses to prolonged, submaximal exercise in hypertensive men. Br J Clin Pharmacol. 1984;17:273–81.
50. Reybrouck T, Amery A, Fagard R, Billiet L. Haemodynamic responses to graded exercise during chronic beta-adrenergic blockade with bunitrolol, an agent with intrinsic sympathomimetic activity. Eur J Clin Pharmacol. 1977;12:333–9.
51. Sundberg S, Gordin A. Influence of beta blockade and intrinsic sympathomimetic activity on hemodynamics, inotropy and respiration at rest and during exercise. Am J Cardiol. 1986;57:1394–9.
52. Clements IP, Offord KP, Baron DW, Brown ML, Bardsley WT, Harrison CE. Cardiovascular hemodynamics of bicycle and handgrip exercise in normal subjects before and after administration of propranolol. Mayo Clin Proc. 1984;59:604–11.
53. Joyner MJ, Freund BJ, Jilka SM, et al. Effects of β-blockade on exercise capacity of trained and untrained men: hemodynamic comparison. J Appl Phisiol. 1986;60:1429–34.
54. Vanhees L, Defoor JG, Schepers D, Lijnen P, Peeters DA, Lacante PH, et al. Effect of bisoprolol and atenolol on endurance exercise capacity in healthy men. J Hypertens. 2000;18:35–43.
55. Bennett M, Cl C, Tatley M, et al. The safety of cardioselective β1-blockers in asthma: literature review and search of global pharmacovigilance safety reports. ERJ Open Res. 2021;7:00801–2020.
56. Lundborg P, Astrom H, Bengtsson C, et al. Effect of β-adrenoceptor blockade on exercise performance and metabolism. Clin Sci. 1981;61:299–305.
57. Kaiser P, Rossner S, Karlsson J. Effects of beta-adrenergic blockade on endurance and short-time performance in respect to individual muscle fiber composition. Int J Sports Med. 1981;2:37–42.
58. Laustiola K, Uusitalo A, Koivula T, et al. Divergent effects of atenolol, prostolol, and propranolol on the peripheral metabolic changes induced by dynamic exercise in healthy men. Eur J Clin Pharmacol. 1983;25:293–7.
59. Hughson RL. Alterations in the oxygen deficit-oxygen debt relationships with β-adrenergic receptor blockade in man. J Phisiol. 1984;349:375–87.
60. Hughson RL, Russell CA, Marshall MR. Effect of metoprolol on cycle and treadmill maximal exercise performance. J Cardiac Rehabil. 1984;4:27–30.
61. McLeod A, Kraus WE, Williams RS. Effects of beta-I-selective and nonselective beta-adrenoreceptor blockade during exercise conditioning in healthy adults. Am J Cardiol. 1984;53:1656–61.
62. Tesch PA, Kaiser P. Effects of beta-adrenergic blockade on O2 uptake during submaximal and maximal exercise. J Appl Physiol. 1983;54:901–5.
63. Kullmer T, Kinderman W. Physical performance and serum potassium under chronic beta-blockade. Eur J Appl Physiol. 1985;54:350–4.
64. Kaiser P, Tesch PA, Thorsson A, Karlsson J, Kaiser L. Skeletal muscle glycolysis during submaximal exercise following acute beta-adrenergic blockade in man. Acta Physiol Scand. 1985;123(3):285–91.
65. Chiasiotis D, Brandt R, Harris RC, Hultman E. Effects of beta-blockade on glycogen metabolism in human subjects during exercise. Am J Phys. 1983;245:E166–70.
66. Sable DL, Brammell HL, Sheehan MW, Nies AS, Gerber J, Lawrence DH. Attenuation of exercise conditioning by beta adrenergic blockade. Circulation. 1982;65:679–84.

67. Svedenhag J, Henriksson J, Juhlin-Dannfelt A, Asano K. Beta-adrenergic blockade and training in healthy men effects of central circulation. Acta Physiol Scand. 1984;120:77–86.
68. Li LL, Lennon DLF, Kochan RG, Nagle FJ, Lardy HA. Enzymatic adaptations to physical training under beta-blockade in the rat. Evidence of a beta-2 adrenergic mechanism in skeletal muscle. J Clin Invest. 1986;78:771–8.
69. Svedenhag J, Henriksson J, Juhlin-Dannfelt A. Beta-adrenergic blockade and training in human subjects: effects on muscle metabolic capacity. Am J Physiol. 1984;247:305–11.
70. Bruno RM, Cartoni G, Taddei S. Hypertension in special populations: athletes. Futur Cardiol. 2011;7:1–11.
71. Van De Water A, Janssens W, Van Neuten J, et al. Pharmacological and hemodynamic profile of nebivolol, a chemically novel, potent, and selective beta 1 adrenergic antagonist. J Cardiovasc Pharmacol. 1988;11:552–63.
72. Munzel T, Gori T. Nebivolol: the somewhat-different beta-adrenergic receptor blocker. J Am Coll Cardiol. 2009;54:1491–9.
73. Gupta S, Wright HM. Nebivolol: a highly selective beta1-adrenergic receptor blocker that causes vasodilatation by increasing nitric oxide. Cardiovasc Ther. 2008;26:189–202.
74. Bian K, Doursout MF, Murad F. Vascular system: role of nitric oxide in cardiovascular diseases. J Clin Hypertens. 2008;10:304–10.
75. Merchant N, Rahman ST, Ferdinand KC, Haque T, Umpierrez GE, Khan BV. Effects of nebivolol in obese African Americans with hypertension (NOAAH): markers of inflammation and obesity in response to exercise-induced stress. J Hum Hypertens. 2011;25:196–202.
76. Flather MD, Shibata MC, Coats AJ, et al. Investigators randomized trial to determine the effect of nebivolol on mortality and cardiovascular hospital admission in elderly patients with heart failure. Eur Heart J. 2005;26(3):215–25.
77. Messias LR, Ferreira AG. Effect of Nebivolol on MIBG parameters and exercise in heart failure with normal ejection fraction. Arq Bras Cardiol. 2016;106:358–66.
78. Lund-Johansen P. Hemodynamic changes in long-term diuretic therapy of essential hypertension. Acta Med Scand. 1970;187:507–18.
79. Hollifield JW. Potassium and magnesium abnormalities: diuretics and arrhythmias in hypertension. Am J Med. 1984;77(5A):28–32.
80. Knochel JP. Neuromuscular manifestation of electrolyte disorders. Am J Med. 1982;72:521–33.
81. Roj BD, Green HJ, Burnett ME. Prolonged exercise following diuretic induced-hypoidratation: effects on thermal strain. Can J Physiol Pharmacol. 2000;78:541–7.
82. Watson G, Judelson DA, Armstrong LE, Yeargin SW, Casa DJ, Maresh CM. Influence of diuretic-induced dehydration competitive sprint and power performance. Med Sci Sport Exerc. 2005;37(7):1168–74.
83. Wald DS, Law M, Morris JK, Bestwick JP, Wald NJ. Combination therapy versus monotherapy in reducing blood pressure meta-analysis on 11.000 participants from 42 trials. Am J Med. 2009;122:290–300.
84. Weir MR, Hsueh WA, Nesbitt SD, Littlejohn TJ III, Graff A, Shojaee A, et al. A titrate-to-goal study of switching patients uncontrolled on antihypertensive monotherapy to fixed-dose combinations of amlodipine and olmesartan medoxomil ± hydrochlorothiazide. J Clin Hypertens. 2011;13:404–12.
85. Volpe M, Christian RL, Ammentorp B, Laeis P. Efficacy and safety of triple antihypertensive therapy with the olmesartan/amlodipine/hydrochlorothiazide combination. Clin Drug Investig. 2012;32:649–64.
86. Corrao G, Parodi A, Zambon A, Heiman F, Filippi A, Cricelli C, et al. Reduced discontinuation of antihypertensive treatment by two drug combination as first step. Evidence from daily life practice. J Hypertens. 2010;28:1584–90.
87. Gupta AK, Arshad S, Poulter NR. Compliance, safety, and effectiveness of fixed-dose combinations of antihypertensive agents: a meta-analysis. Hypertension. 2010;55:399–407.
88. ESC/ESH Guidelines for the management of arterial hypertension. The task force for the management of arterial hypertension of the European Society of Cardiology and the European Society of Hypertension. J Hypertens. 2018;36:1953–2041.

89. Izzo JL, Minesh R, Karan S, Srikakarlapudi S, Osmond PJ. Angiotensin-converting enzyme inhibitors *the*. J Clin Hypertens. 2011;13:667–75.
90. Lang M, Faini A, Caravita S, et al. Blood pressure response to six-minute walk test in hypertensive subjects exposed to high altitude: effects of antihypertensive combination treatment. Eur J Radiol. 2016;219:27–32.
91. Cicero AFG, Grassi D, Tocci G, Galletti F, Borghi C, Ferri C. Nutrients and nutraceuticals for the management of high normal blood pressure: an evidence-based consensus document. High Blood Press Cardiovasc Prev. 2019;26(1):9–25.
92. Borghi C, Tsioufis K, Agabiti-Rosei E, et al. Nutraceuticals and blood pressure control: a European Society of Hypertension position document. J Hypertens. 2020;38(5):799–812.

MIX
Papier aus verantwortungsvollen Quellen
Paper from responsible sources
FSC® C105338

If you have any concerns about our products,
you can contact us on
ProductSafety@springernature.com

In case Publisher is established outside the EU,
the EU authorized representative is:
Springer Nature Customer Service Center GmbH
Europaplatz 3, 69115 Heidelberg, Germany

Printed by Libri Plureos GmbH
in Hamburg, Germany